TREATMENT OF TYPE 2 DIABETES

Edited by **Colleen Croniger**

Treatment of Type 2 Diabetes
http://dx.doi.org/10.5772/58508
Edited by Colleen Croniger

Contributors

Dhastagir Sultan Sheriff, Fatum Elshaari, Alshaari Aa, Elshaari Fa, Kazuko Masuo, Ayse Nur Torun, Carmen Purdel, Mihaela Ilie, Denisa Margina, Blas Gil-Extremera, Ilie-Robert Dinu, Maria Mota, Eugen Mota, Chao Liu, Anca Sirbu, Aura Reghina, Carmen Barbu, Simona Fica, Fuad AlSaraj, Kazuo Kajita, Roberto Pontarolo, Samreen Riaz, Saadia Shahzad Alam

Published by InTech

Janeza Trdine 9, 51000 Rijeka, Croatia

Publishing Process Manager Iva Simcic

Technical Editor InTech DTP team

Cover InTech Design team

First published March, 2015

Printed in Croatia

Additional hard copies can be obtained from orders@intechopen.com

Treatment of Type 2 Diabetes, Edited by Colleen Croniger

p. cm.

ISBN 978-953-51-2032-2

For EU product safety concerns:
IN TECH d.o.o., Prolaz Marije Krucifikse Kozulić 3, 51000 Rijeka, Croatia,
info@intechopen.com or visit our website at intechopen.com.

Meet the editor

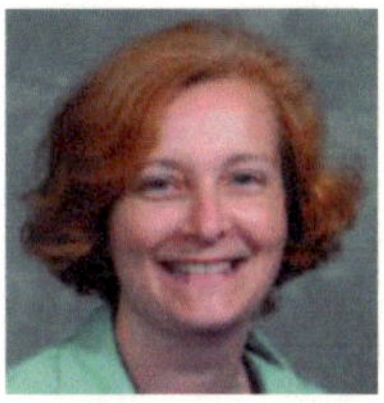

Dr. Colleen Croniger received her graduate degree in Molecular Biology from Case Western Reserve University in Cleveland, Ohio USA. After completing her graduate studies, she studied and learned metabolism from her post-doctoral mentor, Dr. Richard Hanson at Case Western Reserve University. In 2002 Dr. Croniger joined the faculty of the Nutrition Department at Case Western Reserve University. She is an Associate Professor and newly appointed Assistant Dean for Medical Student Research. Her research is focused on obesity, diabetes, nonalcoholic steatohepatitis (NASH) and alcoholic steatohepatitis (ASH) using genetically modified mouse models. Dr. Croniger also teaches graduate and medical students nutrition and metabolism. Dr. Croniger has received the John S. Diekoff Teaching Award for excellence in graduate student teaching. In addition, Dr. Croniger is a member of American Diabetes Association (ADA), American Society for Biochemistry and Molecular Biology (ASBMB) and Research Society on Alcoholism (RSA). Finally, Dr. Croniger is the Metabolic Core director for the Case Western Reserve University Mouse Metabolic Phenotyping Center (MMPC). The MMPC is one of six centers funded by NIH-NIDDK.

Contents

Preface

Obesity and type 2 diabetes are increasing worldwide problems. In this book we reviewed factors that contribute to glucose homeostasis and the pathogenesis of Type 2 diabetes. In addition the book addresses current strategies for treatment of Type 2 Diabetes. It is well accepted that obesity is strongly associated with the development of disease including Type 2 diabetes. In this book, chapters investigate the consequences of weight loss by calorie restriction and by gastric by-pass surgery. The rapid normalization in glucose homeostasis for diabetics after bariatric surgery suggests that remission may be due to mechanisms involving the surgical technique, not just weight loss. This book also addresses the use of statins, incretins and androgen therapy for type 2 diabetics. This is increasingly important since cardiovascular disease is a major complication for type 2 diabetes.

Dr. Colleen Croniger
Associate Professor
Co-Director Case MMPC
Department of Nutrition
Case Western Reserve University
USA

Section 1

Glucose Homeostasis and Diabetes

Chapter 1

The Role of the Kidney in Glucose Homeostasis

Maria Mota, Eugen Mota and Ilie-Robert Dinu

Additional information is available at the end of the chapter

http://dx.doi.org/10.5772/59173

1. Introduction

It is only in recent years that the attention was drawn on the important role of the kidney in glucose homeostasis. Nevertheless, along with the liver, the kidney has an important role in ensuring the energy needs during fasting periods. This organ has a vital role in absorbing the entire quantity of the filtered glucose [1]. Having a glomerular filtration rate of 180 liters per day, it filters approximately 180 grams of glucose per day, bringing its contribution in maintaining normal fasting plasma glucose (FPG) levels [2]. The reabsorption of glucose is ensured by the sodium-glucose cotransporter (SGLT) 2, responsible for the reabsorption of 90% of glucose, and SGLT1, that reabsorbs the remaining glucose [3].

Despite the large amount of data regarding the implication of the kidneys in glucose homeostasis, this organ is often overlooked as a key player in glucose metabolism. But the awareness of the renal mechanisms of glucose control is likely to increase due to the development of new types of glucose-lowering drugs that target this metabolic pathway [4].

2. Short history

2.1. Early non-human studies

The first researchers in this field, Bergman and Drury brought the first clues about the involvement of the kidney in glucose homeostasis in 1938 [5]. They used the glucose clamp technique in order to maintain euglycemia in two groups of rabbits – one functionally hepatectomized and another one functionally hepatectomized and nephrectomized. In the group of hepatectomized and nephrectomized rabbits, the amount of glucose requested in order to maintain euglycemia was very high compared to the one required by the other group

[6] (Figure 1). These data led to the conclusion that the kidneys are an important source of plasma glucose [6].

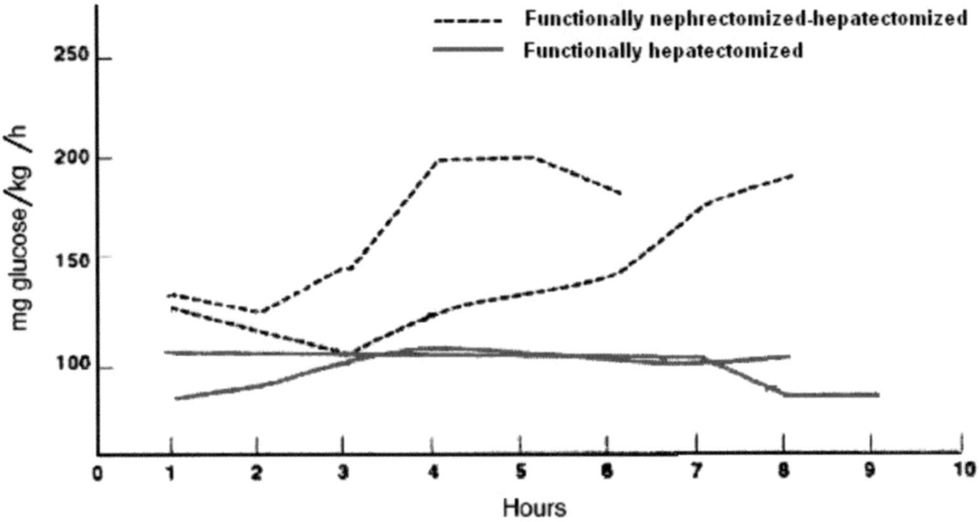

Figure 1. Effect of nephrectomy on glucose needs for maintaining euglycemia in hepatectomized rabbits (Adapted from [6])

A few years later, the study was reproduced by Reinecke in rats. He also determined the arteriorenal venous glucose concentrations in the hepatectomized rats. He found that the glucose levels in renal vein exceeded the arterial levels when the animals became hypoglycemic proving that, under these conditions, the kidneys can release glucose into the circulation [7].

In 1950, Drury et al. injected ^{14}C-labeled glucose into rats that had been hepatectomized or hepatectomized and nephrectomized. His experiment indicated that the kidney represents the source of the glucose produced endogenously and released into the circulation after hepatectomy [8].

In other experiments, Teng proved that the renal cortex of the animal models with diabetes released glucose at a very high rate, but treatment of these animals with insulin could reverse this effect. A few years later, in 1960, Landau was able to prove, having a similar model, that gluconeogenesis from pyruvate was increased by the diabetic kidney [6].

In several experiments, Krebs tried to characterize the substrates that the kidney uses for gluconeogenesis [9], the efficiency of the renal gluconeogenesis in several species [10], and some aspects of the regulation of renal gluconeogenesis [11]. He could also demonstrate that the kidney present a greater amount of gluconeogenic enzymes than the liver, and due to the comparable blood flows (therefore comparable provision of gluconeogenic precursors), Krebs argued that the kidney might be a gluconeogenic organ in vivo as important as the liver [11].

2.2. Early human studies

Studies about human renal glucose metabolism started in the late 1950s. They tried to measure the differences of glucose concentrations between arterial and renal venous blood. By not taking into consideration that the kidney is able to produce and consume glucose in the same time, the fact that many researchers found little or no differences between arterial and venous glucose values led to the conclusion that the kidneys are not able to release glucose [6].

In the mid 1960s, Aber et al. [12] found that kidney can release glucose in patients with pulmonary disease and the quantity of glucose is negatively correlated with arterial pH explaining why the greater the acidosis, the greater the renal glucose release. Several years after, Owen et al. [13] indicated that renal glucose release is increased in very obese patients who fasted for several weeks. These data led to the current textbook idea that the liver is the only source of glucose, in general, except after prolonged fasting or under acidosis.

On the other hand, in subjects that undergo liver transplantation, it may still be observed after removal of the liver, endogenous glucose production [14]. Shortly after the removal of the liver, the production of endogenous glucose decreased only by 50% (Joseph et al.) [14]. Recent research using isotopic measurements have indicated that the kidney can release significant quantities of glucose in postabsorptive normal volunteers.

3. The involvement of kidneys in glucose homeostasis

The plasma glucose concentration is determined by the amount of glucose synthesized, and the one removed from the circulation and metabolized. This concentration must be maintained within a relatively narrow range despite the wide daily fluctuations in glucose ingestion and glucose demands in various tissues [4]. Other substrates such as free fatty acids (FFAs), glycerol, lactate and ketone bodies have greater daily fluctuations. This can be explained by the need of the body to protect himself against hyper- and hypoglycaemia. Hyperglycaemia is associated with both chronic effects (such as nephropathy, retinopathy, neuropathy and premature atherosclerosis) and also acute complications (including diabetic ketoacidosis and hyperosmolar hyperglycaemic state that are associated with higher morbidity and mortality). Hypoglycaemia is also harmful because it can cause neurological events (including coma, seizures), cardiac arrhythmias and death [4].

The regulation of endogenous production of glucose is determined by hormonal and neural factors [15]. In the acute phase, glucoregulatory mechanisms involve insulin, glucagon and catecholamines and they can effect changes in plasma glucose levels in a matter of minutes. Insulin is able to suppress glucose release in both the kidney and liver by direct enzyme activation/deactivation and by reducing the availability of gluconeogenic substrates. Glucagon has no effect on the kidneys, but it stimulates glycogenolysis and gluconeogenesis in the liver [16]. Catecholamines also have multiple acute actions. They can stimulate renal glucose release and glucagon secretion and inhibit insulin secretion [4].

The kidneys are involved in maintaining glucose homeostasis through three different mechanisms: gluconeogenesis; glucose uptake from the blood for its own energy requests and reabsorption into the general circulation of glucose from glomerular filtrate in order to preserve energy [4].

3.1. Renal gluconeogenesis

From the point of view of glucose utilization, the kidney is considered as 2 separate organs; the renal medulla is characterized mainly by glucose utilization and the renal cortex is responsible for glucose release. The separation of these activities represents the consequence of differences in the distribution of numerous enzymes along the nephron. The cells in the renal medulla can use only glucose for their needs (like the brain) and they have enzymes capable of glucose-phosphorylation and glycolysis. They can therefore phosphorylate important amounts of glucose and accumulate glycogen but, because these cells do not have glucose-6-phosphatase or any other gluconeogenic enzymes, they are unable to release glucose into the bloodstream. Moreover, the cells in the renal cortex have gluconeogenic enzymes and they can produce and release glucose into the circulation. However these cells cannot synthesize glycogen because they have little phosphorylating capacity [6].

After a 16-h overnight fast, approximately 10 μmol/(kg /min) of glucose is released into the circulation [17]. Almost 50% of this is the result of glycogenolysis from the liver stocks and the other half is produced by liver and kidney gluconeogenesis. The renal cortex (like the liver) contains gluconeogenic enzymes and it can synthesize glucose-6-phosphate from precursors (lactate, glutamine, glycerol and alanine). Because it contains glucose-6-phosphatase, it is able to release glucose into the blood stream [18] and the human liver and kidneys are the only organs that can perform gluconeogenesis. Therefore, after an overnight fast, the liver produces 75–80% of glucose released into the circulation and the remaining 20–25% is derived from the kidneys [4].

Several studies have indicated that human kidneys and liver provide approximately the same amounts of glucose through gluconeogenesis in postabsorptive period. If the duration of fasting is increased, the glycogen stores are depleted and gluconeogenesis produces all the glucose released into circulation.

An important aspect is that kidney and liver use different gluconeogenic precursors and several hormones have different effects on their release of glucose. Lactate represents the predominant gluconeogenic precursor in both organs, but regarding the aminoacids, the kidney prefers to use glutamine, whereas the liver preferentially uses alanine [19]. Insulin can suppress glucose release in both organs with almost comparable efficacy [20], whereas glucagon stimulates hepatic glucose release only [21]. Catecholamines normally have a direct effect only on renal glucose release [22], but their effect on both hepatic and renal glucose release may be indirect by increasing the quantity of gluconeogenic substrates available and by suppressing insulin secretion. Other hormones, such as growth hormone, cortisol and thyroid hormones can stimulate hepatic glucose release over a great period of time [15]. Their effects on the kidneys regarding glucose release in humans are not completely deciphered.

http://dx.doi.org/10.5772/59173

In the postprandial state the situation changes significantly. Postprandial glucose levels in the plasma are determined by insulin and glucagon levels. After glucose ingestion, plasma glucose levels reach the peak in 60–90 minutes and they return to post-absorptive levels in almost 3–4 h. The plasma insulin increases four times and the plasma glucagon levels decrease by 50% [15]. Meyer et al. indicated that endogenous glucose release is reduced by almost 60% and hepatic glycogenolysis drops to zero in the 4- to 6-h period after meal ingestion [23].This is happening because this period determines the refilling of hepatic glycogen stores and inhibition of endogenous glucose release is able to limit postprandial hyperglycaemia. There is also a reduction in hepatic gluconeogenesis by 82% and glucose molecules generated through hepatic gluconeogenesis are also directed into hepatic glycogen, not only released in the circulation.

Renal gluconeogenesis can increase by approximately twofold and it can represent ~60% of endogenous glucose production in the postprandial state [24]. This mechanism is believed to facilitate the repletion of glycogen stocks in the liver.

A new concept of hepatorenal glucose reciprocity emerged from the differences observed in regulation and interchange between renal and hepatic glucose release [24]. This concept refers to the facts that a pathological or physiological reduction in glucose release by kidney or liver determines a compensatory increase in glucose release of the other one (liver or kidney) in order to avoid hypoglycaemia. This situation occurs in the anhepatic phase during liver transplantation, prolonged fasting, meal ingestion, acidosis and insulin overdoses in diabetes mellitus [24].

3.2. Glycogenolysis

Glycogenolysis is the breakdown of glycogen to glucose-6-phosphate and a hydrolysis reaction (using glucose-6-phosphatase) in order to free glucose. The liver is the only organ that contains glucose-6-phosphatase. So, the cleavage of hepatic glycogen releases glucose, while the cleavage of glycogen from other sources can release only lactate. Lactate, that is generated via glycolysis, is often absorbed by other organs and helps regenerating glucose [6].

3.3. Glucose reabsorption

Apart from the important role in gluconeogenesis and the role of renal cortex in glucose uptake, the kidneys contribute to glucose homeostasis by filtering and reabsorbing glucose. In normal conditions, the kidneys can reabsorb as much glucose as possible, the result being a virtually glucose free urine. Approximately 180 grams of glucose are filtered by the glomeruli from plasma, daily but all of this quantity is reabsorbed through glucose transporters that are present in cell membranes located in the proximal tubules [24].

These glucose transporters have a limited capacity of reabsorption. If this capacity is exceeded, glucose usually appears in the urine. The tubular maximum for glucose (TmG), the term used for the maximum capacity, can vary from 260 to 350 mg/min/1.73 m^2 in healthy subjects. It corresponds to blood glucose levels of 180-200 mg/dL [24]. When the blood glucose is very high and the TmG is reached, the transporters cannot reabsorb all the glucose and glucosuria occurs (Figure 2). Nevertheless, there can be slight differences between the nephrons and the inaccurate nature of biological systems may potentially lead to the development of glucosuria when blood glucose is below TmG. Glucosuria may occur at lower plasma glucose levels in certain conditions of hyperfiltration (eg. pregnancy), but as a consequence of hyperfiltration and not of significant hyperglycemia [25].

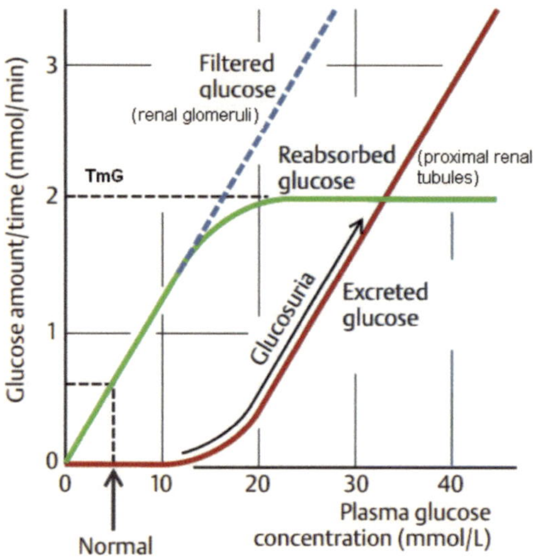

Figure 2. Renal glucose handling. TmG, transport maximum for glucose. Adapted from [26]

In a given day, the kidneys can produce, via gluconeogenesis, 15–55g glucose and it can metabolize 25–35g glucose. Regarding the glucose metabolic pathways, it is obvious that renal reabsorption represents the main mechanism by which the kidney is involved in glucose homeostasis. Therefore, the change in tubular glucose reabsorption may have a considerable impact on glucose homeostasis [4].

3.3.1. Renal glucose transporters

Glucose is a polar compound with positive and negative charged areas; therefore it is soluble in water. Its transport into and across cells is dependent on two specialized carrier protein families: the GLUTs (facilitated glucose transporters) and the SGLTs (sodium-coupled glucose cotransporters). These transporters are responsible for glucose passage and reabsorption in several tissue types, including the proximal renal tubule, blood-brain barrier, small intestine [27]. GLUTs are responsible for the passive transport of glucose across cell membranes, in order to equilibrate its concentrations across a membrane. SGLTs, on the other hand, are involved in active transport of glucose against a concentration gradient by means of sodium-glucose cotransport [27].

There are six members of the SGLT family indicated in Table 1.

Co-transporter	Substrate	Tissue distribution
SGLT1	Glucose, galactose	Intestine, kidney, heart, trachea, brain, testis, prostate
SGLT2	Glucose	Kidney, brain, liver, muscle, heart
SGLT4	Glucose, mannose	Intestine, kidney, uterus, pancreas, liver, brain, lung, trachea
SGLT5	Unknown	Kidney
SGLT6	Glucose, myoinositol	Brain, kidney, intestine
SMIT1	Glucose, myoinositol	Brain, heart, lung, kidney

Table 1. The sodium glucose co-transporter family (adapted from [27])

SGLT2 is considered the most important because, based on animal studies, it is responsible for the reabsorption of 90% of the glucose filtered at the glomerulus [24]. The other 10% of glucose reabsorbed in the proximal tubule is ensured by SGLT1. Of the family of GLUT proteins expressed in the kidneys, GLUT2 is the major transporter and it releases into circulation the glucose reabsorbed by SGLTs in the proximal tubular cells [28].

The renal glucose transport was investigated by analyzing the gene mutations within SGLT family. These can lead to several inherited diseases presenting renal glucosuria that include familial renal glucosuria (FRG) and glucose-galactose malabsorption (GGM). FRG represents an autosomal recessive or autosomal dominant disorder caused by several SGLT2 mutations. Its main characteristic is persistent glucosuria without hyperglycemia or renal tubular dysfunction. Most of the patients with FRG do not have any clinical manifestations; this is why FRG is not commonly described as a "disease" but as a condition known as benign glucosuria. Nevertheless, there is a severe form of FRG, known as type O, where mutations of the SGLT2 gene lead to a complete lack of renal tubular glucose reabsorption. This condition is still associated with a good prognosis. Due to the fact that FRG is mainly asymptomatic, subjects with this condition are discovered through routine urinalysis [24].

GGM represents a more serious disease. It is inherited autosomal recessive and is caused by mutation of the SGLT1 transporter. Its main characteristics are represented by intestinal symptoms. They appear in the first few days of life and determine glucose and galactose malabsorption. The consequences are severe; diarrhea and subsequent dehydration may become fatal unless a special diet (glucose- and galactose-free) is initiated. Some patients with GGM may present glucosuria but it is typically mild, and some other subjects have no sign of urinary glucose excretion. This confirms that SGLT1 has a minor role in renal reabsorption of glucose [24]. The mutations involving the GLUT family are associated with more severe consequences, because these transporters are more widespread throughout the major organ systems. SGLT2 and SGLT1 are located mainly in the renal system, but GLUT2 is present almost everywhere in the organism, having an important role in glucose homeostasis through its involvement in intestinal glucose uptake, renal reabsorption of glucose, and hepatic uptake and release of glucose [24].

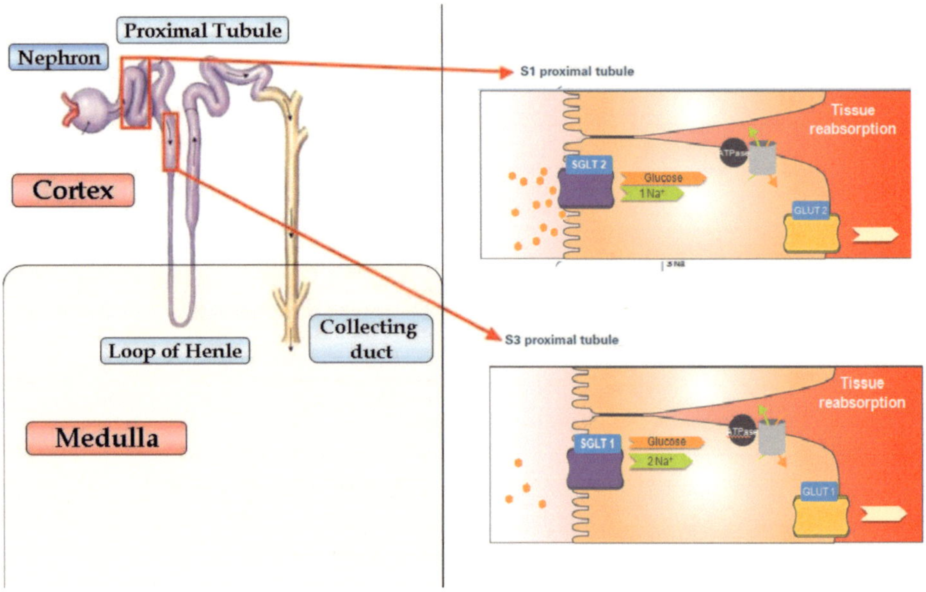

Figure 3. Glucose filtration and reabsorption in the proximal tubule of the kidney (adapted from [28])

Direct *in vivo* experiments of Vallon et al. on gene targeted mice lacking *Sglt2* gene, demonstrated that the SGLT2 protein is responsible for all glucose reabsorption in the proximal tubule and for the bulk of glucose reabsorption in the kidney overall [29]. According to this study, in wild-type mice, 99.7 ± 0.1% of fractional glucose is reabsorbed and in Sglt2−/− mice (not expressing SGLT2), only 36 ± 8% is reabsorbed. It was also found that in Sglt2−/− mice, even if SGLT1 glucose reabsorption is increased (SGLT1 transporters reach their transport maximum), up regulation of SGLT1 expression does not occur (both SGLT1 mRNA and protein expression are reduced by ~40%) when the amount of glucose in proximal tubule is increased. The results of the study of Gorboulev et al. [30] are in correspondence with those of Vallon et al., indicating that wild-type mice do not use the maximal transport capacity of SGLT1 at normoglycemic conditions but when glucose load to the SGLT1 is increased (for instance, diabetes and SGLT2 inhibition), SGLT1 may operate at full transport capacity [30].

Molecular structure of SGLTs has been studied thoroughly on SGLT1, which is the first described member of SGLTs family [31]. SGLT2 is 59% identical to SGLT1 and has almost the same architecture. Its secondary structure consists of 14-transmembrane helices (TM1–TM13) with both the NH2 and COOH termini facing the extracellular side of the plasma membrane [32]. The first kinetic model of Na+/glucose co-transporters was proposed by Parent et al. [33].

4. The kidney in diabetes mellitus

All the metabolic pathways regarding the involvement of the kidney in glucose homeostasis are modified in subjects with diabetes mellitus. Subjects with type 2 diabetes mellitus (T2DM) have an increased renal release of glucose into the circulation in the fasting state [34]. Although one can think that the liver determines increased glucose release into the circulation in diabetes, the liver and the kidneys have comparable increase in renal glucose release (2.60 and 2.21 μmol/(kg min). The kidney can increase its glucose production with 300% compared with the liver that can increase gluconeogenesis only by 30%. Gluconeogenesis, in the kidney, could explain this glucose increase, in the fasting state [34].

In postprandial state, renal glucose release is greater increased in subjects with T2DM than in people without glucose metabolism abnormalities [35]. Meyer et al. studied systemic glucose appearance in subjects with T2DM and individuals with normal glucose tolerance over several hours following ingestion of 75 g glucose. They found that it was significantly greater in diabetic patients than in normal subjects (100.0 ± 6.3 vs. 70.0 ± 3.3 g; $p < 0.001$). The result was determined by a higher endogenous glucose release because the general appearance of ingested glucose was only 7 g greater in the subjects with DM. Almost 40% of the increased endogenous glucose release was caused by increased renal glucose release [35]. This fact was determined mainly by impaired suppression of endogenous glucose release and secondary by reduced initial splanchnic sequestration of ingested glucose. This effect is expected in diabetic patients that have decreased postprandial insulin release and insulin resistance, taking into account that renal glucose release is regulated by insulin [4].

Both renal glucose uptake and glucose production are increased in both the postprandial and post-absorptive states in diabetic patients [35].

It is well known that glucosuria in diabetic patients occurs at different plasma glucose levels compared with the levels where glucosuria can occur in non-diabetic individuals [36]. This is determined by the increased glucose reabsorbtion in subjects with diabetes mellitus. Therefore, the Tm for glucose is increased and glucosuria may occur at higher than normal blood glucose levels. Several studies indicated that the Tm increased from near 350 mg/min in subjects with normal glucose tolerance to approximately 420 mg/min in subjects with diabetes mellitus [36].

As an evolutionary process, the kidney was able to develop a system in order to reabsorb all of the filtered glucose in order to conserve energy especially at a time when energy intake was reduced. Therefore, this may be considered as an adaptive response as the SGLT2 transport increases in response to hyperglycaemia. But, in subjects with diabetes this adaptive response is considered maladaptive, and glycosuria occurs only at very high plasma glucose levels. Thus, instead of allowing the kidneys to excrete excess of glucose, SGLT2 transporters help maintain a higher plasma glucose concentrations [1].

Human and animal studies of renal cells have demonstrated enhanced expression of SGLT2 transporters [37]. Factors like hyperglycaemia, albumin and angiotensin II have been reported to increase the expression of SGLT2 in T2DM [37].

It has also been demonstrated that acidosis increases renal gluconeogenesis and impairs hepatic gluconeogenesis [38]. Therefore one can speculate that the kidney represents an important factor that accelerates gluconeogenesis in diabetic ketoacidosis. Moreover, the exaggerated increase in renal glucose release can be the result of the insufficient suppression of endogenous glucose release postprandial in diabetic patients [39]. These processes can explain the quantity of glycogen stored in diabetic kidneys. A major part of the high renal glucose release found in subjects with diabetes may be determined by increased renal glycogenolysis [6].

5. Diabetic nephropathy

Diabetes represents the most common single cause of end-stage renal disease (ESRD) in the United States and Europe. There can be several factors responsible for this, including an increased prevalence of T2DM, longer life spans among patients with diabetes, and better recognition of kidney disease [40]. Comparing with subjects with type 1 diabetes mellitus, only a smaller fraction of those with T2DM develop ESRD, but due to the increased prevalence of T2DM, these individuals represent more than a half of those with diabetes on dialysis. There are numerous variables in progressing to nephropathy, including racial/ethnic variability because Native Americans, Hispanics and African Americans are at much greater risk of developing ESRD than non-Hispanic white subjects with T2DM [40].

The first clinical signs of nephropathy are represented by low, but abnormal, levels (≥30 mg/day or 20μg/min) of albumin in the urine (previously referred to as microalbuminuria). The detection of albumin in the urine increases the risk of progression to persistent albuminuria, progressive decline in glomerular filtration rate (GFR), increased blood pressure and cardiovascular morbid-mortality. But because T2DM may be present for many years before diagnosis, a higher proportion of individuals with T2DM have microalbuminuria and overt nephropathy shortly after diagnosis. It is known that without treatment, 20-40% of patients with T2DM and microalbuminuria progress to overt nephropathy. Nevertheless, after 20 years from the onset of nephropathy, only 20% will have progressed to ESRD [40]. The explanation comes from the greater risk among subjects with diabetes and chronic kidney disease of dying from cardiovascular disease than progressing to ESRD.

Several clinical trials indicate that the onset and development of diabetic nephropathy may be significantly influenced by numerous interventions including tight glucose control and also use of angiotensin-converting enzyme inhibitors or angiotensin receptor blockers. This is the reason why annual screening for microalbuminuria is critical since it can lead to early diagnosis of nephropathy. Numerous studies, including the well-known Diabetes Control and Complications Trial and United Kingdom Prospective Diabetes Study indicated that intensive glycemic control represent a very important step in reducing the risk of developing microalbuminuria and overt nephropathy [40].

New data from the Action in Diabetes and Vascular Disease: Preterax and Diamicron MR Controlled Evaluation (ADVANCE) trial offers hope regarding the benefic effects of tight glucose control on decreasing the risk of nephropathy [41]. In the ADVANCE trial, after almost 5 years, subjects that were on intensive glycemic control had a 10% relative reduction in the combined outcome of major macrovascular and microvascular events. This was happening mainly because of a 21% relative reduction in the risk of developing nephropathy. The intensive glucose control is also important because it is associated with a 9% reduction in new onset microalbuminuria [41]. Results of this study are of great importance since renal impairment is strongly associated with future risk of major vascular events, and death in patients with diabetes. Nevertheless, the role of modified renal glucose reabsorption in the progression of diabetic nephropathy is not elucidated [4].

6. Therapeutic implications

6.1. SGLT2 inhibitors

SGLT2 is highly specific for (several authors consider that it is found only in) the proximal tubules of the kidney, as compared to SGLT1 or GLUT2, therefore it is a preferred target for more specific renal pharmacologic interventions. Thus, the idea of interfering with the activity of the SGLT2 has gained much attention [2].

Inhibition of SGLT2 transporter 'resets' the reabsorption system by lowering the threshold for glycosuria, resulting the correction of the hyperglycemia [1]. Reduction of the blood glucose level can improve insulin resistance in muscle by increasing insulin signaling, GLUT4 and glycogen synthase activity [1].

The history of SGLT2 inhibitors starts in 1835 when phlorizin was found in the root bark of apple tree [42]. Many years after, it was found to be a non-specific SGLT1 and SGLT2 and it could increase glucosuria and reduce blood glucose levels and normalize insulin sensitivity in a pancreatectomized animal model of T2DM [43]. Nevertheless, it could not become a treatment for diabetes due to numerous side effects. Being non-selective and inhibiting SLGT1 at the intestinal brush border, it can cause serious problems regarding the absorption of dietary glucose. Inhibition of SGLT1 can result in glucose–galactose malabsorption and cause diarrhea, events that occur naturally in SGLT1 deficiency [44]. Moreover, in the intestine, phlorizin is poorly absorbed and is rapidly hydrolyzed to phloretin, a substance that blocks GLUT1, leading to disturbance in glucose uptake in several tissues [45]. Highly-specific inhibitors of SGLT2 have subsequently been developed in order to overcome some of these shortcomings.

Ellsworth et al [46] discovered a group of *C*-aryl glycosides that includes dapagliflozin [47] and canagliflozin [48]. They are resistant to degradation produced by β-glucosidase enzymes in the gastrointestinal tract. Moreover, dapagliflozin has a very high sensitivity for SGLT2 compared to SGLT1, blocking renal glucose reabsorption by almost 40–50%. Using this treatment, they can be excreted up to 80–85 g of glucose per day [47]. Clinical trials evaluating the treatment with dapagliflozin, either as monotherapy or in association with metformin or with insulin in subjects with T2DM have demonstrated its efficacy in reducing glucose and HbA1c levels [3]. Pharmacokinetics and bioavailability of dapagliflozin are not influenced by a high-fat meal and there are no reports regarding any interactions with several other drugs used in the treatment of T2DM [3].

Human trials analyzing canagliflozin are more limited than for dapagliflozin. It has been indicated that both drugs have similar therapeutic characteristics [3]. Canagliflozin could induce an important, dose-dependent decrease in the mean renal glucose threshold to approximately 60 mg/dl (3.33 mmol/l) [49].

There are numerous other SGLT2 inhibitors including sergliflozin, remogliflozin, ipraglifozin and empagliflozin. Some of them, such as ipraglifozin and empagliflozin, are being tested in phase III trials and are promising very good results while other compounds have disappointed in clinical trials due to possible side effects (sergliflozin) or to susceptibility to hydrolysis by β-glucosidase enzymes (sergliflozin and remogliflozin) [3].

As already mentioned, patients diagnosed with FRG often gave higher urinary glucose excretion of almost 120 g per day. It remains unclear why treatment with SGLT2 inhibitors cannot achieve the same levels of glycosuria even when the maximal doses are used. Moreover, SGLT2-null mice can only reabsorb up to a third of the filtered glucose [29], but subjects taking dapagliflozin reabsorb ~50% at the highest doses. Moreover, the nonselective inhibitor phlorizin completely blocks reabsorption. One possible explanation may be that SGLT1 has a greater role in the kidney than it was previously imagined [50]. There are some theories that include antisense nucleotide technology to knock out SGLT2 in order to achieve a higher degree of blockade of glucose reabsorption than SGLT2 inhibition. Preliminary data in human subjects with T2DM with moderate or severe renal impairment indicate that SGLT2 inhibition determines proportionally less glycosuria than in subjects with preserved renal function [51]. These findings confirm that a low GFR in subjects with T2DM is accompanied by a comparable loss of tubular absorptive capacity that represents the anticipated consequence of nephron loss [3].

The approach of lowering hyperglycaemia in T2DM by blocking glucose reabsorption has many attractions. One of them is represented by the activity of SGLT2 inhibitors that is not dependent on pancreatic β-cell function, which deteriorates over time. This is the only class of drugs that present this mechanism of action. Other drugs such as the insulin secretagogues [glinides, sulphonylureas, dipeptidyl peptidase-4 (DPP-4) inhibitors and glucagon-like peptide 1 (GLP-1) agonists] and insulin sensitizers (thiazolidinediones and metformin) depend on insulin secretion. The insulin independence of their action indicates that the risk of hypoglycaemia is very low [6].

As a consequence, the liver can react to the induced glycosuria by increasing glucose release. The mechanism for increased liver glucose excretion is not well understood. The relative small decrease in plasma glucose but also insulin concentrations after massive glycosuria may stimulate endogenous glucose release. Other additional mechanisms are not excluded. Moreover, glucose output is usually not decreased enough to attain and maintain normal glucose values in patients with T2DM treated with SGLT2 inhibitors [52]. Adaptation of glucose metabolism to massive glycosuria needs further investigation.

Osmotic diuresis accompanies glycosuria. It is usually detected an increase in urine output with acute SGLT2 inhibition; while chronic administration of SGLT2 inhibitors is accompanied by an excess urine volume of 200–600 ml per day. As a consequence, haematocrit increases are noted but they are moderate and clinical signs of volume depletion, such as tachycardia and orthostatic hypotension, are rarely met [52].

http://dx.doi.org/10.5772/59173

SGLT2 inhibitors determine glucose and sodium reabsorption blocking and natriuresis also occurs. Changes in serum sodium concentration are not frequent with chronic SGLT2 inhibition because at the nephron level, reduced sodium reabsorption in the proximal segment determines the increase of sodium delivery to the juxtaglomerular apparatus, and the inhibition of the renin-angiotensin-aldosterone system (RAAS) occurs. In experimental diabetic rats fed a high-salt diet [53], SGLT2 inhibition could prevent blood pressure increase. This effect may be countered by an activation of the RAAS if volume depletion appears as a consequence of excessive diuresis. SGLT2 inhibition in patients with T2DM also determines the reduction of blood pressure levels (by 2–5 mmHg) [52]. The possible explanations may be the enhanced natriuresis and RAAS deactivation [3]. Because most of the individuals with T2DM also present high blood pressure, this effect is of great importance in clinical practice.

Several phase III clinical trials of dapagliflozin reported the decrease of serum uric acid concentrations [54]. Sodium and urate are handled together in several physiological circumstances, and also in response to several drugs such as diuretics and antihypertensives. Several sodium-dependent phosphate transporters may also excrete urate into the urine. Therefore, the excretion of urate determined by SGLT2 inhibitors is explained by this mechanism. GLUT9 might represent an alternate explanation. GLUT9 represents an antiporter that exchanges glucose for uric acid; his two isoforms act together to reabsorb glucose from the tubule lumen in exchange for uric acid [55].

Another important effect of SGLT2 inhibition is weight loss. Clinical trials in patients with T2DM have reported a decrease of 2.5–4.0% of body weight [52]. At first, this weight loss is predominantly due to fluid depletion, but soon after that appears the loss of subcutaneous and visceral depots of adipose tissue. This effect is caused by an important caloric loss through the urine. Nevertheless, body weight loss remains constant after several months of treatment [3].

Clinically, the most frequent and undesired effect of SGLT2 inhibitors is represented by high incidence of genitourinary infections. These infections were observed more frequent in women than in men taking SGLT2 inhibitors and tend to occur in susceptible subjects; these include postmenopausal women, history of urinary tract infections or poor hygiene. Interestingly, studies with dapagliflozin in addition to metformin reported a not significant difference in incidence of genitourinary infections between individuals in the placebo and treatment groups [56], while in subjects receiving dapagliflozin in addition to insulin, the difference was significant [57]. This might explain a possibly increased risk of this adverse effect in patients with advanced T2DM (when immune function may be defective) [3].

The incidence of genitourinary infections tends to decrease in time, with long-term treatment, when the adaptation to the treatment is installed or exclusion of susceptible individuals over time appears. More important, infections of the upper urinary tract, that tend to be more severe than those of the lower urinary tract, are not frequent, although the reported patient exposure is presently too limited to rule out this adverse event [56].

Another reported event was a very small, but consistent, increase in PTH levels (<2.0 ng/l) together with increased plasma phosphate concentration. The increased PTH might indicate a mild form of secondary hyperparathyroidism but the available studies so far offer very few data regarding the long-term effects of SGLT2 inhibitors on bone metabolism, making room for other clinical studies on this important issue.

There have been reports regarding several cases of bladder cancer and breast cancer, in subjects with T2DM receiving treatment with dapagliflozin [58]. Trials with large numbers of patients with different SGLT2 inhibitors are required to assess any associated increased risks of breast or bladder cancer [3].

Theoretical safety and tolerability concerns also include impairment in renal function [54]. Although, until now, there are no data indicating that the SLGT2 inhibitors would determine or be responsible for deterioration of renal function, the few clinical studies investigating these drugs have relatively short duration (6-12 months). Moreover, several authors are speculating that SGLT2 inhibitors may play an important role in preventing diabetic nephropathy. First, improved glycaemic control decreases the risk of diabetic nephropathy and other diabetic complications [40]. Second, by increasing the quantity of sodium in the juxtaglomerular apparatus, the use of SGLT2 inhibitors may determine a protective effect on the kidney, independently of glucose decreased.

In T2DM, the high quantity of glucose and sodium absorbed in the proximal tubule reduces the quantity of sodium to be delivered to the juxtaglomerular apparatus. Thus, the glomerulo-tubular feedback reflex is activated; this leads to high renal plasma flow, increased intra-glomerular pressure and elevated GFR. All these processes can induce normal salt delivery to the juxtaglomerular apparatus; however this can result in increased intra-glomerular pressure. All these alterations in renal hemodynamic lead to renal hypertrophy and eventually the result is represented by diabetic nephropathy [59]. SGLT2 inhibitors may prevent diabetic nephropathy by inhibiting the glomerulo-tubular feedback reflex and, therefore increasing sodium delivery to the distal nephron [1]. Nevertheless, this therapy is contraindicated in patients with estimated GFR (eGFR) <45 mL/min/1.73 m^2 and must be used at lower doses at eGFRs of 45-60 mL/min/1.73 m^2 [60]. New clinical trials are expected to evaluate the efficacy and safety of SGLT2 inhibitors.

The pathogenesis of type 2 diabetes combines numerous defects in many tissues. Therefore, there is no single antidiabetic drug that can compensate all the metabolic disturbances, and a good treatment for diabetes will require the use of multiple drugs in combination. Having a unique pharmacokinetic and a special mechanism of action, the SGLT2 inhibitors can be used not only as monotherapy [61] but also in combination with currently available antidiabetic agents [62,63].

7. Conclusions

Although not traditionally discussed, the kidneys play a very important role in maintaining glucose homeostasis by gluconeogenesis and glucose reabsorption, the latter being mediated by active (SGLT) and passive (GLUT) transporters. Only recently, excessive renal glucose reabsorption was taken into consideration regarding its importance in the physiopathology of

T2DM. In hyperglycemia, the kidneys may play an exacerbating role by reabsorbing excess glucose, bringing their contribution to chronic hyperglycemia. Knowing the kidneys' role in glucose homeostasis and the effect of glucose dysregulation on the kidneys is very important for the optimal management of T2DM and prevention of associated renal complications. The numerous metabolic defects found in T2DM imply the use of several therapies. SGLT2 inhibitors represent a new promising class of drugs for the treatment of T2DM.

Author details

Maria Mota[1*], Eugen Mota[2] and Ilie-Robert Dinu[2]

*Address all correspondence to: mmota53@yahoo.com

1 Department of Diabetes, Nutrition, Metabolic Diseases, University of Medicine and Pharmacy Craiova, Romania

2 Department of Nephrology, University of Medicine and Pharmacy Craiova, Romania

References

[1] DeFronzo RA, Davidson JA, Del Prato S. The Role of the Kidneys in Glucose Homeostasis: A New Path Towards Normalizing Glycaemia. Diabetes Obes Metab 2012;14: 5–14

[2] Cersosimo E, Solis-Herrera C, Triplitt C. Inhibition of Renal Glucose Reabsorption as a Novel Treatment for Diabetes Patients. J Bras Nefrol 2014;36(1): 80–92

[3] Ferrannini E, Solini A. SGLT2 Inhibition in Diabetes Mellitus: Rationale and Clinical Prospects. Nat Rev Endocrinol 2012;8(8): 495-502

[4] Gerich JE. Role of the Kidney in Normal Glucose Homeostasis and in the Hyperglycaemia of Diabetes Mellitus: Therapeutic Implications. Diabet Med 2010;27: 136 –142

[5] Bergman H, Drury DR. The Relationship of Kidney Function to the Glucose Utilization of the Extraabdominal Tissues. Am J Physiol 1938;124: 279–284

[6] Gerich JE, Meyer C, Woerle HJ, et al. Renal Gluconeogenesis: Its Importance in Human Glucose Homeostasis. Diabetes Care 2001;24: 382-391

[7] Reinecke R. The Kidney as a Source of Glucose in the Eviscerated Rat. Am J Physiol 1943;140: 276–285

[8] Drury D, Wick A, MacKay E. Formation of Glucose by the Kidney. Am J Physiol 1950;165: 655–661

[9] Krebs H, Hems R, Gascoyne T. Renal gluconeogenesis. IV. Gluconeogenesis from Substrate Combinations. Acta Biol Med Germ 1963;11: 607–615

[10] Krebs H, Yoshida T. Renal Gluconeogenesis. II. The Gluconeogenic Capacity of the Kidney Cortex of Various Species. Biochem J 1963;89: 398–400

[11] Krebs H. Renal Gluconeogenesis. Adv Enzyme Reg 1963;1: 385–400

[12] Aber G, Morris L, Housley E. Gluconeogenesis by the Human Kidney. Nature 1966;212: 1589–1590

[13] Owen O, Felig P, Morgan A, et al. Liver and Kidney Metabolism During Prolonged Starvation. J Clin Invest 1969;48: 574–583

[14] Joseph SE, Heaton N, Potter D, et al. Renal Glucose Production Compensates for the Liver During the Anhepatic Phase of Liver Transplantation. Diabetes 2000;49: 450–456

[15] Gerich JE. Physiology of Glucose Homeostasis. Diabetes Obes Metab 2000;2: 345–350

[16] Stumvoll M, Meyer C, Kreider M, et al. Effects of Glucagon on Renal and Hepatic Glutamine Gluconeogenesis in Normal Postabsorptive Humans. Metabolism 1998;47: 1227–1232

[17] Stumvoll M, Meyer C, Mitrakou A, et al. Renal Glucose Production and Utilization: New Aspects in Humans. Diabetologia 1997;40: 749–757

[18] Schoolwerth A, Smith B, Culpepper R. Renal Gluconeogenesis: A Review. Miner. Electrolyte Metab 1988;14: 374–361

[19] Stumvoll M, Meyer C, Perriello G, et al. Human Kidney and Liver Gluconeogenesis: Evidence for Organ Substrate Selectivity. Am J Physiol 1998;274: E817–E826.

[20] Cersosimo E, Garlick P, Ferretti J. Insulin Regulation of Renal Gglucose Metabolism in Humans. Am J Physiol 1999;276: E78–E84.

[21] Babata L, Pedrosa M, Garcia R. Sustained Liver Glucose Release in Response to Adrenaline Can Improve Hypoglycaemic Episodes in Rats under Food Restriction Subjected to Acute Exercise. International Journal of Endocrinology, 2014. doi: 10.1155/2014/969137

[22] Meyer C, Stumvoll M, Welle S, et al. Relative Importance of Liver, Kidney, and Substrates in Epinephrine Induced Increased Gluconeogenesis in Humans. Am J Physiol Endocrinol Metab 2003; 285: E819–E826.

[23] Meyer C, Dostou JM, Welle SL, et al. Role of Human Liver, Kidney, and Skeletal Muscle in Postprandial Glucose Homeostasis. Am J Physiol Endocrinol Metab 2002;282: E419–E427

[24] Marsenic O. Glucose Control by the Kidney: an Emerging Target in Diabetes. Am J Kidney Disease 2009;53(5): 875–883

[25] Moe OW, Wright SH, Palacín M. Renal Handling of Organic Solutes. In: Brenner BM, Rector FC. (eds.) Brenner & Rector's The Kidney. Vol. 1. 8th ed. Philadelphia, PA: Saunders Elsevier; 2008. p214-247

[26] Silbernagl S, Despopoulos A, ed. Color Atlas of Physiology. New York: Thieme; 2009

[27] Wright EM, Hirayama BA, Loo DF. Active Sugar Transport in Health and Disease. J Int Med. 2007;261(1): 32-43

[28] Komoroski B, Vachharajani N, Boulton D, et al. Dapagliflozin, a Novel SGLT2 Inhibitor, Induces Dose-dependent Glucosuria in Healthy Subjects. Clin Pharmacol Ther. 2009;85(5): 520-526

[29] Vallon V, Platt KA, Cunard R et al. SGLT2 Mediates Glucose Reabsorption in the Early Proximal Tubule. J. Am Soc Nephrol 2011;22: 104–112

[30] Gorboulev V, Schürmann A, Vallon V et al. Na+-D-glucose Cotransporter SGLT1 is Pivotal for Intestinal Glucose Absorption and Glucose-dependent Incretin Secretion. Diabetes 2012;61: 187–196

[31] Wright E, Loo D, Hirayama, B. Biology of Human Sodium Glucose Transporters. Physiol Rev 2011;91: 733–791

[32] Turk E, Kim O, le Coutre J et al. Molecular Characterization of Vibrio Parahaemolyticus vSGLT:a Model for Sodium-coupled Sugar Cotransporters. J Biol Chem 2000;275: 25711–25716

[33] Andrianesis V, Doupis J. The Role of Kidney in Glucose Homeostasis - SGLT2 Inhibitors, a New Approach in Diabetes Treatment. Expert Rev Clin Pharmacol 2013;6(5): 519-539

[34] Meyer C, Stumvoll M, Nadkarni V, et al. Abnormal Renal and Hepatic Glucose Metabolism in Type 2 Diabetes Mellitus. J Clin Invest 1998;102: 619–624

[35] Meyer C, Woerle HJ, Dostou JM, et al. Abnormal Renal, Hepatic, and Muscle Glucose Metabolism following Glucose Ingestion in Type 2 Diabetes. Am J Physiol Endocrinol Metab 2004;287: E1049–E1056

[36] Mogensen CE. Maximum Tubular Reabsorption Capacity for Glucose and Renal Hemodynamcis During Rapid Hypertonic Glucose Infusion in Normal and Diabetic Subjects. Scand J Clin Lab Invest 1971;28: 101–109

[37] Rahmoune H, Thompson PW, Ward JM, et al. Glucose Transporters in Human Renal Proximal Tubular Cells Isolated from the Urine of Patients with Non-Insulin-Dependent Diabetes. Diabetes 2005;54: 3427–3434

[38] Exton J: Gluconeogenesis. Metabolism 21:945–990, 1972

[39] Ferre P, Pegorier J-P, Williamson D, et al. Interactions in Vivo Between Oxidation of Non-Esterified Fatty Acids and Gluconeogenesis in the Newborn Rat. Biochem J 1979;182: 593–598

[40] Molitch ME, DeFronzo RA, Franz MJ, et al. Nephropathy in Diabetes. Diabetes Care. 2004;27(1):S79-S83

[41] ADVANCE Collaborative Group; Patel A, MacMahon S, Chalmers J, et al. Intensive Blood Glucose Control and Vascular Outcomes in Patients with Type 2 Diabetes. N Engl J Med. 2008;358(24): 2560-2572

[42] Ehrenkranz JR, Lewis NG, Kahn CR, et al. Phlorizin: a Review. Diabetes Metab Res Rev 2005;21: 31–38

[43] Rossetti L, Smith D, Shulman GI, et al. Correction of Hyperglycemia with Phlorizin Normalizes Tissue Sensitivity to Insulin in Diabetic Rats. J Clin Invest 1987;79: 1510–1515.

[44] Wright EM. I. Glucose Galactose Malabsorption. Am J Physiol 1998;275: G879–G882

[45] Isaji M. Sodium–glucose Cotransporter Inhibitors for Diabetes. Curr Opin Investig Drugs 2007;8: 285–292.

[46] Ellsworth BA, Meng W, Patel M, et al. Aglycone Exploration of C-arylglucoside Inhibitors of Renal Sodium-dependent Glucose Transporter SGLT2. Bioorg Med Chem Lett 2008;18: 4770–4773.

[47] Meng W, Ellsworth BA, Nirschl AA et al. Discovery of Dapagliflozin: A Potent, Selective Renal Sodium-Dependent Glucose Cotransporter 2 (SGLT2) Inhibitor for the Treatment of Type 2 Diabetes. J Med Chem 2008;51: 1145–1149.

[48] Nomura S, Sakamaki S, Hongu M et al. Discovery of Canagliflozin, a Novel C-Glucoside with Thiophene Ring, as Sodium-Dependent Glucose Cotransporter 2 Inhibitor for the Treatment of Type 2 Diabetes Mellitus. J Med Chem 2010;53: 6355–6360

[49] Sha S, Devineni D, Ghosh A, et al. Canagliflozin, a Novel Inhibitor of Sodium Glucose Co-Transporter 2, Dose Dependently Reduces Calculated Renal Threshold for Glucose Excretion and Increases Urinary Glucose Excretion in Healthy Subjects. Diabetes Obes Metab 2011;13: 669–672

[50] Hummel CS, Lu C, Loo DD, et al. Glucose Transport by Human Renal Na+/D-glucose Cotransporters SGLT1 and SGLT2. Am J Physiol Cell Physiol 2011;300: C14–C21

[51] Kadokura T, Saito M, Utsuno A, et al. Ipragliflozin (ASP1941), a Selective Sodiumdependent Glucose Cotransporter 2 Inhibitor, Safely Stimulates Urinary Glucose Excretion without Inducing Hypoglycemia in Healthy Japanese Subjects. Diabetol Int 2011;2:172–182

[52] Ferrannini E, Ramos S J, Salsali A, et al. Dapagliflozin Monotherapy in Type 2 Diabetic Patients with Inadequate Glycemic Control by Diet and Exercise: A Random-

ized, Double-Blind, Placebo-Controlled, Phase 3 Trial. Diabetes Care 2010;33: 2217–2224.

[53] Osorio H, Bautista R, Rios A. et al. Effect of Phlorizin on SGLT2 Expression in the Kidney of Diabetic Rats. J Nephrol 2010;23: 541–546

[54] List JF, Woo V, Morales E, et al. Sodium-glucose Cotransport Inhibition with Dapagliflozin in Type 2 Diabetes. Diabetes Care 2009;32: 650–657

[55] Doblado M, Moley KH. Facilitative Glucose Transporter 9, a Unique Hexose and Urate Transporter. Am J Physiol Endocrinol Metab 2009;297: E831–E835

[56] Bailey CJ, Gross JL, Pieters A, et al. Effect of Dapagliflozin in Patients with Type 2 Diabetes who Have Inadequate Glycaemic Control with Metformin: A Randomized, Double-Blind, Placebo-Controlled Trial. Lancet 2010;375: 2223–2233.

[57] Wilding JP, Norwood P, T'joen C, et al. A Study of Dapagliflozin in Patients with Type 2 Diabetes Receiving High Doses of Insulin Plus Insulin Sensitizers: Applicability of a Novel Insulin-Independent Treatment. Diabetes Care 2009;32: 1656–1662.

[58] FDA. FDA Briefing Document. NDA 202293. Dapagliflozin Tablets, 5 and 10 mg. Advisory Committee Meeting, July 19, 2011 [online]. http://www.fda.gov/downloads/AdvisoryCommittees/CommitteesMeetingMaterials/Drugs/EndocrinologicandMetabolicDrugsAdvisory Committee/UCM262994.pdf (accesed 1 August 2014)

[59] Nelson RG, Bennett PH, Beck GJ et al, for The Diabetic Renal Disease Study Group. Development and Progression of Renal Disease in Pima Indians with Non-insulin-dependent Diabetes Mellitus. N Engl J Med 1996;335: 1636–1642.

[60] Williams ME, Garg R. Glycemic Management in ESRD and Earlier Stages of CKD. Am J Kidney Dis. 2014;63(2 Suppl 2): S22-38

[61] Wilding John P.H.,The role of the kidneys in glucose homeostasis in type 2 diabetes: clinical implications and therapeutic significance through sodium glucose co-transporter 2 inhibitors, Metabolism (2014), doi: 10.1016/j.metabol.2014.06.01

[62] Farhard M.H., Mazan A., John E.G., SGLT2 inhibitors in the treatment of type 2 diabetes. Diabetes Research and Clinical Practice 2014;104: 297-322

[63] Andrianesis V., Doupis J., The role of kidney in glucose homeostasis – SGLT2 inhibitors, a new approach in diabetes treatment, Expert Rev. Clin. Pharmacol. 2013; 6(5): 519-539.

Chapter 2

Thiamine and the Cellular Energy Cycles — A Novel Perspective on Type 2 Diabetes Treatment

Saadia Shahzad Alam and Samreen Riaz

Additional information is available at the end of the chapter

http://dx.doi.org/10.5772/59224

1. Introduction

Cellular survival is dependant upon the energy pathways ingrained within them. Their comprehension is imperative in understanding the role of their component enzymes in type 2 diabetes treatment and the inextricable linkage of a few of them to thiamine. The Glycolytic pathway is an ancient metabolic, cytosolic pathway that converts glucose into pyruvate under anaerobic conditions and further into lactate or ethanol. The free energy released from this forms high energy compounds ATP and NADH.Under aerobic conditions CO2 and substantially more ATP is produced [1]. The pathway of glycolysis comprises of 2 clear divisions (Fig 1). After glycolysis, further aerobic processing of glucose is conducted through the Kreb Cycle, synonymous with tricarboxylic acid or citric acid cycle (Fig 2). Intracellularly the mitochondria serve as site of citric acid cycle and oxidative phosphorylation activities.

The overall chemical reaction of the tricarboxylic acid cycle is:

$$\text{Acetyl-CoA} + 3\text{NAD}^+ + \text{FAD} + \text{GDP} + \text{P}_i + 2\text{H}_2\text{O} \rightarrow 2\text{CO}_2 + 3\text{NADH} + \text{FADH}_2 + \text{GTP} + 2\text{H}^+ + \text{HSCoA}^2 \quad (1)$$

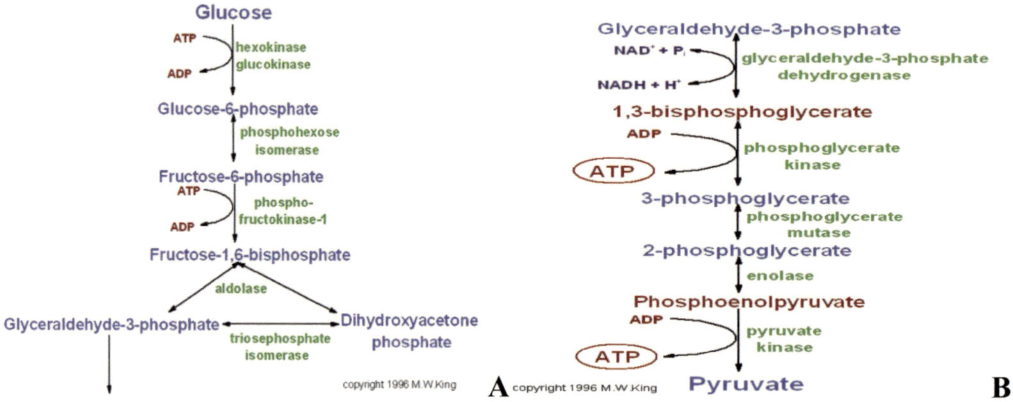

Adapted from Michael W. King, Ph.D / IU School of Medicine / miking at iupui.edu / © 1996–2011.

Figure 1. (A) Phase1 (Priming Phase) of Embden Meyerhoff Pathway; (B) Phase 2 (Energy Yielding Phase) of Embden Meyerhoff Pathway; A & B: A Schematic Pathway of glycolysis from glucose to pyruvate.and its connection to the reductive pentose pathway and citric acid cycle.

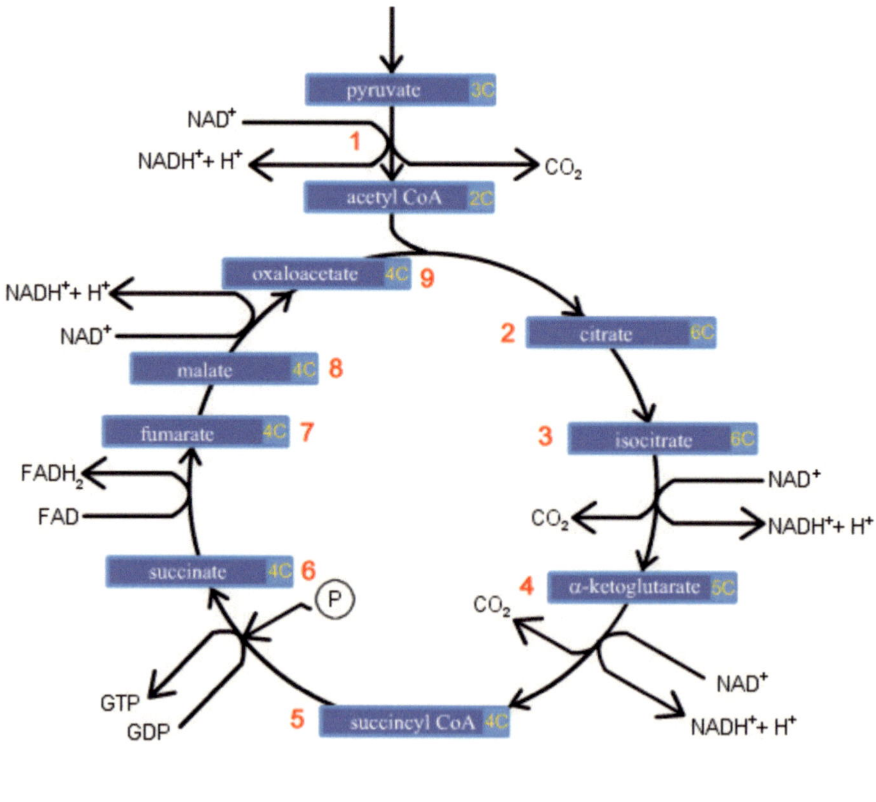

Figure 2. Krebs cycle (www. library.thinkquest.org)

http://dx.doi.org/10.5772/59224

2. The mitochondrial catalytic repertoire

The pyruvate dehydrogenase complex: Both prokaryotic and eukaryotic species carry among others, conglomeration of proteins into a mega, specifically arranged multienzyme structural complex termed (a "metabolon").

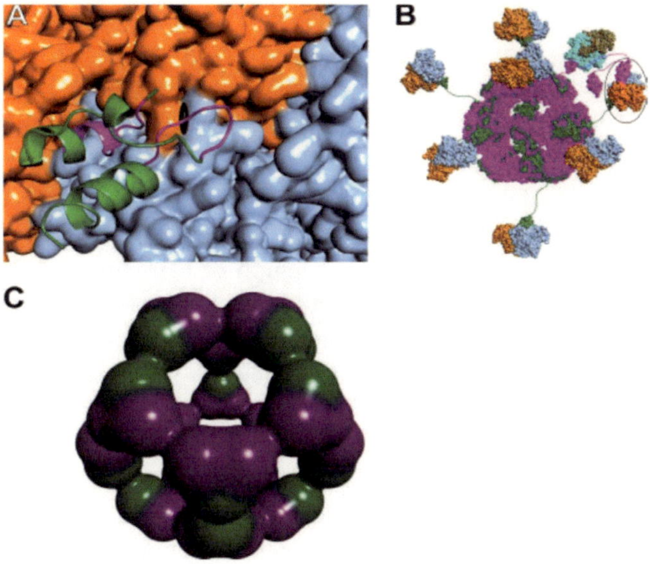

Figure 3. Protein-protein Interactions in the Native human PDC. Adapted from Brautigham (2006)

a. Close-up view of E3BD (ribbons representation) bound to E3 (surface) (Brautigham 2006). One monomer of E3 is colored orange, and the other is blue. The approximate position of the dyad axis of the E3 dimer is shown by the black symbol and arrow. Most of E3BD is colored green, but those residues with atoms that would clash with a second bound E3BD are shown in purple.

b. Schematic model of the native human PDC. The dodecahedral 60-meric core of the human PDC is modeled using the structure of the catalytic domain of B. tearothermophilus E2 (Izard 1999). The E2p polypeptides are colored magenta, with E3BP polypeptides colored green. The E3 dimers are shown in blueand orange, with a single E3BD bound per dimer of E3 (Brautigham 2006), as indicated by the data. In this model, it is possible for 20 E3 dimers to bind; only 7 are shown for clarity. A single E1p heterotetramer docked to the E1pBD of E2p is represented, subunits shown in tan and cyan. The structure of the human versions of E1p bound to E1pBD is unknown; shown here is the structure from B. stearothermophilus (Frank 2004). The circled E3 has an LBD of E. coli E2p docked to the active site. E2p and E3BD are therefore noncovalently cross-linked via their mutual interaction with E3.

c. Possible arrangement of E2p and E3BP components in a 40/20 core.Shown is a dodecahedral arrangement of 20 heterotrimers composed of 2 E2p proteins (purple) and one E3BP (green)(Brautigham 2008). Of these enzyme complexes of the metabolon, the pyruvate dehydrogenase complex is highly evolutionarily conserved mitochondrial α-ketoacid dehydrogenase complex, along with the branched-chain α-ketoacid dehydrogenase complex (BCKDC), and the α-ketoglutarate dehydrogenase complex (KGDC) [4, 5]. The complex has 3 main components with multiple subunits and multiple names.(Fig 3)

The heterotetramer **PDEI p PYRUVATE DEHYDROGENASE (EC1.2.4.1)** comprises of 2 alpha and 2 beta subunits [6]. Its alpha 1 subunit is designated as PDE1A-2,(pyruvate dehydrogenase (lipoamide) alpha2). Its gene PDHA2 is located on chromosome 4 having length of 1383 bp/460 aa [7, 8] Whereas the alpha 2 subunit is designated asPDH E1-A type1 (i.e.) synonym PHE1A. Its gene PDHA1 is located on chromosome X which has length of 15922 bps [9] and a mol.wt of 160KDa. The Pyruvate dehydrogenase E1 component subunit beta, or pyruvate dehydrogenase (lipoamide) beta mitochondrial, synonym, PDE1-B, has gene located on chromosome 3 having length of 6198 bp [10-12]. The key function of the complex E1alpha subunit containing the active site is to be the rate limiting enzyme, unidirectionally funneling intermediate metabolites from glucose breakdown to either the oxidative metabolic pathways or fatty acid and cholesterol synthesis [13]. **PDE2p** contains **dihydrolipoyl transacetylase enzyme activity (EC2.3.1.12)** encoded by DLAT Dihydrolipoamide acetyl tranferase gene, present on human chromosome 11 band q23.1. It has mol wt 200 KDa [14]. Interestingly, this long arm region of chromosome 11 often presents with translocations in cellular genetic abnormalities [15]. **PDE3/GCSL/LAD/PHE3 (EC 1.8.1.4)** component contains the dihydrolipoyl dehydrogenase activity. E3 activity is encoded by the DLD located on chromosome 7 and length 28799 [16]. It has a mol.wt of 110 KDa. This protein has four different sites: the flavin adenine dinucleotide binding site, the nicotinamide adenine dinucleotide binding site, the centre site and the interface site. The protein forms a homodimer with the FAD and NAD binding regions on one unit and the interface domain of the other unit forming the active centre [17].

2.1. Structural association of the 3 units

The human pyruvate dehydrogenase multi enzyme complex (PDC) is a nuclear encoded mitochondrial matrix 9.5 megadalton catalytic organization of copies of three catalytic components i.e. heterodimeric pyruvate dehydrogenase (E1p 30copies) (thiamine diphosphate (ThDPdependant), homodimeric dihydrolipoyl transacetylase (E2p12 copies) and dihydrolipoamide dehydrogenase dimer (E3) (FAD containing) residing in the inner mitochondrial membrane [4](Fig. 3). The (E1p) and E3subunits surround a 60-meric dodecahedral core of 40 copies of E2p and 20 copies of a monomeric non catalytic component, E3-binding protein (E3BP), which specifically tethers E3 dimers to the pyruvate dehydrogenase complex [18]. Each E2p subunit contains two consecutive lipoic acid-bearing domains (LBDs), termed as L1 and L2, one subunit binding domain (SBDp) which binds E1p and the inner-core/catalytic domain containing the E2 p active site responsible for the self assembly of the core which connects with the other independent domains by unstructured linkers [3](Fig.3). Similarly, each E3BP subunit consists of a single LBD (referred to as L3), the E3-binding domain (E3BD) and the noncatalytic inner core domain. It is presumed that the lipoyl bearing domains LBDs (L1, L2, and L3) and 60 subunits of the transacetylase seem to form a free circulation of lipoyl groups among which the acetyl groups are freely exchanged [18] and shuttle between the active sites of the three catalytic components of the PDC during the oxidative decarboxylation cycle [19]. Unspecified copies of each PDC regulatory enzyme pyruvate dehydrogenase kinases and pyruvate dehydrogenase phosphatases are also strung non-covalently to the core by the LBD2 [5, 20].

The active site synchronization over a distance of 20 Angstroms via proton wire through an acidic tunnel in the protein, keeps the active sites in an alternating activation state [22]. Phosphorylation of the heterotetrameric ($\alpha2\ \beta2$) E1p component is essential for the inactivation of the human PDC which occurs at 3 serine residues of the alpha subunit. Two of these sites are located in the conserved phosphorylation loop A [6] which forms one wall of the active site channel and helps to anchor ThDP to its active site.Site 3 is in the phosphorylation loop B which provides coordination to magnesium is chelated by the ThDP potassium. Phosphorylation of any of the 3 sites inactivates E1p and drastically reduces the affinity for pyruvate [24]. Disordered loops of E1p arise from phosphorylation and result in downregulation of the PDC activity. Binding of the cofactor ThDP induces ordering of both the loops which then can mediate decarboxylation and reductive acetylation of the pyruvate. Phosphorylation of PDC is crucial in regulating carbohydrate and lipid metabolism [14, 25]. Starvation and diabetes increase phosphorylation that inactivates PDC, leading to impaired glucose oxidation [26, 27]. On the other hand prevention of PDC phosphorylation by specific PDK inhibitor, dichloracetate increases reactive oxygen species levels in the mitochondria leading to cellular apoptosis and the inhibition of tumour growth [28, 29]. Therefore the regulation of PDC flux by reversible phosphorylation is a potential target for obesity and cancer [30, 31].Finally the expression of PDK2and PDK4 is down regulated by insulin in the long term [32, 33]. In the animal model, downregulation of skeletal muscle pyruvate dehydrogenase in the rat model before and after the onset of diabetes mellitus has been observed [34]. Dephosphorylation/activation of the PDC is ascribed to two Mg and Ca dependant genetically and biochemically distinct isoforms of pyruvate dehydrogenase phosphatase PDP heterodimeric (PDP1&PDP2), which are important regulators of PDC activity. PDP1 has both a catalytic (PDPc) subunit bound to the inner mitochondrial membrane and a regulatory (PDPr) subunit [35]. Both PDP1 components are targeted by insulin which enhances PDPc activity and lessens PDPr negative control resulting in enhanced overall PDP1 efficiency.These effects are at the core of insulin signaling of PDH [36]. PDP2, recently discovered in rat tissues consists of a catalytic subunit insensitive to Ca, 10 fold less sensitive to Mg than PDP c is also considered a target in insulin signaling [37, 38]. In humans too, down regulation of PDP in obese subjects is a malfunction that signals insulin resistance [39].

2.2. Diseases produced by defective PDC

As the PDC has prime significance in intermediary metabolism, mutations in the genes encoding for PDCsubunits produce severe clinical phenotypes [40]. Congenital defects in E1p in the X linked gene lead to lactic acidemias, encephalopathies, neuronal dysfunction in infancy [40]. Mutations in the E2, E3BP cause primary biliary cirrhosis leading to liver failure [41, 42], autoimmune hepatitis [43] and neurodegenerative conditions such as Alzheimer's disease. Combined enzyme deficiencies of α-ketoacid dehydrogenase complexes pyruvate dehydrogenase complex, BCKDC and ketoglutarate dehydrogenase complexes have been observed due to genetic changes in human E3 [44] resulting in lactic acidemias and maple syrup urine disease [45-47]. Other anamolies of the PDC include autoantibodies leading to paediatric biliary cirrhosis [47].Additionally, the aberrant down-regulation of pyruvate dehydrogenase complex activity by reversible phosphorylation has been shown to be contributory to hyperglycemic states observed in type-2 diabetes [25], increasing the chances of pyruvate dehydrogenase complex as a therapeutic target for a 150 million people affliction i.e. diabetes). Failure of functioning of the pyruvate dehydrogenase complex and specially of its E1p subunit due to lack of thiamine vitamin B1 would therefore inevitably lead to poor handling of glucose and its substrates and could manifest as deleterious effects in type 2 diabetics. The human 2 ketoglutarate dehydrogenase complex while extensively studied has not yet been reconstructed in vitro and reliance on other mammal models persists [5, 48](Fig 4).

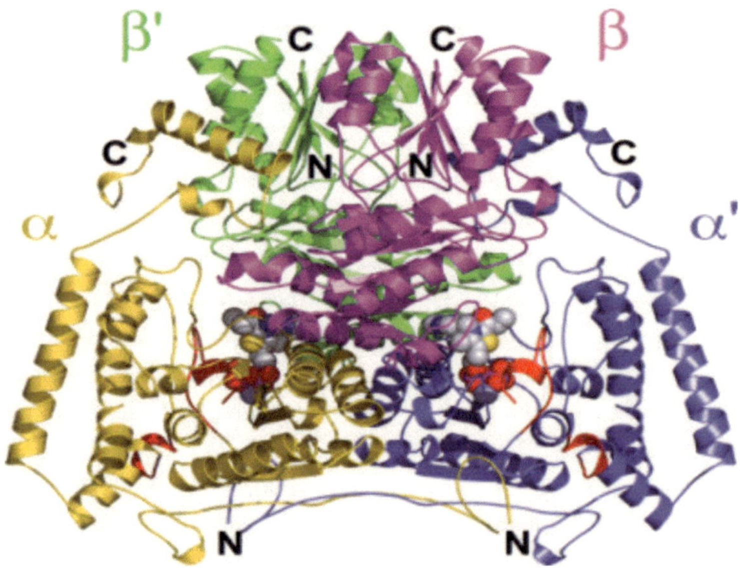

Figure 4. Representative Model for Human 2 Ketoglutarate Dehydrogenase Complex: All figures of molecular structures were created with the program PyMol (DeLano Scientific, San Carlos, CA). Jun Li. The Journal of Biological Chemistry, 2007;282, 11904-913.

2.3. Structure of alphaketoglutarate dehydrogenase complex

This 4 to 10 mega Dalton supramolecular complex is organized around a polyhedral form of a cubic core of 24/60 lipoate bearing dihydrolipoyl succinyltransferase E2 subunits (8 trimers) arranged with octahedral (432) symmetry [5] associated with non covalently attached multiple copies of dihydrolipoamide E1k and dihydrolipoamide E3K individually held via its E1/E3 binding domains which serve as scaffolds for the E2 core. There is also biochemical evidence of E3 binding to the aminoacid terminal region of E1 terminal allowing for separation of a stable E1-E3 submolecular complex from the E2 core [49].Also attached are regulatory kinase and phosphatase units [50]. Further lipoyl bearing domains LBDs of the E2 core are attached serving as swing arms impart substrate chanelling by sequentially visiting the different active sites in each of the three E1, E2 and E3 catalytic components [51] to transfer acyl groups to the active site of E2 leading to oxidative decarboxylation of the alpha ketoacids [51].The complex has 3 main enzymatic components with multiple subunits & copies and varied names: oxoglutarate dehydrogenase (lipoamide); EC: 1.2.4.2 (E1k), dihydrolipoamide S-succinyltransferase; EC:2.3.1.61 (E2k) and dihydrolipoamide dehydrogenase; EC:1.8.1.4 (E3k) [52].

1. **Alpha ketoglutarate dehydrogenase/2 oxoglutarate dehydrogenase E1k heterotetramer** (2 alpha and 2 betachains) (53) component has 6 copies (lipoamide) polypeptide enzyme having mol wt 115.94 kDa (from nucleotide sequence) and sequence length 34160 aminoacids.It is encoded by the OGDHgene localized on chromosome 10, 54290aa & 7 at p13-p14 [54] containing 22 exons spanning 102483 bpairs [55, 56]. It contains a thiamine diphosphate cofactor and catalyzes thiamine diphosphate dependant decarboxylation of 2 oxoglutarate and subsequent reductive acylation of the oxidized lipoyl moiety LBD (lip-LBD-S2) which is covalently bound to the E2 component dihydrolipoamide succinyl transferase [5]. Thiamine diphosphate is tightly but not covalently bound to the 2-oxoglutarate dehydrogenase component [57] ThDP remains an essential cofactor and alphaketoglutarate dehydrogenase complex in the form of homo dimers alpha2, homo tetramers alpha 4 or heterotetramers alpha 2 beta 2 contain ThDP binding pockets that constitute two or four active sites for this enzyme which operate independently without an obligatory alternating mechanism in the E1b component [58] and overall activity is abolished at 50% phosphorylation (1 of 2 sites) within each active channel similar to PDC [59].

2. **Dihydrolipoamide S-succinyltransferase E2k** core has 24 /60 copies containing lipoyl active site as well as active sites for E1 and E3 subunits based on similar mammalian PDC structural studies and molecular wt of 64.5 KDa [5]. It is encoded in gene DLST located on chromosome 14 q24.2-q24.3 with a length of 21815 base pairs [60]. This inner core plays an essential role in mediating the E1 catalyzed decarboxylation of 2 oxoglutarate and reductive acylation of the lipoyl moiety and E3 catalyzed reoxidation of the dihydrolipoyl moiety.

3. Located in the mitochondrial lumen, **Dihydrolipoamide dehydrogenase E3k** or E3component a flavoprotein (dimer) has 12 copies, a sequence length of 28796 aminoacids and is 54.15kDa in weight. It is encoded in the DLD gene localized to 7q31-q32 [61], its function is to catalyze the transfer of electrons from dihydrolipoamide to $NAD^+$and bears close

structural and functional approximation to the PDE3 component of pyruvate dehydrogenase and its full complex contains 6 dimers [5].

The alphaketoglutarate dehydrogenase complex EC 1.2.4.2 also termed as oxoglutarate dehydrogenase complex, acts on alphaketo-glutarate/2 oxoglutarate a key intermediate in the krebs cycle converting to succinyl co A, produces NADH and CO2 in an irreversible reaction [62] KGDHC catalyzes a vital step in the Krebs cycle, which is also a step in the metabolism of the potentially excitotoxic neurotransmitter glutamate. It allows amino acids to enter the citric acid cycle and produce energy; this is a reversible reaction in which glucose which enters the cycle can leave it to make amino acids thus linking amino acid pathways to the citric acid cycle. It also participates in lysine degredation and tryptophan metabolism. Alpha-KGDH is vital for maintaining NADH supply to the respiratory chain and is limited only when alpha-KGDH is also inhibited by ROS. In addition being a key target, it is also able to generate ROS during its catalytic function which is regulated by the NADH/NAD+ratio [63]. Its cofactors are TPP bound to E1, lipoic acid covalently bound to lysine on E2 which accepts the hydroxyethyl carbanion from TPP as an acetyl group, coenzyme A which is substrate for E2 and accepts the acetyl group from it, FAD bound to the E3 subunit reduced by lipoamide and NAD which is substrate for E3 and reduced by FADH2 [64]. Basic short term regulation of KGDHC is through adenosine diphosphate ADP, P (i) and Ca2+; these positive effectors increase manifold the affinity of ketoglutarate dehydrogenase complex to alpha-ketoglutarate. While KGDHC inhibitors are NADH, adenosine triphosphate, succinyl-CoA, and thioredoxin protects KGDHC from self-inactivation during catalysis [65]. Alpha-KGDH is also sensitive to oxidative stress and a number of metabolites modify the activity of KGDHC, including inactivation by 4-hydroxynonenal. In the human brain, comparison of KGDHC activity to other enzymes of energy metabolism like aconitase, phospho-fructokinase and the electron transport complexes shows it to be lower than all of them. Therefore impairment of KGDHC function is likely to disturb brain energy metabolism and result in brain disease [66]. In Wernickes encephalopathy there is AKGDH and thiamine deficiency associated with increased oxidative stress markers, lipid peroxidation resulting in neuronal cell death in pons, thalamus and cerebellum [67, 69]. In general, the clinical manifestations of KGDHC deficiency relate to the severity of the deficiency. A range of disorders have been recognized: varying from psychomotor retardation in childhood, to intermittent neuropsychiatric disease with ataxia and other motor disabilities, such as Friedreich's and other spinocerebellar ataxias [70], as well as neural diseases where mental deficits are also visible such as Parkinson's disease, and Alzheimer's disease (AD) [70]In Parkinsons Disease which has been deeply investigated, KGDHC Activity is reduced, coupled to elevated levels of monoamine oxidase B [71] and cytosolic accumulation of cytochrome c which inturn activates other pathways, including cell death cascades and enzyme inhibition which alters Ca2+homeostasis [72] The KGDHC enzyme is further a target for ubiquitination-dependent degradation in mitochondria by binding of Siah2, the RING finger ubiquitin-protein isopeptide ligase 2, encoded by gene siah2 [73]. Diabetes mellitus, thiamine dependent megaloblastic anaemia and sesorineural deafness associated with deficient alpha ketoglutarate dehydrogenase activity have also been reported [74]. There exist 2 wings,oxidative and reductive of the pentose phosphate pathway(Fig 5). The oxidation steps, utilizing glucose-6-phosphate (G6P) as the substrate, occur at the beginning of the pathway and generate 2 moles of NADPH. The reactions catalyzed by glucose-6-phosphate dehydrogenase (G6PD) and 6-phosphogluconate dehydrogenase are essential for the conversion of hexoses to pentoses [75].

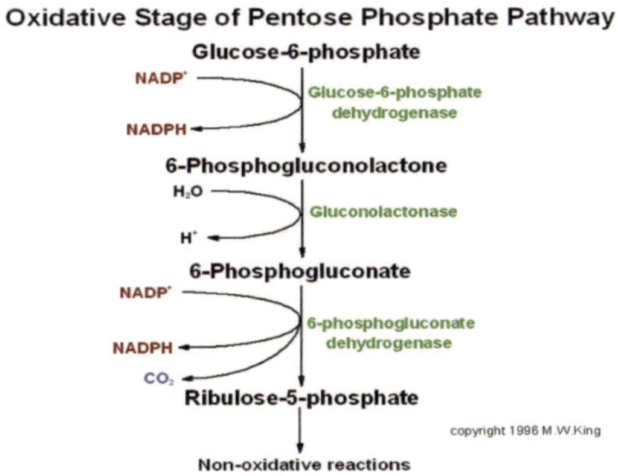

A) Digrammatic Representation of the Oxidative Stage of Hexose Monophosphate Shunt

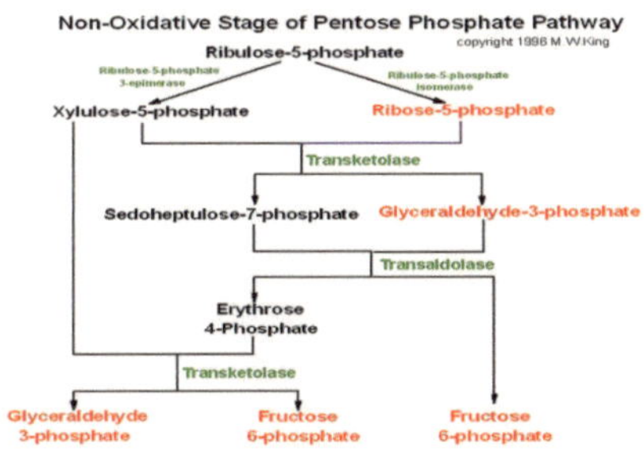

B) Reductive or Non Oxidative Stage of the Hexose Monophosphate Shunt

Figure 5. (A): Digrammatic Representation of the Oxidative Stage of Hexose Monophosphate Shunt and (B) Reductive Stage of the Hexose Monophosphate Shunt

The non-oxidative reactions of the pentose phosphate pathway are mainly functioning to produce ribose 5 phosphate, and equally significantly to convert dietary 5 carbon sugars into both 6 (fructose-6-phosphate) and 3 (glyceraldehyde-3-phosphate) carbon sugars which can then be utilized by the pathways of glycolysis [76].

2.4. Functions of the pentose phosphate pathway in normal and diseased conditions

The Pentose phosphate pathway (PPP) is primarily energy forming, and non mitochondrial with only a cytoplasmic enzymatic presence entrusted to utilizing 6 carbon sugars, and producing in turn 5 carbon sugars for the synthesis of neucleotides, nucleic acids and reducing equivalents in the form of NADPH. The pentose phosphate pathway is a metabolic redox estimator and regulates transcription during the anti-oxidant response, as a shift from primary carbon metabolism, is fastest in oxidative stress [77]. NADPH cofactor serves as reducing equivalent in the endoplasmic reticulum lumen for fatty acid and steroid biosynthesis in hepatic and, adipose tissue, adrenal cortex [78]. High levels of PPP enzymes are in neutrophils and macrophages as they utilize NADPH to produce ROS to destroy engulfed microbes in a process termed as respiratory burst [79]. G6PD deficiency effects red blood cell viability dependent on PPP generated NADPH, a glutathione reducer, the absence of which results in hemolysis seen with certain drugs and diseases like malaria which cause oxidative stresss [80]. Cancer cells are known to access successfully the glucose flux in the pentose phosphate pathway supporting NADPH and reactive oxygen species production and glutathione reduction [81] responding to both incremental and decremental reactive oxygen species [82]. Electron leakage from the mitochondrial electron transport remains essential (through the action of ribonucleotide reductase) in generating deoxyribonucleiotides from nucleotides as well producing ROS in collusion with oncogenes [83] and molecular oxygen [84] promoting genetic damage in normal cells and therapy resistance in cancerous cells [85].Malignant cells also use reduced glutathione [81] or NADPH to combat oxidative stress and to support the oxidation of fatty acids in detached cells [86]. **Transketolase** is the premier cytosolic enzyme of the reductive pentose phosphate pathway. Its 3 genes TKT, Transketolase like TKTLI and Transketolase like TKTL2 encode for proteins with transketolase activity.All of them participate in the reductive pentose pathway reactions catalyzing transfer of a 2 carbon fragment from a ketose donor to an aldose (acceptor substrate) [87].

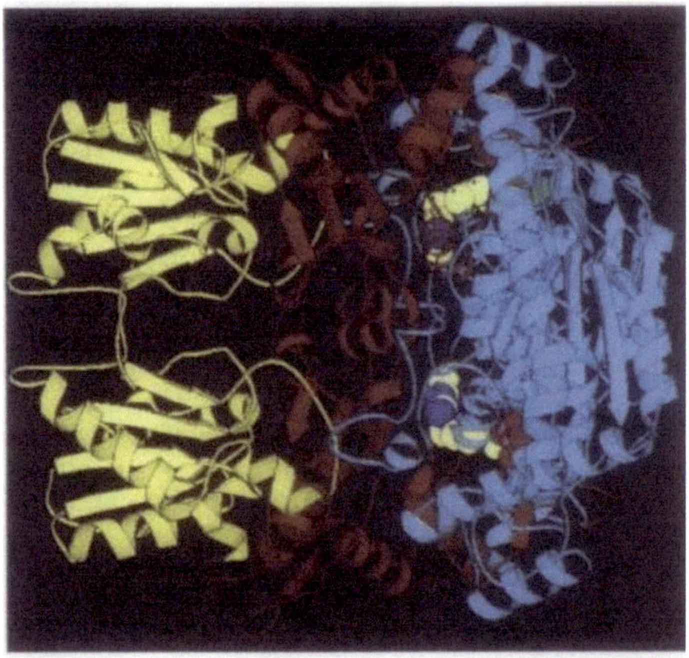

Adapted from Kochetov2005, Lindquist 1992

Figure 6. Schematic View of Transketolase Dimer Showing its Different Components. The 3 components are colour differentiated: N terminal domain, light blue, middle domain, light brown & C terminal domain yellow.The bound cofactor ThDP is shown as a CPK model and Ca++ion in green

Transketolase: synonymous with TKT1 &TK is composed of and encoded by the TKTgene located on chromosome 3 (30390 bp) [89-91]. **Transketolase like protein 1:** named as TKT2, TKR, TK 2, Transketolase 2, Transketolase-related protein has molwt of 60-70 KDaltons depending on splice variation encoded by the TKTL1 gene located on chromosomeX Length: 25052 bp [92, 93]. **Transketolase like protein 2** termed TK is composed of 913 aminoacids encoded by gene TKTL2 located on chromosome 4 having length of 2742 bp [94].

TKT Structure: Transketolase (TK) is a homodimer [95] (Fig 6) and the least structurally complicated member of thiamine diphosphate (ThDP)-dependent enzymes group containing PDHC & OGDHC [96]. Each monomer consists of three distinct regions the N terminal or PP binding region, the middle or pyrimidine binding region and C terminal region [87]. The first 2 regions are associated with coenzyme binding while the role of the third remains unknown [85, 97].

Thiamine Binding Site: TKT has two active centres with one THDP molecule attached to a binding motif [98, 99] and a bivalent cation (Ca affinity more than Mg [100]) tightly bound at each centre by noncovalent interactions [101]. Thiamine binding site is located within a deep furrow which allows only the C2 atom of the thiazolium ring to be exposed to the donor substrate [101]. A highly conserved starter sequence glycine-aspartate-glycine GDG and concluding sequence asparagine-asparagine (NN) represent this site between residues 154 and 185 [101]. Further the interactions of the non-covalently bound coenzyme ThDP-magnesium with the protein component are at five critical sites containing arginines (Arg 101, Arg 318, Arg 395, Arg 401 and Arg 474and Asp155) [101] contribute to dimer formation, stability or catalytic activity [102, 96]. The dimerization process involves initial binding of magnesium to the aspartate in the starter sequence which inturn interacts with the pyrophosphate molecule of the thiamine diphosphate through hydrogen bonding [101], followed by one transketolase monomer engaging the pyrophosphate moiety and the other with the thiazolium and pyrimidine rings of ThDP [88, 97]. The importance of this interaction is reflected in the noticeable refractoriness in Wernickes encephalopathy to thiamine treatment alone in hypomagnesemic alcoholics [103]. This enzyme has a 2 stage catalytic cycle central to which is the TPP molecule, initiated by the deprotonation in its thiazolium ring due to interaction with Glu 418 of apotransketolase.

2.5. Role of transketolase in disease and therapy

Transketolase enzyme genetic variants and depreciated enzyme activities have been noted in neurodegenerative diseases like Wernickes Korsakoff syndrome and Alzheimers disease [104]. Upregulation of the TKT L1 gene has been found in a number of malignant disorders resulting in enhanced total transketolase activity and cellular proliferation in human colon cancer [105], thyroid [106], cervical [107], ovarian cancer [108], nephroblastoma and adenocarcinoma. Its increased expression is found to be a potential diagnostic biomarker for breast cancer [109] and prognostic biomarker for nasopharyngeal [110] and laryngeal squamous cell carcinoma [111]. The reason may lie in the role of tranketolase in the reductive pentose pathway which remains a source a carbons such as in ribose required for neucleotide synthesis, NADPH and reduced glutathione in addition to aromatic acids and fatty acids required for cellular growth in general and explosive growth in particular. Transketolase has begun to emerge as a target in the cellular immune response in multiple sclerosis [112]. Human transketolase can be used in structure-based drug design as target for inhibition in the treatment of cancer [113] and in the search for new transketolase inhibitors as non permanently charged thiamine analogs,which are substrates for the thiamine activator thiamine pyrophosphokinase. These pyrophosphate analogs antagonize the ability of transketolase in vitro [113]. In diabetes mellitus type 2 experimental model, the role of transketolase in the reductive pentose pathway and its activation by administration of lipid soluble thiamine derivative benfotiamine is well documented and undeniable [114] and further clinical research is ongoing.

2.6. Pharmacotherapeutics of type 2 diabetes

Treatment is done using 4 categories of oral antidiabetic drugs.

1. Insulin secretagogues: Sulfonylureas, meglitinides, D-phenylalanine derivatives

2. Those reducing insulin resistance:

  i. Biguanides

  ii. Thiazolidinediones (glitazones)

3. Those decreasing carbohydrate absorption from the gut: Alpha Glucosidase inhibitors.

2.7. Insulin secretagogues

i. Sulfonylureas:

These act by stimulating insulin release from pancreatic B cells. Sulfonylureas may also act by decreasing hepatic insulin clearance [115]. They increase insulin concentration often failing to improve first phase insulin release in response to a glycemic challenge. There is secondary failure and tachyphylaxis to sulfonylurea therapy following prolonged use. Their adverse effects are hypoglycaemia, GIT disturbances, cholestatic jaundice, agranulocytosis, aplastic and hemolytic anemia, generalized hypersensitivity and dermatological reactions [116]. There is also a debate on associated cardiovascular mortality – due to blockage of KATP channels of the hearts and vascular tissues [117]. Second generation sulfonylurea glimepiride is useful as single therapy in previously drug naïve patients and also in combination with non-secretagogue medication [118]. Glimepiride may be linked to lower incidence of hypoglycaemia [119] and may improve insulin sensitivity [120]. It also has an insulin sparing action [121].

ii. Meglitinides:

Like the sulfonylureas, meglitinides also stimulate insulin secretion.

iii. D-phenylalanine derivatives:

Nctaglinide is the latest insulin secretagogue to become available. It selectively enhances early insulin release providing excellent meal time glucose control while reducing total insulin exposure [122]

iv. Biguanides:

These agents don't cause hypoglycemia and are thus called euglycemic agents. Current proposed mechanisms of biguanides include glycolysis simulation in tissues, reducing glucose absorption from GIT with increased glucose to lactate conversion, reduced hepatic and renal gluconeogenesis, in the GI tract and reduction of plasma glucagon levels [123]. Most frequent toxicity are gastrointestinal (anorexia,nausea,vomiting,abdominal discomfort and diarrhea). It is contra indicated in patients with hepatic disease or in conditions predisposing to tissue anoxia because of risk of lactic acidosis [124].

v. Thiazolidinediones (glitazones):

They are also considered to be euglycemic and are effective in 70% users. Three drugs have been used clinically from this group (Troglitazone, Rosiglitazone and Pioglitazone). Troglitazone a severely hepatotoxic and its removal from public use is well known. These are selective agonists for nuclear peroxisome proliferator – activated receptor – gamma (PPAR GAMMA) whose activation enhances insulin responsive genes that regulate carbohydrate and protein metabolism [125]

vi. Alpha Glucosidase Inhibitors:

Competitive inhibitors of intestinal alpha glucosidases namely acarbose and miglitol decrease the post meal digestion and assimilation of simple and complex carbohydrates such as starch and disaccharides [126]. These are effective also in prediabetic individuals and successfully restored β cells function. Therefore, diabetes prevention may be a further indication for their usage [127].

3. New drugs for type 2 diabetes

3.1. Currently available

The Incretin hormones released by the gut, gastric inhibitory peptide (GIP) and Glucagon like peptide1 (GLP-1) (liraglutide) stimulate insulin secretion upon nutrient entry into the gut, suppression of glucagon release,slow gastric emptying and decrease food intake [128, 129]. Therefore, they have an antidiabetogenic potential. Incretin mimetics e.g. Exenatide LAR from exendin 4 is currently in use and most resistant to DPP4 degredation. GIP has also been shown enhancing β cell proliferation and inhibiting apoptosis in islet cell lines [130, 131]. Additionally functional GIP receptors have been identified on adipocytes and shown to stimulate glucose transport, accelerating fatty acid synthesis and stimulating lipoprotein lipase activity in animal models [131, 133, 134]. Several novel GIP analogues have been developed which act as stronger GIP agonists, showing resistance to degradation by Dipeptidyl Peptidase-4 (DIPP-4) [135] and demonstrating increased insulinotropic and blood glucose lowering activity [135]. Dipeptidyl peptidase Inhibitors (vildagliptin & sitagliptin) suppress breakdown of Glucagon like peptide1 (GLP-1) show great potential and are undergoing clinical testing. Antihyperglycemic synthetic analogs of amylin a hormone which are produced by the pancreas to lower blood sugar levels are available in injectable form and require close monitoring. Dapagliflozin a renal glucose reabsorption inhibitor reduces glycemic reabsorption independent of insulin, promises to be a new drug for type 2 diabetes treatment [136]. Testosterone replacement therapy in diabetic hypogonadal men decreases insulin resistance [137] probably by protective effect on pancreatic beta cells through its action on inflammatory cytokines [138].

3.2. Experimental new drugs

A vanadium and allixin based drug [139] and macrophage migration inhibitory factor MIF blocking inhibitory synthetic oral drug reducing blood sugar levels was tried in the mouse model and found to be effective in both the type 1&2 diabetc model [140]. Lisofylline, a fat metabolism inhibitor which prevents buildup of ceramide a by product of fat metabolism in mouse skeletal muscle decreased the insulin resistance and thus appears to be a novel new approach for type 2 diabetes [141]. It also has the ability to protect insulin producing cells by inhibiting cytokines produced by immune cells leading to apoptosis and cellular dysfunction and is thus effective in type1 diabetes [142]. LXR agonists have shown potential and require further testing in human and model systems [143]. Growth factors and protein kinase C inhibitors may act as innovative therapies for diabetic retinopathy [144].

3.3. Surgical interventions

Recently a type of gastric bypass surgery has been successful in normalizing blood sugar in a small number of normal to moderately obese type 2 diabetics [145, 146]. This surgery may possibly reduce death rate by 40% from all causes in morbidly obese people [147].

3.4. Micronutrient approaches to treatment of diabetic complications

People with diabetes have reduced antioxidant capacity which lays the basis for usage of antioxidant vitamins such as β carotene or vitamin C or E. A reduced level of ascorbic acid (Vitamin C) leaves the body more at mercy of the detrimental effects of aldose reductase, an enzyme responsible for many diabetic complications, such as cataracts and peripheral neuropathy [148]. Quercetin is another powerful aldose reductase inhibitor. It has been shown to inhibit aldose reductase by upto 50% [149]. Vitamin E is a free radical scavenger. It may play a preventive role in diabetic retinopathy by decreasing DAG levels, normalizing protein kinase C activation, normalizing blood flow in retinal and renal microvasculature and restoring NO mediated endothelium dependent relaxation [150, 151]. Renal and retinal vascular flows and responses were normalized in individuals who had diabetes of less than 10 years duration with high dose oral vitamin E therapy given for short periods while unchanged glycaemic control was observed [152].

Magnesium and chromium deficiency have been associated with poor diabetic control, insulin resistance, macro vascular disease and hypertension [153] and decreased glucose tolerance respectively [154]. Reduction of neuronal damage in diabetics by inhibiting glutamate dehydrogenase via vitamin B6 therapy has also been observed [155].N-Reduced glutathione precursor NAcetyl Cysteine is a gene expression and cellular metabolism modulating antiox-

http://dx.doi.org/10.5772/59224

idant and its role in prevention of β cell oxidatory damage by acting as NFKB (a genetic regulator) inhibitor and subsequent deintensification of inflammatory responses is well documented [156]. Trace element vanadyl sulfate that behaves like insulin normalized hyperglycemic levels in diabetic animals and decreased the insulin need by upto 75% [157]. In human with Type 2 diabetes, low doses of vanadyl sulfate enhanced insulin responsive glucose uptake, glycogen production and decreased endogenous glucose formation. This resulted in reduced lipid oxidation and plasma free fatty acids levels [158]. Alpha lipoic Acid has powerful antioxidant activity, insulinomimetic action and provides protection from insulin resistance linked diabetic stress while improving glucose utilization [159]. Hyperglycemia reduction in diabetic rats was observed along with improvement in GSH levels with selenium therapy [160].Calcium AEP has benefited both type 1 and type 2 diabetics as it is alpha cell membrane integrity factor required for cellular membrane function. The hormone dehydroepiandrosterone (DHEA) undergoes a decrease in levels with aging that many researchers have linked to impair glucose metabolism. It was found to be as effective in reducing body fats and maintaining insulin responsiveness as exercise [161]. Thiamine is also now showing potential as therapy for type 2 diabetes.

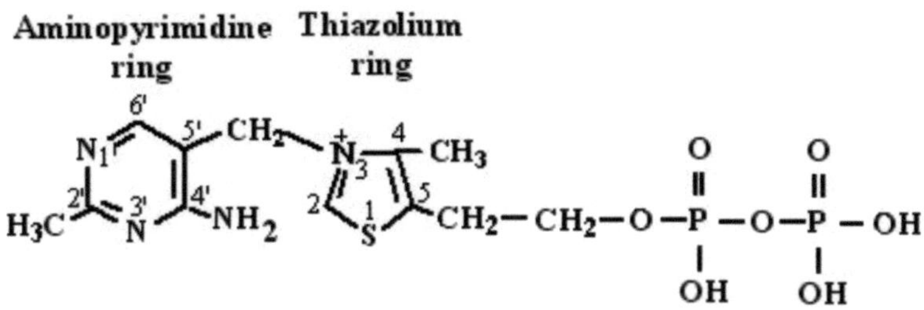

Figure 7. Structure of thiamine diphosphate molecule.

Thiamine (termed aneurin or antineuritic vitamin initially) was the premier discovery of the B vitamins and thus ranked vitamin B1(Fig 7). It has relative temperature, acid stability and water solubility containing a pyrimidine ring and a thiazole nucleus linked with a methylene bridge. Thiamine is an essential micronutrient with a dietary reference intake (DRI) for normal healthy subjects of 1.1 mg/day for females and 1.3 mg/day for males [162]. Found in range of foodstuffs such as cereal grains. Its rich sources are brown rice, bran, oat meal, flax, poultry, egg yolks, beef, pork, liver, nuts, fruits and vegetables such as oranges, asparagus, kale, cauliflower, potatoes [163].UK law demands compulsary fortification of flour with thiamin of not less than 0.24mg/100g flour to replace losses during milling. In Pakistan no compulsory fortification is done and the general public consumes milled white flour which is easily available and probably thiamine deficient. Thiamine is naturally found in 4 forms in varying degrees of phosphorylation in TMP thiamine monophosphate, TPP thiamine pyrophosphate or diphosphate and TTP=thiamine triphosphate. It is commercially available as salt in its mononitrate HCl (also natural byproduct) and relatively inaccessible semi lipid soluble form S-acyl derivative benfotiamine and truly lipid soluble thiamine disulphide derivatives sulbutiamine and fursultiamine. Out of these, Thiamine HCl is the water soluble, easily accessible and commonly used vitamin supplement available with the trade name Benerva.

3.5. Pharmacokinetics

3.5.1. Thiamine absorption in normal conditions

Thiamine is released from its administered form by phosphatase and pyrophosphatase in the proximal part of the small intestine, following which absorption occurs mainly from this site with some from the stomach and the colon; thiamine absorbed in the colon may originate from intestinal microflora. Its absorption is hindered by alcohol consumption and folic acid deficiency [164].High affinity organic anion transporters THTR1 [165], THR2 for thiamine and reduced folate transporter RFC-1 transports both folic acid thiamine monophosphate (TMP) intracellularly [166, 168] at normal physiological concentrations. At high expression levels RFC1 also transports TPP out of the cells [167]. At higher concentrations thiamine crosses cell membranes in its open unionized form of the thiazolium ring even by passive diffusion.THTR2 is placed on the luminal surface of the gastrointestinal epithelial cells and THTR1 is on the basolateral surface mainly but not exclusively [169]. THTRI is expressed widely in human tisseues with particular high expression in skeletal muscles, placenta, heart liver and kidney [168, 170].Mutations in the SLC19A2 (D93H, S143F and G172D) cause malfunctioning of the thiamine transporter THTR1, thiamine deficiency and thiamine responsive megaloblastic anaemia (TRMA) [171, 172]. THTR2 is widely expressed most abundantly in placenta, kidney and liver [173]. Also highly expressed RFC-1, is in human tissues including mitochondrial membranes [168, 174]. It has affinities for TMP and TPP of 26μM and 32μM respectively [167, 168]. Cellular efflux is the probable reason for the presence of thiamine in plasma and cerebrospinal fluid [175-177].Thiamine in the glomerular filtrate is reabsorbed by the renal brush border membrane high affinity transporters where influx is increased by an outward directed H+gradient [178] RFC-1 is expressed on the apical and basolateral surface of the proximal tubular epithelial cells [179]; it may mediate the reuptake of TMP and provide a solution to the normal absence of TMP in the urine. Proton antiport membrane transport may operate in both intestinal and renal proximal tubular thiamine uptake [180]

3.5.2. Assessment of thiamine status

Erythrocytes contain approximately 90% of total thiamine in the blood and therefore conventionally their transketolase levels have generally been considered to be the measure of thiamine status in the body [181].Thiamine deficiency is assessed conventionally by measuring the percentage below complete saturation of the thiamine dependant enzyme transketolase (TK) in RBCs-"thiamine effect". The normal value of the thiamine effect in human subjects is in the range 0-15%, mild deficiency is 15-25% and severe thiamine deficiency >25% [182]. Latest research has however questioned its reliability as thiamine transporters THTR1 and RFC1 in erythrocytes are upregulated in thiamine deficieny and RBC TK levels are not decreased in tandem [183]. Furthermore it doesn't account for changes in TK expression in RBC and other precursor cells. The expression of TK is decreased in thiamine deficiency [184]. Currently assessment of mononuclear TK activity and plasma thiamine concentration determination using HPLC flourimetric determination with respect to normal healthy controls gives greater insight into thiamine status [185-187]. More recently in capillary enzyme reaction and capillary electrophoresis methods are emerging as potential alternative monitoring and determining techniques for thiamine in samples [188].

3.5.3. *Thiamine metabolism within the cells*

When TMP enters cells by RFC-1 it is hydrolyzed to thiamine by phosphatases [168]. Thiamine deficiency decreased the activity of TPPK [189] and was implicated in decreased hepatic levels of TPP with normal levels of thiamine in STZ diabetic rats [190].Within mitochondria TPP is slowly hydrolyzed to TMP by phosphatases which may leave the mitochondria via the same transporter. High concentrations of thiamine monophosphate inhibit thiamine pyrophspho-kinase activity noncompetitively [191] and inhibit the entry of TPP into the mitochondria competitively [189]. A small amount of TPP is further phosphorylated to thiamine triphosphate (TTP) by thiamine pyrophosphate kinase and hydrolyzed to TPP by TPPphosphatase [192] [168]. Plasma half life is relatively short (2days) [193] but its tissue half life is approximately 9-18 days [194]. Thiamine is stored largely in skeletal muscle and the highly perfused organs such as heart, brain, liver and kidneys [163]. Subcellularly only 10% of total TPP is available for binding to transketolase most of it is associated with the mitochondria [185].Thiamine and its acid metabolites are are excreted primarily in the urine [195].

4. Pharmacodynamics of thiamine

Thiamine diphosphate binds to a evolutionarily highly conserved domain located in a deep cleft in the active sites of the thiamine dependant enzymes resulting in the activity of these enzymes [196]. The physiological function of thiamine is mainly fulfilled by TPP (TDP). Structurally the basis of thiamine action and activation of all ThDP-dependent enzymes lies in thiamine catalysis and deprotonation of the thiazolium ring and contribution of the aminopyrimidine side chain in this effect [197-198] while the pyrimidine ring with its dual proton donor and acceptor capability functioning as a proton transfer system. On the basis of these chemical alterations TPP functions as coenzyme for mitochondrial enzymes pyruvate dehydrogenase (PDH [199] and α ketoglutarate dehydrogenase [200] of the citric acid cycle.

4.1. Symtoms of severe thiamine deficiency

Thiamine derivatives and thiamine dependant enzymes are universally present in all cells of the body thus a thiamine deficiency would seem to affect all organ systems especially the heart and the nervous system due to their high oxidative metabolism as witnessed in its severest form as beriberi (dry, wet or infantile) [195]. Symptoms occur rarely include tachycardia, warmth, flushing, irritability, sweating, nausea, restlessness and allergic reactions. Pharma-cokinetic interactions at the level of drug metabolism include microsomal enzyme induction by prolonged anticonvulsant pheytoin resulting in decreased plasma levels of thiamin in patients with seizure disorders such as epilepsy. The water soluble thiamine HCl form is safe in humans in oral doses less than or equal to several hundred milligrams via oral route. A UK EVM found that a small clinical trial in Alzheimers patients revealed no adverse effects of thiamineHCl at daily oral intakes of 6000 to 8000mg for five to six months. A randomized double blind placebo controlled trial was conducted in India for therapy of primary dysmenorrhea, a daily oral dose of 100mg thiamine was given to 556 females for 60-90 days and no adverse effects were noted.In extremely rare cases of allergic sensitivity were noted solely in patients using thiamine by the parenteral route and were probably due to the injection vehicle and it not been reported to be carcinogenic or mutagenic. No known genetic microsomal variations increase susceptibility to thiamine toxicity [214].

5. Thiamine and diabetes

Experimental evidence suggests that thiamine transport maybe abnormal in diabetes.In experimental diabetes, these was diminished intestinal absorption of thiamine and TMP. Mild deficiency of thiamine in diabetes may induce increased expression of THR1 as found in frank thiamine deficiency. In streptozocin induced diabetic rats with supportive insulin therapy to regulate hyperglycemia, 54% decreased plasma thiamine concentration was reported in contrast to normal controls [190]. This was induced in the diabetic state despite high dietary intake (9 fold) in excess of DRI for rats. The primary cause was marked increased renal clearance of thiamine which was increased by 8 fold. In streptozotocin-induced diabetic rats, there was decreased transketolase expression and activity in renal glomeruli, liver, skeletal muscle and RBCs after 12 weeks of diabetes was found associated with progressive increase in the renal clearance of thiamine and increased albuminuria with duration of diabetes, suggesting that abnormal renal handling of thiamine may occur early in the process of impairment of renal function in diabetes [190]. In experimental diabetes, similar low plasma thiamine concentration was associated with low TK activity and expression in renal glomeruli.Reduced activity of PDH was also noticed due to thiamine depletion. Similar impairment of thiamine-related metabolism may occur in the diabetic retina and peripheral nerves predisposing these tissues to the adverse effects of hyperglycaemia.

5.1. Effect of thiamine therapy in diabetes: On glycemic control in experimental and animal model

Thiamine therapy was found to decrease hyperglycemia in cirrhosis, insulin resistance of muscle and inadequate insulin secretion by β cells. In thiamine responsive megaloblastic anaemia too hyperglycemia is linked to impaired insulin secretion due to mutated high affinity thiamine transporter. Therapeutic intervention by thiamine in both cases is likely to involve improved β cell metabolism and insulin secretion. This effect was not noticed in permanent insulin deficiency of the STZ diabetic rat model where most of the pancreatic β cells are damaged or destroyed and resultantly no improvement in glycemic control is observed. It is not yet known if thiamine or benfotiamine improve glycemic control in type 2 diabetic animal model.

5.2. Mild thiamine deficiency in diabetics and improved post therapy thiamine status in clinical studies

Mild thiamine deficiency has been observed in diabetics in different international studies.There is paucity of data on thiamine and thiamine dependant enzyme status in clinical diabetes mellitus. In Japan a study of 46 diabetic patients (7 type 1, 39 type 2) with moderate glycemic control (glycated hemoglobinA1c 9%) found lower diabetic RBC TK activity in 79% of patients and a concomitant decrease in thiamine level in 76% of diabetics. Oral thiamine supplementation 3-80mg/day increased thiamine levels (20 patients) and TK activity (15 patients). In a larger Israel study of 100 type 2 diabetic patients (glycated HbAic 9.2%), TK activity was lower than the minimum normal range in 18% of diabetics. A smaller Italian study of 10 type 1 diabetic children with normal renal function found plasma thiamine concentration to be decreased by 34% with respect to normal healthy controls and was normalized in a placebo controlled intervention with lipophilic thiamine derivative benzoxymethyl thiamine (50mg/day).

5.3. Intervention of high dose thiamine therapy in biochemical dysfunction in diabetes and the prevention of microvascular dysfunction, neuropathy, dyslipidemia complications

Microvascular disease (nephropathy, retinopathy and neuropathy) a common debilitating manifestation of chronic diabetes mellitus, has no effective therapy. Hyperglycaemia in diabetic subjects is an essential element for development of both microvascular and macrovascular complications risk factor DCCT 2003. High doses of thiamine and its derivative S-benzoylthiamine monophosphate (Benfotiamine) are proposed as a new therapy to counteract biochemical dysfunction leading to the development of microvascular complications [114]. High dose thiamine and Benfotiamine may counter the development of microvascular complications by activation of the reductive pentosephosphate pathway. Interestingly by activation of the hexosamine pathway the glucose-mediated induction of lipogenic enzymes, glycerophosphate dehydrogenase (GPDH), fatty acid synthase (FAS) and acetyl-CoA carboxylase, was stimulated in liver and adipocytes(Fig 8). In turn, this diverts metabolic flux away from the hexosamine pathway, decreased lipogenesis and correct diabetic dyslipidaemia as shown below (Fig 8).

Drugs such as cerivastatin decreased total and LDL cholesterol, triglycerides, microalbuminuria and increased HDL cholesterol in type 2 diabetic patients. However, normal levels of these metabolite were not achieved. Interestingly pharmacologically combined therapy of vit B1, B6 and B12 did not augur well in diabetics having diabetic nephropathy and substantial adverse outcomes associated with high dose vitamin B6, B9 and B12 co-supplementation in patients with advanced diabetic nephropathy was brought to light Recently concluded Diabetic Intervention with Vitamins to Improve Nephropathy (DIVINE) study produced an unexpected accelerated decline in renal function. The reasons could have been multipronged ranging from toxic accumulation of folate and B12 in patients of diabetic nephropathy with low GFR or competitive inhibition of TMP and TPP transport at the level of RFC1 transporter by high dose folate at key sites such as the kidney and vascular cells thus adversely affecting sharing of thiamine between tissues rich in thiamine and those deficient in it [183].

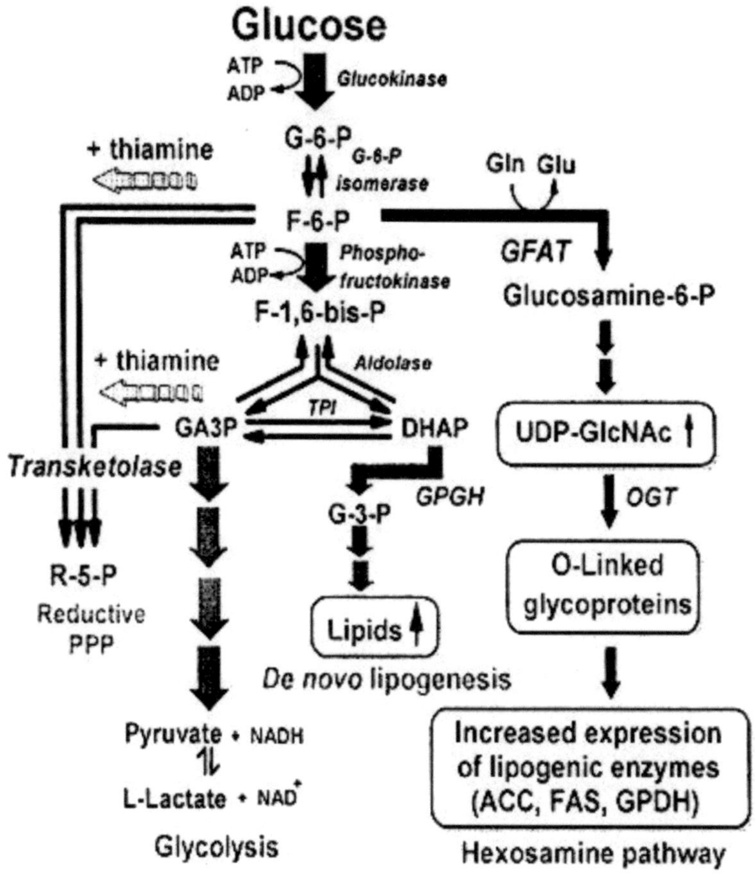

Figure 8. Metabolic Mechanism for Supression of Hepatic Lipogenesis in Diabetes by Thiamine.Adapted from PJ Thornalley 2006

6. Summary

Thus final summarization of these studies indicates that high dose thiamine repletion may decrease the risk of micro and macrovascular disease and counter incipient nephropathy in diabetes. The effect of thiamine occurred independent of control of hyperglycaemia, blood pressure and statin/fibrate therapy, suggesting that high dose thiamine therapy may produce improvements in the prevention of dyslipidaemia and diabetic nephropathy in addition to those produced by current therapy for control of hyperglycaemia, blood pressure, cholesterol and lipids. Since dyslipidemia and microalbuminuria are reversible in type 2 diabetic patients, it is possible that high dose thiamine therapy might improve renal function and metabolic control through reduction in biochemical dysfunction and improvement in thiamine dependant enzyme activities in diabetic patients with existing dyslipidaemia and microalbuminuria. However, it appears that there may be noticeable variations in these parameters on the basis of geographical, racial and pharmacogenetic factors. So the need of the hour was an indepth study as a double blind placebo controlled clinical trial to study the effect of high dose thiamine therapy on biochemical profile and activities of thiamine dependant enzymes in type 2 diabetic patients in our multiracial population in Pakistan.

7. Therapeutic implications

Based on the data above, the first ever randomized, double blinded, placebo controlled clinical intervention trial registered with the World Health Organization involving high dose B1 therapy was conducted by Dr.Saadia ShahzadAlam of the Pharmacology Deptt (Co-Principal Investigator 1) of Federal Postgraduate Medical Institute Lahore for a period of 5 months to study the effect of high dose thiamine therapy on biochemical profile and activities of thiamine dependant enzymes on type 2 diabetics in the Pakistani population. This trial was also pioneering internationally on the subject of diabetic nephropathy and the effect of thiamine supplementation on it. 40 type 2 micoalbuminuric diabetic patients at the Diabetes Clinic of Shaikh Zayed Hospital Lahore were administered 300mg/day (100mg tablets Administration of 300mg B1 TDS) / placebo for 3 months followed by a 2 month washout period. The results of this trial were quite interesting and have been published internationally, plasma thiamine levels of both thiamine and placebo groups were significantly depleted as compared to normal controls. There were significant baseline derangements of incipient diabetic nephropathy (microalbuminuria), glycemic control parameters FBS and glycated hemoglobin, lipid profile including total cholesterol, HDL, LDL, triglycerides and VLDL in type 2 microalbuminuric diabetics as compared to healthy individuals. Following 3 months 300 mg/day thiamine administration there was significant improvement of urinary albumin excretion, and preservation of glomerular filtration rate suggested that these occurred due to thiamine replenishment and decreased glycated hemoglobin and LDL cholesterol levels were observed in the washout period as a delayed effect. Additionally following thiamine therapy significant reduction in plasma levels of sVCAM-1, noticeable and an inverse linkage between thiamine therapy and vWF was apparent in this group as compared to placebo, suggested noticeable benefit with reduction in the risk factors of type 2 diabetes. Significant changes in other serum and urinary biomarkers profile were also observed in type 2 diabetics following thiamine therapy in a simultaneously carried out proteomic study. Three thiamine dependant enzymes PDE3, PDE1β, AKGDHE1 and Transketolase were determined to be dysfunctional at baseline in type 2 microalbuminuric diabetic patients in comparison to normal healthy controls, and improved in both activity and gene expression with high dose thiamine therapy While importantly no hepatic or renal adverse effects were encountered prior, during therapy or as a residual effect, post washout thus fortifying the previously established human safety track record of thiamine.[200]. We hope that these findings would contribute to knowledge regarding the role of thiamine therapy at 300mg/day dosage on biochemical profile and molecular aspects of those vital thiamine dependant enzymes and help in providing improved, safe and more effective treatment for type 2 diabetic patients with incipient nephropathy, dyslipidemia with expected decrease risk of heart disease and kidney failure.

Acknowledgements

I am grateful to Higher Education Comission of Pakistan for funding the project,Prof.M.Waheed Akhtar principal investigator of the project and co-supervisor, Prof.Paul J Thornalley, Dr.Naila Rabbani as Co Principal Investigator 2 of the project and Prof.Abdul Hameed Khan my Ph.D supervisor.

Author details

Saadia Shahzad Alam[1*] and Samreen Riaz[2]

*Address all correspondence to: saadia.pharma@gmail.com

1 Pharmacology Department, Federal Postgraduate Medical Institute, Lahore, Pakistan

2 Department of Microbiology and Molecular Genetics, University of the Punjab, Lahore, Pakistan

References

[1] Jeremy M. Berg, John. L. Tymoczko. The Glycolytic Pathway. Biochemistry 6th Edition 2006,435-57.

[2] David L. Nelson, Michael M. Cox. The Citric Acid Cycle. Lehninger Principles of Biochemistry 5th edition. 620-35.

[3] Brautigam CA, Wynn RM, Chuang JL et al. Structural insight into interactions between dihydrolipoamide dehydrogenase (E3) binding proteins of human pyruvate dehydrogenase complex. Structure, 2006; 14(3): 611-21.

[4] Patel MS, and Roche T.E.Molecular biology and biochemistry of pyruvate dehydrogenase complexes. FASEB J, 1990; 4: 3224-33.

[5] Reed RL. A trial of research lipoic acid to alpha-keto acid dehydrogenase complexes. J Biol Chem, 2001; 276(42): 38329-336.

[6] Cizak EM, Korotchkina LG, Dominiak PM, Sidhu S, and Patel MS. Structural basis for flip-flop action of thiamine pyrophosphate-dependent enzyme relevated by human pyruvate dehydrogenase. J.Biol. Chem, 2003; 278:21240-246.

[7] Dahl NH, Brown RM, Hutchison WM, Maragos C, Brown GK. A testis-specific form of the human pyruvate dehydrogenase E1 alpha subunit it coded for by an intronless gene on chromosome 4. Genomics 1990; 8(2):225-32.

[8] Fitzgerald J, Hutchison WM, Dahl HH. Isolation and characterization of the mouse pyruvate dehydrogenase E1 alpha genes. Biochem Biosphy Acta 1992; 1131(1); 83-90.

[9] Borglum AD, Flint T, Hansen LL, Kruse TA. Refined alphalocalization of the pyruvate dehydrogenase E1 alpha gene (PDHA1) by linkage analysis. Hum Genet, 1997; 99:80-82.

[10] Weimann S, weil B, Wellenreuther R, Gassenhuber J, Glassl S et al. Toward a catalog of human genes and Proteins: sequencing and analyzing of 500 novel complete protein coding human cDNAs. Genome Res 2001; 11(3):422-35.

[11] Koike K, Urata Y, Koike M. Molecular cloning and characterization of human pyruvate dehydrogenase beta subunit gene. Proc Natl Acad Sci USA, 1990; 87:5594-97.

[12] Koike K, Urata Y, Matsuo S, Koike M. Characterization and nucleotide sequence of the gene encoding the human pyruvate dehydrogenase alpha subunit. Gene, 1990; 93: 307-11.

[13] Brown GK, Otero LJ, LeGris M, Brown RM. Pyruvate dehydrogenase deficiency. J Med Genet,1995; 31: 875–79.

[14] Harris RA, Bowker-kinley MM, Huang B, Wu P. Regulation of the activity of the pyruvate dehydrogenase complex. Adv Enzyme Regul. 2002; 42:249-59.

[15] Leung PS, Watanabe Y, Munos S, Teuber SS, Patel MS, et al. Chromosome location and RFLP analysis of PDC-E2: the major autoantigen of primary biliary cirrhosis. Autoammunity, 1993; 14(4):335-40.

[16] Scherer SW, Otulakowski G, Robinson BH, Tsui LC. Lacalization of the human dihydrolipoamide dehydrogenase gen (DLD) to7q31-q32. Cytogenet Cell Genet, 1991; 56(3-4):176-177

[17] Wang YC, Wang ST, Li C, Liu WH. Chen LY, Liu TC. The role of N286 and D320 in the reaction mechanism of human dihydrolipoamide dehydrogenase E3 center domain. J Biomed Sci, 2007; 14(2): 203-10.

[18] Roche, TE, Hiromasa Y, Turkan A, et al. Essential role of lipoyl domains in the activated function and control of pyruvate dehydrogenase Kinases and phosphatase isoform 1. Eur J Biochem. 2004;270: 1050-56

[19] Perham RN. Domains, motifs, and linkers in 2-oxo acid dehydrogenase multienzyme complexes: a paradigm in the design of a multifunctional protein. Biochem 1991; 30:8501-12.

[20] Roche TE, Hiromasa Y. Pyruvate dehydrogenase kinase regulatory mechanisms and inhibition in treating diabetes, heart ischemia, and cancer. Cell Mol Life Sci. 2007; 64 (7-8):830-49.

[21] Wieland, OH, Patzelt, C, Loffler GX. Active and inactive forms of pyruvate dehydrogenase in rat liver. Effect of starvation and insulin treatment of pyruvate dehydrogenase interconversion. Eur J Biochem, 2007; 26:426-33

[22] Wieland OH. The mammalian pyruvate dehydrogenase complex: structure and regulation. Revs Physiol, Biochem Pharmacol, 1983; 96: 123-1 70.

[23] Kolobova E, Tuganova A, Boulatnikov I, Popov KM. Regulation of pyruvate dehydrogenase activity through phosphorylastion at multiple sites. Biochem. J, 2001; 335(Pt1):69-77.

[24] Korotchkina LG, Patel MS. Mutagenesis study of the phosphorylation sites of recombinanat human pyruvate dehydrogenase site specific regulation. J Biol. Chem, 1995; 270(24): 14297-304

[25] Sugden MC, Holness MJ. Recent advances in mechanisms regulating glucose oxidation at the level of pyruvate dehydrogenase complex by PDKs. Am J Physiol Endocrinol Metab, 2003; 284(5):E855-62.

[26] Holness MJ, Kraus A, Harris RA, Sugden MC. Targeted upregulation of pyruvate dehydrogenase kinase (PDK)-4 in slow-twitch skeletal muscle underlies the stable modification of the regulatory characteristics of PDK induced by high-fat feeding. Diabetes, 2000; 49:775-81.

[27] Kwon HS, Huang B, Unterman TG, Harris RA. Protein Kinase B-alpha inhibits human pyruvate dehydrogenase kinase 4-gene induction by dexamethasone through inactivation of FOXO transcription factors. Diabetes, 2004; 53:899-10

[28] Bonnet S, Archer Sl, Allalunis, et al. A Mitochondria-K+channel axis is suppressed in cancer and its normalization promotes apoptosis and inhibits cancer growth. Cancer Cell, 2007; 104:9445-50.

[29] Cairns RA, Papandreou I, Sutphin PD, Denko NC. Metabolic targeting of hypoxia and HIF1 in solid tumors can enhance cytotoxic chemotherapy. Proc Natl Acad Sci USA, 2007; 104: 9445–50

[30] Pan JG, Mak TW. Metabolic Targeting as an Anticancer Strategy: Dawn of New Era? Sci STKE. 2007,e14.

[31] Sugden MC. PDC Deletion. The way to a man's heart disease. Am J Physiol Heart Circ Physiol, 2008; 295:H917-H19.

[32] Roche TE, Baker JC, Yan X, et al. Distinct regulatory properties of pyruvate dehydrogenase kinase and phosphatase isoforms. Prog Nucleic Acid Res Mol Bio, 2001; 70:33-75

[33] Wu P, Peters JM, Harris RA. Adaptive increase in pyruvate dehydrogenase kinase 4 during starvation is mediated by peroxisome proliferator activated receptor alpha. Biochem Biosphy Res Commun, 2001; 287:391-96.

[34] Bajato G, Murakami T, Nagasaki M, Tamura N, Harris RA, et al. Downregulation of the skeletal muscle pyruvate dehydrogenase complex in the Otsuka Long-Evans Tokushima fatty rat both before and after the onset of diabetes mellitus. Life Sci, 2004; 75(17):2117-2130.

[35] Karpova T, Danchunk S, Kolobova E, Popov KM. Characterization of the isoenzymes pyruvate dehydrogenase phosphate implications for the regulations of pyruvate dehydrogenase activity. Biochem Biosphy Acta, 2003; 1652: 126-135.

[36] Turkan A, Gong X, Peng T, Roche TE. Structural requirement with in the lipoyl donail for the Ca2+-dependent binding and activation of pyruvate dehydrogenase phosphatase isoform 1or its catalyst subunit. J. Biol Chem, 2002; 227:14976-985

[37] Caruso, M, Maitan MA, Bifulco G, et al. Activation and mitochondrial translocation of protein kinase C are necessary for insulin stimulation of pyruvate dehydrogenase complex activity in muscle and liver cells. J Biol Chem,2001; 276:45088-97.

[38] Huang HM, Zhang H, Xu H, Gibson GE Inhibition of the dehydrogenase complex alters mitochondrial function cellular calcium regulation. Biochem Biophy Acta,2003; 1637: 119-26.

[39] Piccinini M, Mostert M, Alberto G, Ramondetti C, Rosa F. Novi, et al. Down-regulation of pyruvate dehydrogenase phosphate in obese subjects is a defect signals insulin resistance. Obes Res, 2005; 13: 678-86.

[40] Robinson BH, MacKay N, Petrova-Benedict R, Ozalp I, Coskun T, et al. Defects in the E2 lipoyl transacetylase and the X-lipoyl containing component of the pyruvate dehydrogenase complex in patients with lactic acidemia. J Clin Invest,1990; 85(6):1821–24

[41] Braun S, Berg C, Buck S, Gregor M, Kelin R. Catalytic domain of PDC-E2 contain epitopes recognized aby antimitochondrial antibodies in primary biliary cirrhosis." W J Gastro. WJG, 2010; 16(8): 973-81.

[42] Mackay IR, Whittingham SF, Fida S et al. Thepeculiar autoimmunity of primary biliary cirrhosis. Immunol. Rev; 2000; 174: 26–37.

[43] O'Brien C, Joshi S, Feld JJ, Guindi M, Dienes HP, et al. Long-term follow up of antimitochondrial antibody-positive autoimmune hepatitis.Hepatology (Baltimore, Md.) 2008; 48(2): 550-56.

[44] De kok A, Hengeveld AF, Martin A, Westphal AH. The pyruvate dehydrogenase multi-enzyme complex from Gram-negative bacteria. Biochem Biosphys Acta, 1998; 1385(2):353-366

[45] Chuang DT, Shih VE, Scriver CR, Beaudet AL, Sly WS, Velle D, Childs B, Kinzler KW, Vogelstein B. Maple Syrup urine disease (branched-chain ketoaciduria). In the metabolic and the molecular bases of inherited disease.2001;(2).NewYork: McGraw-Hill, 1971-2005.

[46] Odievre M-H, Chretien D, Munnich A, Robinson BH, Dumoulin R, Masmoudi S, Kadhom N, Rotig A, Rustin P, Bonnefont J-P. A novel mutation in the dihydrolipoamide dehydrogenase E3 subunit gene (DLD) resulting in an atypical form of a-ketoglutarate dehydrogenase deficiency. Hum Mut, 2005.

[47] B Melegh, G Skuta, L Pajor, G Hegedu¡s, B Sumegi. Autoantibodies against subunits of pyruvate dehydrogenase and citrate synthase in a case of paediatric biliary cirrhosis. Gut, 1998; 42:753–56

[48] Zhou ZH, McCarthy DB, O'Connor CM, Reed LJ, Stoops JK. The remarkable structural and functional organization of the eukaryotic pyruvate dehydrogenase complexes.Proc Natl Sci USA,2001; 98(26):14802-07.

[49] McCartney RG, Rice JE, Sanderson SJ, Bunik V, Lindsay H, et al. Subunit interactions in the mammalian α-ketoglutarate dehydrogenase complex. Evidence for direct association of the α-ketoglutarate dehydrogenase and dihydrolipoamide dehydrogenase components. J. Biol. Chem, 1998; 273(37):24158–64.

[50] Mainul Islam, Wallin R, Wynn R, Myra Conway M, Fujii H, et al. A Novel Branched-chain Amino Acid Metabolon Protein-Protein Interactions In a Supramolecular Complex. J Biol Chem, 2007; 282(16): 11893–903

[51] Parham RN. Swinging arms and swinging domains in multifunctional enzymes: catalytic machines for multistep reactions. Annu Rev Biochem, 2000; 69, 961-1004.

[52] Shi Q, Karuppagounder SS, Xu H, Pechman D, Chen H, et al. Responses of the mitochondrial alpha-ketoglutarate dehydrogenase complex to thiamine deficiency may contribute to regional selective vulnerability. Neurochem Int, 2007; 50(7-8):921-31.

[53] Fries M, Jung HI, Perham RN. Reaction mechanism of the heterotetrameric (α2β2) E1 component of 2-oxo acid dehydrogenase multienzyme complex. Biochemistry, 2003; 42(23): 6996-02.

[54] Szabo P, Cai X, Ali G, Blass JP. Localization of the gene (OGDH) coding for the E1 component of the alpha ketoglutarate dehydrogenase complex to chromosome 7p13-p11.2. Genomics, 1994; 20(2): 324-6.

[55] Koike K. The gene encoding human 2-oxogluterate dehydrogenase: structural organization and mapping to chromosome. Gene, 1995; 159(2), 261-66.

[56] Koike K. Cloning, structure, chromosomal localization promoter analysis of human 2-oxogluterate dehydrogenase gene. Biochem Biosphy Acta, 1998; 1385(2): 373-84.

[57] Scheu KFR, and Blass JP. The alpha-ketoglutarte dehydrogenase complex. Oxidative/ energy metabolism in Neurodegenerative Disorders, 1999; 893:61-78.

[58] Jun Li, Mischa Machius, Jacinta L. Chuang, R. Max Wynn, and David T. Chuang. The Two Active Sites in Human Branched-chain Keto AcidDehydrogenase Operate Inde-

pendently without anObligatory Alternating-site Mechanism. J Biol Chem, 2007; 282(16): 11904–913

[59] Li J, Wynn, RM, et al. Cross-talk between thiamin diphosphate binding and phosphorylation loop conformation in human branched-chain alpha-keto acid decarboxylase/dehydrogenase. J Biol Chem, 2004; 279: 32968-78.

[60] Nakano K, Takase C, Sakamoto T, Ohta S, Nakagawa S, et al. An unsplicted cDNA for human dehydrolipoamide succinyltransferase: characterization and mapping of the gene to chromosome 14q24.2-q24.3. Biochem Biosphy Res Commun, 1993; 192(2): 527-33.

[61] Scherer SW, Otulakowski G, Robinson BH, Tsui LC. Lacalization of the human dihydrolipoamide dehydrogenase gen (DLD) to7q31..q32. Cytogenet Cell Genet, 1991; 56(3-4):176-177.

[62] De kok A, Hebgeveld AF, Martin A, Westphal AH. The pyruvate dehydrogenase multi-enzyme complex from Gram-negative bacteria.Biochem Biosphys Acta, 1998; 1385(2):353-366

[63] Tretter L, Adam-Vizi V. Alpha ketoglutarate dehydrogenase: a target and generator of oxidative stress. Philos Trans R Soc Lond B Biol Sci, 2005; 360: 2335-45.

[64] Donald Voet, Judith G. Voet, charlotte W. Pratt, 1999. Fundamentals of Biochemistry. John Wiley & sons, Inc Voet & voet.

[65] Strumilo S. Short term regulation of the alpha ketoglutarate dehydrogenase complex by energy-linked and some other effectors. Biochemistry, 2005;70: 726-729.

[66] Gibson GE, Park LCH, Sheu KFR, Blass JP, Calingasan NY. Neurochem Int, 2000;36: 97-112.

[67] Shi Q, Risa O, Sonnewald U, Gibson GE. Mild reaction in the activity of the alpha ketoglutarate dehydrogenase complex elevates GABA shunt and glycolysis. J Neurochem, 2009;109: 214-221.

[68] Shi Q, Karuppagounder SS, Xu H, Pechman D, Chen H, Gibson GE. Responses of the mitochondrial alpha-ketoglutarate dehydrogenase complex to thiamine deficiency may contribute to regional selective vulnerability.Neurochem Int, 2007;50(7-8): 921-31.

[69] Des Jardins,Roger. F. Butterworth.Role of mitochondrial dysfunction and oxidative stress in the pathogenesis of selective neuronal loss in Wernickes encephalopathy.Mol Neurobiol,31: 1-3,17-25

[70] Mastrogiacomo, LaMarche J, Do S, Lindsay G, Bettendorff L, et al. Immunoreactive Levels of α-ketoglutarate Dehydrogenase Subunits in Friedreich's Ataxia and Spinocerebellar Ataxia Type 1. Neurodegeneration, 1996;5(1): 27-33.

[71] Kumar MJ, Nicholls DG, Andersen JK. Oxidative alpha ketoglutarate dehydrogenase inhibition via subtle elevations in monoamine oxidase B levels results in loss of spare

respiratory capacity: implications for parkinson's disease. J Boil Chem, 2003;278: 46432-439.

[72] Huang HM, Zhang H, Xu H, Gibson GE "Inhibition of the dehydrogenase complex alters mitochondrial function cellular calcium regulation." Biochem Biophys Acta, 2003;1637: 119-126.

[73] Habelhah H, Laine A, Erdjument Bromage H, Tempst P, Gershwin ME, et al. Regulation of 2-oxoglutarate (alpha ketoglutarate) dehydrogenase stability by the RING finger ubiquitin ligase siah. J Biol Chem, 2004;279: 53782-788

[74] Abboud M, Alexander D., Najjar S. Diabetes mellitus, thiamine-dependentmegaloblastic anemia, and sensorineural deafness associated with deficient α-ketoglutarate dehydrogenase activity,J Paeds; 107(4): 1A-28A.

[75] Zubay G.Biochemistry.1983.Addison-Wesley Publishing Company,Inc.

[76] Christopher K, Mathews KE, Holde V, Kevin GA: The Pentose Phosphate Pathway Biochemistry 3rd edition, 511-20.

[77] Antje Krüger and Markus Ralser. The pentose phosphate pathway is a metabolic redox sensor and regulates transcription during the anti-oxidant response. Sci Signaling, 2011;4(167):pe17

[78] Seckl JR, Walker BR. Minireview: 11beta-hydroxysteroid dehydrogenase type 1-a tissue-specific amplifier of glucocorticoid action. Endocrinology,2001;142 (4): 1371–76.

[79] ImmunologyatMCG1/cytotox http://lib.mcg.edu/esimmuno/ch/cytotox.htm

[80] Cappadoro M, Giribaldi G, O.Brien E, et al. Early phagocytosis of glucose-6-phophate dehydrogenase (G6PD)-deficiency erythrocytes parasitized by plasmodium falciparum may explain malaria protection in G6PD deficiency. Blood,1998 ;92(7): 2527-34.

[81] Schafer ZT, Grassian AR, Song L, Jiang Z, Gerhart-Hines Z, Irie HY, Gao S, Puigserver P, Brugge JS: Antioxidant and oncogene rescue of metabolic defects caused by loss of matrix attachment. Nat, 2009;461:109-113

[82] Wang J, Yi J. Cancer cell killing via ROS: to increase or decrease,that is the question. Cancer Biol Ther, 2008;1875-84.

[83] Vafa O, Wade M, Kern S, Beeche M, Pandita TK, Hampton GM, Wahl GM: c-Myc can induce DNA damage, increase reactive oxygen species, and mitigate p53 function: a mechanism for oncogene-induced genetic instability. Mol Cell, 2002, 9:1031-44.

[84] Trachootham D, Alexandre J, Huang P: Targeting cancer cells by ROS-mediated mechanisms: a radical therapeutic approach? Nat Rev Drug Discov,2009, 8:579-591.

[85] Ishikawa K, Takenaga K, Akimoto M, Koshikawa N, Yamaguchi A, Imanishi H, Nakada K, Honma Y, Hayashi J: ROS-generating mitochondrial DNA mutations can regulate tumor cell metastasis. Science, 2008; 320:661-64.

[86] DeBerardinis RJ, Mancuso A, Daikhin E, Nissim I, Yudkoff M, Wehrli S, Thompson CB: Beyond aerobic glycolysis: transformed cells can engage in glutamine metabolism that exceeds the requirement for protein and nucleotide synthesis. Proc Natl Acad Sci USA, 2007; 104:19345-350

[87] Kochetov, Sevpstyanova IA: Binding of the coenzyme and formation of the transketolase active center. JUBMB Life, 2005; 57 (7): 491-97

[88] Lindquist, G Schneider, U Ermler and M Sundstrom. Three dimensional structure of transketolase, a thiamine diphosphate dependent enzyme, at 2.5 A resolution. EMBO J,1992;11(7): 2373-79.

[89] McCool BA, Plonk SG, Martin PR Singleton CK. Cloning of human transketolase cDNAs and comparison of the nucleotide sequence of the codin region in wernicke-Korsakoff and non-wernicke-Korsakoff individuals.J Biol Chem, 1993;268 (2): 1397-04.

[90] Abedinia M, Lapsys NM, Layfield R,Jones SM, Nixon PF, Mattick JS. Nucleotide and predicted amino acid sequence of a cDNA clone encoding part of human transketolase. Biochem Biosphy Res Commun, 1992;183 (3): 1159-66.

[91] Lapsys NM, Layfield R, Baker E, Callen DF, Sutherland GR. Chromosomal location of the human transketolase gene. Cytogenet cell Genet, 1992;61(4):274-75

[92] Coy JF, Dressler D, Wilde J, Schubert P: Mutations in the transketolase-like gene TKTL1: clinical implications for neurodegenerative disease, diabetes and cancer.Clin Lab, 2005; 51(5-6):257-73.

[93] Coy JF, Dubel S, Kioschis P, Thomas K, Micklem G. "Molecular cloning of tissue-specific transcripts of a transketolase-related gene: implications for the evolution of new vertebrate genes." Genomics, 1996;32(3);309-16. : 8838793

[94] Weimann S, weil B, wellenreuther R, Gassenhuber J, Glassl S. Toward a catalog of human genes and Proteins: sequencing and analyzing of 500 novel complete protein coding human cDNAs. Genome Res, 2001;11(3):422-35.

[95] Booth, C. K., & Nixon, P. F. Reconstitution of holotransketolase is by a thiamin-diphosphate-magnesium complex.Eur J Biochem, 1993;218: 261-65.

[96] Cristian Obiol-Pardo and Jaime Rublo-Martines. Homology modeling of human transketolase: description of critical sites useful for drug design and study of the cofactor binding mode. J Mol Graph Model, 2009;27:723-34.

[97] Nikkola, M., Lindqvist, Y., and Schneider, G. Lindqvist, Y., and Schneider, G. Refined Structure of Transketolase from Saccharomyces cerevisae at 2.0 Å resolution (1994) J Biol Chem., 238, 387-04.

[98] M. Reynen, H. Sahm, Comparison of the structural genes for pyruvate decarboxylase in di€erent Zymomonas strains, J. Bacteriol, 1988; 170: 3310-3313

[99] Hawkins, C. F., Borges, A., and Perham, R. N. A common structural motif in thiamin pyrophosphate-binding enzyme. FEBS Lett, 1989; 255: 77-82

[100] Kochetov GA, Sevostyanova IA.Functional non equivalence of transketolase active centers.IUBMB Life. 2010 Nov;62(11):797-802

[101] James J.WangL. Aspartate 155 of human transketolase is essential for thiamine diphosphate-megnesium binding, and cofactor inding is required for dimer information.Biochemica et Biophys Acta, 1997;1341:165-72.

[102] Martin,P.R., Pekovich,S.R., McCool, B.A., and Singleton C.K. Molecular Genetics of transketolase and its role in the pathogenesis of the Wernicke-Korsakoff syndrome Metab Br Dis, 1995;10: 189-94

[103] Traviesa, D. C. Magnesium deficiency: a possible cause of thiamine refractoriness in Wernicke–Korsakoff encephalopathy. Journal Neurol Neurosur Psych, 1974;37, 959–962.

[104] Coy JF, Dressler D, Wilde J, Schubert P. Mutations in the transketolase-like gene TKTL1: clinical implications for neurodegenerative disease, diabetes and cancer.Clin Lab, 2005;51(5-6):257-73.

[105] Hu LH, Yang JH, Zhang DT, Zahng S, Wang L, Cai PC, Zheng JF, Huang JS: The TKTL1gene influences total transketolase activity and cell proliferation in human colon cancer LoVo cells. Anticancer Drugs, 2008: 18: 427-33.

[106] Zerilli M, Amato MC, Martorana A. Increased expression of transketolase-like-1 in papillary thyroid carcinomas smaller than 1.5 cm in diameter is associated with lymph-node metastates.Cancer, 2008;113:936-44.

[107] Kohrenhagen N,Voelker HU, Suchmidt M, Kapp M, Lrockenberger M, et al. Expression of transketolase-like 1 (TKTL1) and p-Akt correlates with the progression of cervical neoplasia.Mol cell Proteomics, 2008;7: 2337-2349.

[108] Krockenberger, Honig A, Rieger L. Transketolase-like 1 expression correlates with subtypes of ovarian cancer and the presence of distant metastates. Int J Gynecol Cancer, (2007);17: 101-106.

[109] Foeldi M, Stickeler E, Bau L, Kretz O, Watermann D, et al. Transketolase protein TKTL1 overexpression: A potential biomarker and the repeutic target in breast cancer. Oncol Rep, 2007;17: 841-45.

[110] ZhangW L, ZhouYH, L. Xiao et al., "Biomarkers of nasopharyngeal carcinoma," Progress in Biochemistry and Biophysics, 2008;35(1) : 7–13.

[111] Voelker H U,Hagemann C,Coy J. (2008) Expression of transketolase-like 1 an activation of Akt in grade IV glioblastoma as compared with grades II and III astrocytic gliomas.Am J Clin Pathol,130:50-57.

[112] Lovato L, Cianti R, Gini B, Marconi S, Bianchi L, et al. : Transketolase and 2′,3′-cyclic-nucleotide 3′ –phosphodiesterase type I isoforms are specially recognized by IgG autoantibodies in multiple sclerosis patients. Mol cell proteomics 2008; 7(12):2337-49

[113] Thomas AA, Le Huerou Y, De Meese J, Gunawardana I, Kaplan T, et al. Synthesis in Vitro and in Vivo activity of thiamine antagonist transketolase inhibitors. Bioorg Med Chem Lett,2008;18: 2206-10.

[114] Hammes HP, Du X, Edelstein D: Benfotiamine blocks three major pathways of hyperglycemic damage and prevents experimental diabetic retinopathy. Nat Med, 2003; 9:294-99.

[115] Goodman Gillman. Insulin, Oral Hypoglycaemic agents and the endocrine pancreas. The Pharmacological Basis of Therapeutics Tenth Edition, 2006;61:1686-10.

[116] Katzung B.G.Basic and clinical pharmacology Eighth edition. Pancreatic Hormones and Anti DiabeticDrugs. 2004;711-34.

[117] Schwartz,TheodoreB.Meinert,CurtisL.The UGDP Controversy: thirty-four years of contentious ambiguity laid to rest.Perspectives in Biology and Medicine,2004; 47(4) : 564-74

[118] Starlix package insert. East Hanover, NJ, Novartis Pharmaceuticals Corporation, Dec. 2000.

[119] Holstein A, Plaschke A, Egberts EH. Lower incidence of severe hypoglycemia in type 2 diabetic patients treated with glimepride versus glibenclamide. Diabetology 43: A40.

[120] Volk A, Maerker E,Rett K, Haring HY, Overkamp D1, et al. :Effects on peripheral insulin sensitivity.Diabetologia, 2000;43:A39

[121] Campbell RK. Glimerpiride role of a new sulfonylurea in the treatment of type 2 diabetes mellitus. Ann Pharmacother, 1998;32:1044-52

[122] Hollander PA, Schwartz SL, Gatli MR, Haas S, Zheng H, et al. Natenglinide but not glyburide, selectively enhances early insulin release and more effectively controls post meal glucose excursions with less total insulin exposure. Diabetes, 2000;49:447

[123] Katzung B.G.Basic and Clinical pharmacology Eighth edition. Pancreatic Hormones and AntiDiabeticDrugs, 2009;727-47.

[124] Goodman Gillman. Insulin, Oral Hypoglycaemic agents and the the pharmacology of endocrine pancreas. The Pharmacological Basis of Therapeutics Eleventh Edition, 2006;60:1686-10.

[125] Brown&Bennet. Diabetes mellitus, insulin,oral anti diabetes agents,obesity.Clinical Pharmacology Ninth Edition. 2004;8:679-695

[126] Lebovtiz HE. Alpha glucosidase inhibitors as agents in the treatment of diabetes. Diabetes Rev, 1998;6: 132.

[127] Chiasson JL, et al. Acarbose for prevention of type 2 diabetes mellitus: the STOP-NIDDM randomized trial. Lancet, 2002;359: 2072.

[128] Holst JJ, Gromada J. Role of incretin hormones in the regulation of insulin secretion in diabetic and nondiabetic humans. Am. J. Physiol Endocrinol Metab, 2004;287:E1953-59.

[129] Deacon CF. Circulation and degradation of GIP and GLP-1. Horm Metab Res, 2004;36:761–65

[130] Ehses JA, Pelech SL, Pederson RA, and McIntosh CH. Glucose-dependent insulinotropic polypeptide activates the Raf-Mek1/2-ERK1/2 module via a cyclic AMP/cAMP-dependent protein kinase/Rap1-mediated pathway. J Biol Chem,2002;277: 37088-097.

[131] Trümper A, Trümper K, and Hörsch D. Mechanisms of mitogenic and antiapoptotic signaling by glucose-dependent insulinotropic polypeptide in beta(INS-1)-cells. J Endocrinol, 2002;174: 233-46

[132] Eckel RH, Fujimoto WY, Brunzell JD: Gastric inhibitory polypeptide enhanced lipoprotein lipase activity in cultured preadipocytes. Diabetes, 1979;28 :1141–42.

[133] Beck B, Max JP. Gastric inhibitory polypeptide enhancement of the insulin effect on fatty acid incorporation into adipose tissue in the rat. Regul Pept, 1983;7:3–8.

[134] Oben J, Morgan L, Fletcher J, et al Effect of the entero-pancreatic hormones, gastric inhibitory polypeptide and glucagon-like polypeptide-1 (7–36) amide, on fatty acid synthesis in explants of rat adipose tissue. J Endocrinol 1991;130:267–72.

[135] Gault VA, Irwin N, Green BD, McCluskey JT, Greer B, Bailey CJ, Harriott P, O'Harte FP, Flatt PR: Chemical ablation of gastric inhibitory polypeptide receptor action by daily (Pro3)GIP administration improves glucose tolerance and ameliorates insulin resistance and abnormalities of islet structure in obesity-related diabetes. Diabetes, 2005;54 :2436 –46.

[136] Bailey CJ, Gross JL, Pieters A, Bastien A, List JF. Effect of dapagliflozin in patients with type 2 diabetes who have inadequate glycaemic control with metformin: a randomized, double-blind, placebo-controlled trial. Lancet,2010;375(9733):2223-33.

[137] Traish AM, Saad F, Guay A. The dark side of the testosterone deficiency: II. Type 2 diabetes and insulin resistance. J Androl, 2009;30(1):23-32.

[138] Zitzmann M. Testosterone deficiency, insulin resistance and the metabolic syndrome. Nature Reviews Endocrinology, 2009;5(12): 673-81.

[139] Makoto Hiromura et al. Glucose lowering activity by oral administration of bis (allixin) oxidovanadium (IV) complex in streptozotocin-induced diabetic mice and gene expression profiling in their skeletal muscles. Metallomics,2009.

[140] Yuriko Sanches-Zamora, Luis I Terrazas, Alonso Vilches-Flores,Emmanuel Leal, Imelda Juarez, et al. Macrophage migration inhibitory factor is a therapeutic target in treatment of non-insulin dependent diabetes mellitus. The FESEB Journal,2010.

[141] FrangioudakisG, Garrard,J RaddatzK, NadlerJ.L, MitchellT.W, C. Schmitz-Peiffer. Saturated and n-6 polyunsaturated-fat diets each induce ceramide accumulation in mouse skeletal muscle: Reversal and improvement of glucose tolerance by lipid metabolism inhibitors. Endocrinology,2010;151(9): 4187.

[142] Zandong Yang, University of Virginia Health System. Drug Shows Promise in Preventing Type 1 Diabetes. ScienceDaily, 2003.

[143] Takeshi Ogihara, Jen-Chieh Chuang. Liver X Receptor Agonists Augment Human Islet Function through Activation of Anaplerotic Pathways and Glycerolipid/Free Fatty Acid Cycling.J Biol Chem,2010;285(8): 5392-04.

[144] Aiello LP,Cahill MT,Cavallerano JD. Growth factors and protein kinase C inhibitors as novel therapies for the medical management diabetic retinopathy.EyeSci J Roy Coll Opthamol, 2004;18:117-125.

[145] Adams TD, Gress RE, Smith SC, et al. Long-term mortality after gastric bypass surgery. N E J M, 2007;357(8):753-61.

[146] Cohen RV, Schiavon CA, Pinheiro JS, Correa JL, Rubino F. Duodenal-jejunal bypass for the treatment of type 2 diabetes in patients with body mass index of 22-34Kg/m2: a report of 2 cases: Sur Obes& Related Dis, 2007;3(2): 195-97

[147] Vasonconcelos,Alberto. "Could type 2 diabetes be reserved using surgery?" New scientist, 2007;2619: 11-13.

[148] Cuningham JJ. The glucose/insulin system and vitamin C: implications in insulin dependent diabetes mellitus. J. Am Coll Nutr, 1998;17:105-8.

[149] Chaudhry PS, Cabrera J, Juliani HR, Varma SD. Inhibition of human lens aldose reductase by flavonides, sulindac and indomethacin. Biochem Pharmacol, 1983;32:1995-98.

[150] Kunisaki M, Bursell SE, Clermont AC. Vitamin E prevents Diabetes induced abnormal retinal blood flow via the diacylglycerol protein kinase c pathway. Am J Physiol, 1995;269: E239-E46.

[151] Keegan A, Walbank H, Cotter MA, Cameron NE. Chronic vitamin E treatment prevents defective endothelium-dependent relaxation in diabetic rat aorta. Diabetologia, 1995; 38:1475-78.

[152] Bursell SE, Clermont AC, Aiello LP, Aiello LM, Schlossman DK, et al. High dose vitamin E supplementation normalizes retinal blood flow and creatinine clearance in patients with type 1 diabetes. Diabetes Care, 1999; 22:1245-51.

[153] Tosiello L, (1996) Hypo magnesemia and diabetes mellitus: A review of clinical implications, arch Intern Med;156:1143-48.

[154] Mooradian AD, Failla M, Hoogwerg B. Selected vitamins and minerals in diabetes (technical review). Diabetes Care, 1994; 17:464-79.

[155] Nair AR, Biju Mp, Paulose CS. Effect of pyridoxine and insulin administration on brain glutamate dehydrogenation activity and blood glucose control in streptozotocin-induced diabetic rats. Biochem biophy Acta, 1998;1381:351-54.

[156] Ho E, Chen G, Bray TM. Supplementation of N-acetylcysteine inhibits NFKappa B activation and protects against alloxan-induced diabetes in CD-1 mice. FASEB, 1999;13:1845-54.

[157] Poucheret P,Verma S,Grinpas MD. Vanadium and Diabetes.Mol Cell Biochem, 1998;188:73-80.

[158] Cam MC, Rodrigues B, McNeill JH. Distinct Glucose lowering and Beta cell protective effects of vanadium and food restriction in streptozotocin diabetes. Eur J Endocrinol, 1999;141: 546-54.

[159] Rudich A, Tirosh A, Potashnik R, Khamaisi M, Bashan N. Lipoic acid protects against oxidative stress induced impairment in insulin stimulation of protein kinase B and glucose transport in 3T3-L1 adipocytes. Diabetologia, 1999;42:949-57.

[160] Mukherjee B, Anbazhagan S, Roy A, Ghosh R, Chatterjee M. Novel. Implications of the potential role of selenium on antioxidant status in streptozotocin-induced diabetic mice. Biomed Pharmacother, 1998;52: 89-95.

[161] Han DH, Hasen PA, Chen MM, Holloszy JO. DHEA treatment reduces fat accumulation and protects again insulin resistance in male rats.J Gerontol A Biol Sci Med Sci, 1998;53:B19-24.

[162] Provisional report by UK Expert Group on Vitamins andMinerals. August 2002. (http://www.food.gov.uk/foodindustry/Consultations/ukwideconsults/evmconsulteg). Safe Upper Levels of Vitamins and Minerals, Expert Group on Vitamins and Minerals, 2003.

[163] Combs, G.F. Jr. The vitamins: fundamental aspects in nutrition and health. 3rd edition. Ithaca, NY: Elsevier academic Press (2008).

[164] Mahan LK, Escott-Stump S, Krause's food, nutrition, and diet therapy. 10th ed. Philadelphia: W.B. Saunders Company, 2000.

[165] Dutta B, Huang W, Molero M, Kekuda R, Leibach FH, et al. Cloning of the human thiamine transporter, a member of the float transporter family. J Biol Chem, 1999;274: 31925-29.

[166] Matherly LH. Molecular and the celluar biology of the human reduced folate carrier. Progr Nucleic Acid Res Mol Biol, 2001;67:131-62.

[167] Zhao RB, Gao F, Wang YH, Diaz GA, Gelb BD, et al. Impact of the reduced folate carrier on the accumulation of active thiamine metabolites in murine leukemia cells. J Biol Chem, 2001; 276:1114-18.

[168] Zhao RB, Gao F and Goldman ID. Reduced folate carrier transports thiamine monophosphate: an alternative route for thiamine delivery into mammalian cells.Am J Physiol Cell Physiol, 2002; 282:C1512-C17

[169] Said HM, Balamurugan K, Subramanian VS, and Marchant JS. Expression and fuctional contribution of hTHTR-2 in thiamine absorption in human intestine. Am J Physiol. Gastrointest. Liver Physiol, 2004;286: G491-G98.

[170] Reidling JC, Said HM. In vitro and in vivo characterization of the minial promoter region of the human thiamin transporter SLC 19A2. Am J Physiol Cell Physiol, 2003;285:C633-C41.

[171] Balamurugan K, and Said HM. Functional role of specific amino acid reduces in human thiamine transporter SLC19A2: mutational analysis. Am. J. Physiol-Gastrointest. Liver Physiol, 2002;283: G37-G43.

[172] Fleming JC, Tertaglini E, Steinkamp MP, Schordret DF, Chon N. The gene mutated in thiamine-responsive anaemia with diabetes and deafness (TRMA) encodes a functional thiamine transpoter. Nat Gen, 1999;22:305-12.

[173] Eudy JD, Spiegelstein O, Barber RC, Wlodarczyk BJ, Talbot J. Identification and characterization of the human and mouse SLC19A3gene: A novel member of the reduced folate family of micronutrient transporter gene. Molec. Gene Metab, 2000;71: 581-590.

[174] Trippet TM, Garcia S, Manova K, Mody R, Cohen-Gould L. Localization of a human reduced folate carrier protein in the mitochondrial as well as the cell membrane of the leukemia cells. Cancer. Res, 2001;61:1941-47.

[175] Babaei-Jadidi R, Karachalias N, Ahmed N, Battah S, Thornalley PJ. Prevention of incipient diabetic nephropathy by high-dose thiamine and benfotiaminne. Diabetes, 2003;52:2110-20.

[176] Chin E, Zhou J and Bondy C. Antomical and development patterns of facilitative glucose transporter gene-expression in the rat kidney.J.Clin. Invest, 1993;91: 1810-15.

[177] Tallaksen C. M., Bohmer T., Karlsen J. and Bell H. Determinationof thiamin and its phosphate esters in human blood, plasma,and urine. Meth. Enzymol, 1997;279, 67–74.

[178] Gastaldi G, Coya E, Verri A, Laforenza U, Faellin A and Rindi G. Transport of thiamine in rat renal brush border membrane vesicles. Kidney Int. 2002;57: 2043-54.

[179] Morshed KM, Ross DM, and McMartin KE. Folate transport proteins mediate the bidirectional transport of 5-methyltetrahydrofolate in cultured human proximal tubule cells. J Nutrit,1997;127: 1137-47.

[180] Rindi G and Laforenza U. Thiamine intestinal transport and related issues: recent aspects. PSEBM, 2000;224:246-255.

[181] Smeets, E.S.J., Muller, H.,and Wael, J.D. X. A NADH-transketolase dependent essay in erythrocyte hemolysate. Clin. Chim. Acta. 2000;33: 379-86.

[182] Brady JA, Rock CL, And Horneffer MR. Thiamine status diuretic medications and the management of congestive heart failure. J. Am. Diet. Assoc, 1995;95: 541-44.

[183] Thornalley PJ, Babaei-Jadidi R, Al Ali H et al. High prevalence of low plasma thiamine concentration in diabetes linked to marker of vascular disease.Diabetologia, 2007;50:2164-70.

[184] Pekovich SR, Martin PR, Singleton CK. Thiamine deficiency decreases steady-state transketolase and pyruvate dehydrogenase but not a-ketoglutarate dehydrogenase mRNA levels in three human cell types..J Nutr, 1998;128: 683-87.

[185] Bettendorff L, Peters M, Jouan C, Wins P., Schoffeniels E. Determination of thiamine and its phosphate esters in cultured neurons and astrocytes using an ion-pair reversed-phase high-performance liquid chromatographic method. Annal. Biochem, 1991;198(1): 52-59.

[186] Losa R, Sierra MI, Fernandez A,Blanco D, Buesa JM. Determination of thiamine and its phosphorylated forms in human plasma, erythrocytes and urine by HPLC. JPBA, 2005;37(5):1025-29.

[187] Lu J, Frank EL. Rapid HPLC measurement of thiamine and its phosphate esters in whole blood.Clin Chem, 2008;5495:901-06.

[188] Shabangi M, Sutton JA. Separation of thiamine and its phosphate esters by capillary zone electrophoresis and its application to the analysis of water soluble vitamins. Journal of Pharma Biomed analysis, 2005; 38(1): 66-71.

[189] Barile M, Valenti D, Brizio C, Quagliariello E and Passarella S. Rat liver mitochondria can hydrolyse thiamine pyrophosphate to thiamine monophophate which can cross the mitochondrial memberane in carrier-mediated process. FEBS Lett, 1998;435:6-10.

[190] Babaei-Jadidi R, Karachalias N, Kupich C, Ahmed N, Thornalley PJ. High dose thiamine therapy counters dyslipidaemnia in streptozotocin-included diabetic rats. Diabetologia, 2004;47:2235-46.

[191] Wakabayashi Y. Purification properties of porcine thiamine pyrophosphokinase. Vitamins,1978;52: 223-36.

[192] Makarchikov AF, Lakaye B, Gulyai IE, Czerniecki J, Coumnas B. Thiamine triphosphate and thiamine triphosphatase activities: from bacteria to mammals. Cell Molec Life sci, 2003;60 :1477-88.

[193] Weber W, Kewitz H. Determination of thiamine in human plasma and its pharmacokinetics. Eur J Clin Pharmocal, 1985;28:213-19.

[194] Ariaey-Nejad MR, Balaghi M, Baker EM, Sauberlich HE. Thiamin metabolism in man. Am J Clin Nutr, 1970;23:764-778.

[195] Tanphaichitr V, Shills ME, Olsen JA, Shike M et al. Thiamin In: Modern nutrition in health and disease. Lippincott Williams & Wilkins, 9th ed. 1999. Baltimore.

[196] University of California Santa Cruz Genome Browser(UCSC) http://genome.ucsc.edu.

[197] Schneider, G., and Lindqvist, Y. Crystallography and mutagenesis of transketolases: Mechanistic implications for enzymatic thiamine catalysis. Biochem Biosphy Acta, 1998;1385: 387-98.

[198] Schellenberger, A. Sixty years of thiamine diphosphate biochemistry. Biochem Biosphy Acta, 1998;1385:177-86.

[199] Cizak EM, Korotchkina LG, Dominiak PM, Sidhu S, and Patel MS. Structural basis for flip-flop action of thiamine pyrophosphate-dependent enzyme relevated by human pyruvate dehydrogenase.JBiolChem, 2003;278:21240-246.

[200] Sheu KFR, Blass JP. The alpha ketoglutarate complex. Ann NY Acad Sci, 1999; 893: 61-78.

Chapter 3

Pathogenesis of Type 2 Diabetes Mellitus

Fuad AlSaraj

Additional information is available at the end of the chapter

http://dx.doi.org/10.5772/59183

1. Introduction

The natural history of type 2 diabetes (T2DM) has been well described in multiple populations. Patients with T2DM have inherited genes from parents that make their tissues resistant to insulin. Insulin resistance (IR) in muscle and liver and β-cell failure represent the core pathophysiologic defects in development of T2DM. Age, genes, IR, lipotoxicity, glucotoxicity, amyloid deposition and abnormal incretin are factors playing a role in progressive β-cells dysfunction. The progressive decline in insulin secretion, decrease of the pancreatic β- cell mass and function and the presence of IR will contribute in changing the state of the dysglycemia from normal to, impaired fasting glucose (IFG), impaired glucose tolerance (IGT) and end with overt diabetes [1].

2. Glucose metabolism

Excessive hepatic glucose output is an important factor in the fasting hyperglycemia of patients with T2DM. Following administration of isotope in healthy subjects and in patients with T2DM, the overall hepatic glucose output was an increase by twofold and the gluconeogenesis more than threefold in patients compare with the controls. This finding demonstrated the increased in gluconeogenesis is the predominant mechanism responsible for increased hepatic glucose output in patients with T2DM and it is correlated with fasting plasma glucose level. [2]. Insulin controls the hepatic glucose production and promotes glucose utilization by the skeletal muscle. There is a correlation between the hepatic glucose production and the fasting glucose, in normal subjects, the postabsorptive hepatic glucose production is increased. But in patients with T2DM, the main causes are increased mostly by gluconeogenesis and to less extent by glycogenolysis by the liver. The Increased production of gluconeogenic precursors (lactate, alanine, and glycerol) and hyperglucagonemia with increased hepatic FFA acid oxidation might be responsible for glucogenesis. There is also a reduction in suppression of hepatic glucose production after carbohydrate ingestion which plays a role in the impairment in postprandial glucose homeostasis in T2DM [3].

The increased of the glycogenolysis and the decreased in the hepatic glucose uptake by glucagon will produce hyperglycemic phenotype associated with insulin deficiency and IR. In the overnight fasted, it is essential in countering the suppressive effects of basal insulin to maintain appropriate levels of glycogenolysis, fasting hepatic glucose production and blood glucose. Glycogenolysis is also increased by the counter-regulatory hormones response to hypoglycemia and in exercise [4]. Insulin and glucagon secretion are determined by plasma glucose concentration which is widely fluctuated according to the demand such as exercise and supply as taking high carbohydrate meal. In the resting postabsorptive state, the glycogenolysis and gluconeogenesis are equal or in balance in hepatic glucose release. This is a key regulated process. In the postprandial state, suppression of liver glucose output and stimulation of skeletal muscle glucose uptake are the most important factors. Under stressful conditions, the counter-regulatory hormones of the hypoglycemia secretion are increased with increased of the sympathetic nervous system activity. Their actions to increase hepatic glucose output and to suppress tissue glucose uptake are partly mediated by increases in tissue fatty acid oxidation. In T2DM, the fasting hyperglycaemia resulted from increased gluconeogenesis while, the postprandial hyperglycemia occurs due to impaired suppression of glycogenolysis and impaired skeletal muscle glucose uptake [5].

In normal subjects the fasting plasma glucose levels are constant from day to day. This constancy is due to a close co-ordination between glucose production by the liver and glucose uptake in peripheral tissues. In T2DM, fasting hyperglycemia to less extent is correlated with increased hepatic glucose production due to impaired hepatic sensitivity to insulin. But, it is largely due to reduced insulin secretion and increased glucagon secretion. Though the basal immunoreactive insulin and glucagon levels in patients with T2DM may appear normal compared with the normal subjects, the islet function testing at matched glucose levels reveals impairments of the basal, steady-state, and stimulated insulin and glucagon secretion due to a reduction in β- cells secretory capacity and a reduced ability of glucose to suppress glucagon release. Islet α- and β-cells functions are reduced by more than 50% in T2DM by the time that clinical fasting hyperglycemia develops (140 mg/dL) [6]. The efficiency of glucose uptake by the peripheral tissues is also impaired due to a combination of decreased insulin secretion and defective of the cellular insulin action [6, 7]. The defective in first phase glucose induced insulin secretion is followed by fasting hyperglycemia and the progressive failure in pancreatic β-cells function is matched by rising glucose levels to maintain basal and second-phase insulin output. The glucose is not only directly regulated insulin synthesis and secretion. But, moderated all other islet signals, including other substrates, hormones, and neural factors. In T2DM the defects are in first-phase insulin secretion and in the deficiency of the ability of glucose to potentiate other islet nonglucose β-cell secretagogues. In T2DM patients, the resulting hyperglycemia does not correct the first phase of insulin secretion defect. However, it compensates for the defective glucose potentiation, maintains nearly normal basal insulin levels and insulin responses to nonglucose secretagogues [8].

The major primary reduction of suppression in the output of the endogenous hepatic glucose release and the minor effect of the splanchnic glucose sequestration in these patients are the cause of increasing in systemic glucose delivery which subsequently responsible for the postprandial hyperglycemia [9, 10].

The fasting hyperglycemia is mainly caused by the increased of thc released hepatic glucose production. This mechanism is increased in psotabsorptive state and exhibits a positive correlation with fasting glucose level [3, 7 11].

The increase of the glucogenesis in the postprandial state represents the primary mechanism responsible for impaired suppression of hepatic glucose production [3]. The increased in the rate of glucose release by the liver results in part from impaired hepatic sensitivity to insulin, but it is largely due to reduced insulin secretion and increased glucagon secretion [6]. The degree of fasting hyperglycemia in a given patient with T2DM is closely related to the degree of impaired pancreatic β-cells responsiveness to glucose.

The fasting insulin secretion in normal subject and in patients with T2DM is comparable. But, there is a marked impairment of insulin secretion in patients with DM in relation to the degree of hyperglycemia. This is demonstrating the closed feedback loop operating between glucose levels and pancreatic β-cells which regulates the relationship of insulin secretion and hepatic glucose production [11]. The glucose uptake by peripheral tissue is impaired due to a combination of decreased insulin secretion and defective in cellular insulin action [6, 7].

The amyloid deposition process is associated with disproportionate hyperproinsulinemia. The amylin in transgenic mice develops islet amyloid deposits and hyperglycemia. This is suggestive the process of amyloid fibril formation impairs the function of the β-cells and eventual death. The progressive loss of β-cell function in T2DM, initially reflected by the loss in first-phase insulin secretion, followed by a decrease in the maximal capacity of glucose to potentiate all non-glucose signals. Finally, a defective steady-state and basal insulin secretion develops, leading to complete β-cells failure requiring insulin therapy [12].

The conclusion is, T2DM is characterized by a steady-state re-regulation of plasma glucose concentration at an elevated level in which islet cells dysfunction play a necessary role [7].

3. Insulin secretion, function and impairment

Insulin is synthesized and produced by β- cells in the pancreas. It is a peptide hormone regulates the metabolism of fat and carbohydrate in the body. It helps glucose absorption from the circulation by fat tissue and skeletal muscles. Figures 1 [13] and 2 [14].

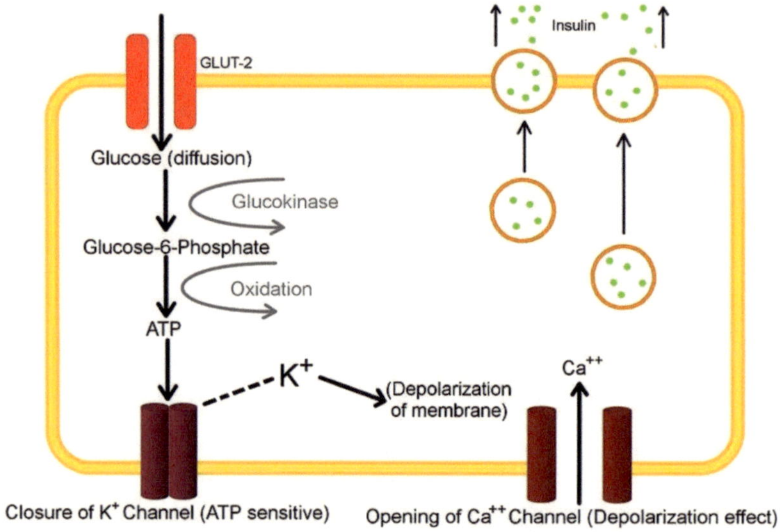

Figure 1. Insulin secretion [13].

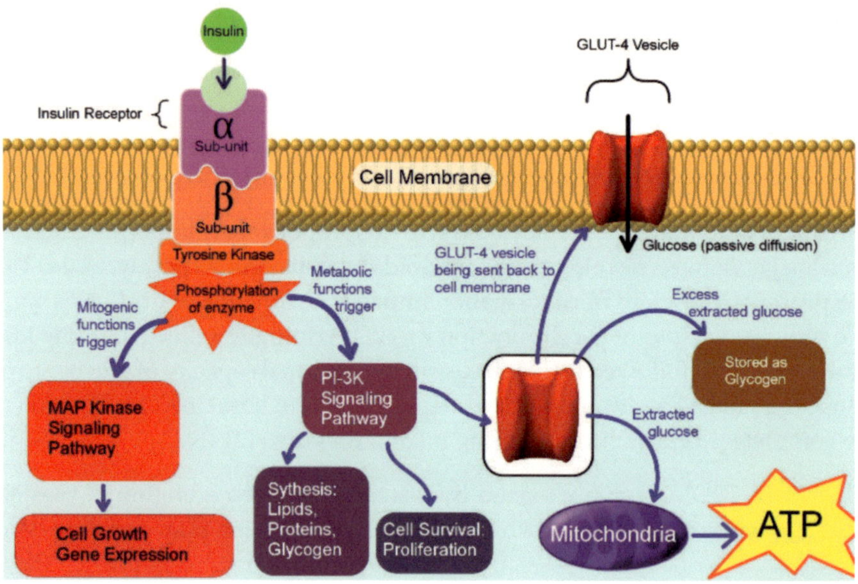

Figure 2. Insulin functions [14].

Pancreatic β-cells secrete insulin in two phases, first and second phase (biphasic manner). The loss of first phase is an independent predictor of T2DM onset. In patients with T2DM, the restoration of this phase suppresses the hepatic glucose output and improves the blood glucose concentration [15]. There are many metabolic abnormalities precede the clinical picture of

http://dx.doi.org/10.5772/59183

T2DM as demonstrated in a study of normal first- degree subjects who had relatives with T2DM. Following intravenous glucose infusion, these subjects showed a reduced first phase insulin secretion with decreased ability of the β-cells to respond to successive increase or decrease in glucose with mild elevation in 2hours post challenge glucose level [16]. In patients with T2DM, the earliest detectable defect and exhaustion of β- cells function appeared in the reduction of the first-phase insulin secretion. This phase is brief burst and spike lasting for about 10 minutes followed by plateau second phase lasted for 2-3 hours. The reductions in both phases occur equally early and precede development of IR [17]. The fasting plasma insulin concentration is often a marker of insulin sensitivity (IS) and the changing in acute insulin secretion following glucose challenge is an early observation of progressive pancreatic defect. Glucotoxicity and lipototoxicity are contributor factors in progressive and the continuous decline in pancreatic function [1, 18].

Insulin is secreted from the secretory cells by priming reaction. Each cell contains thousands of secretory vesicles/granules. Less than <5% of these cells exist to release the readily pool insulin by exocytosis followed by minimal latency of immediate releasable pool of insulin. The bulk of granules in the cell (>95%) exist in a non-releasable reserve pool of insulin, which must undergo a series of ATP-, Ca^{2+}-, and temperature-dependent reactions to release insulin [19].

The prevalence of Gestational diabetes (GDM) is 2-3% of all pregnant women. GDM women have the same second –phase insulin response as women with normal oral GTT. But, the first phase-insulin secretion is reduced with intravenous glucose and has a later peak rise with OGTT. Both groups showed a decreased in IS by 50-70%, this is back to normal in postpartum period in women with normal OGTT but this is not in women with GDM. In the same period, the latter group also demonstrated a persistent and excessive proinsulin secretion. Women with GDM have also a substantial increase in insulin secretion with OGTT or a meal compared to the same women in postpartum period. But this rise is less in women with GDM compared with pregnant women who retain normal OGTT [20].

The glycemic progression from normal to IGT mainly due to IR and from this state to overt DM depends primarily on β-cells failure in addition to progression to severe IR. Two studies, San Antonio and Hoorn Study showed the high fasting proinsulin reflects the β-cells dysfunction and the progression to DM. IR is determined by fasting hyperinsulinemia and lower glucose removal. Therefore, the 2 hours blood glucose level following oral glucose load is the most powerful in prediction of development of T2DM. IR and progressive β-cells dysfunction are the two important defects in development of the disease [21]. IFG and IGT are intermediate states in glucose metabolism that exist between normal GT and overt diabetes are related to these defects in addition to the reduction in early-phase insulin secretion. But, subjects with IGT also have impaired late-phase insulin secretion. The latter group also demonstrated a significant higher muscle IR and low hepatic IR while subjects with IFG have severe hepatic IR with normal or near-normal muscle IS [22]. The insulin secretion and glucose homeostasis in the first phaase insulin secretion is determined by a complex pathawy of multiple signals including hypoxia inducible factor 1α, von Hippel-Lindau, factor inhibiting HIF, nicotinamide phospho-ribosyl-transferase, and the sirtuin family in addition to many other novel regulatory factors are crucial [15].

4. Insulin resistance

Patients with T2DM have high whole body glucose production and glucogenesis but low glycogenolysis compared with normal subjects. In patients with IR, there is impairment of glucose transport and insulin signaling in target tissues with release of inflammatory markers from the adipose tissue [23, 24]. The glucose, FFA, autonomic nerves, fat-derived hormones and the gut hormone glucagon-like peptide-1 (GLP-1) are mediators sending signals to the β-cells to respond to IR. The maintenance of normal glucose and lipid metabolism is by the reciprocal relation of IR to IS and insulin secretion. Hyperbolic relation is the best description of the curvilinear relation between IS and secretion. This relation is impaired with failure of these signals to act on β-cells to secret insulin ends with subsequent development of dysglycemia (Impaired Fasting glucose- IFG, impaired Glucose tolerance –IGT and DM) [25].

Obesity is the most common cause of IR and T2DM. Simply being overweight (BMI >25) raises the risk of developing T2DM by a factor of 3 [26].

The main components of IR are dysglycemia, dyslipidemia, obesity, hypertension and hyperinsulinemia. Therefore, it is the key feature of metabolic syndrome (MS) and vascular complications (cardiovascular and stroke). IR components once are acquired, those with genetic predisposition will develop the full picture of the disorder suggesting the final phenotypic expression involves both genetic and acquired influences. The most important environmental factor in IR is central obesity which is mainly caused by intake of high fat, and refined carbohydrate without physical activity. These are exacerbated by genetic predisposition but IR could be reduced with minimizing dietary intake and regular exercise [27].

The three potential mechanisms of the controlling glucose metabolism in the skeletal muscles are the glycogen synthase, the hexokinase and the major insulin-stimulated glucose transporter GLUT4. Therefore, defects in glycogen synthesis in the skeletal muscles playing a major role in the pathogenesis of IR [28]. The decrease in the ability of normal responding skeletal muscles to circulating insulin levels or concentrations is main principle of development of IR which could precede the overt T2DM by 10 to 20years [28].

T2DM is characterized by increased hepatic glucose output, increased peripheral resistance to insulin action (due to receptor and postreceptor defects) and impaired insulin secretion.

Two major variants of insulin receptor abnormalities associated with acanthosis nigricans, hyperinsulinemia and marked hyperandrogenism. The classic type A IR syndrome, which is due to genetic defect in the insulin-signaling system such as mutation in the insulin receptor gene [29] and type B IR syndrome, which results from autoantibodies to the insulin receptor [30].

Many factors could enhance IR include, obesity, inflammation and inflammatory markers, defects in genes and drugs. These will be demonstrated further in this chapter.

5. The role of obesity and inflammatory markers in insulin resistance and T2DM

Obesity has a substantial negative effect on life expectancy and longevity. It reduces the length of life in severely obese people by an estimation of 5 to 20 years. This negative effect should be addressed in the health public policy [31]. Obesity, IR, and T2DM are growing health concerns, and the incidence and the prevalence of these diseases are increasing worldwide [32, 33]. Obesity will cause a decline in life expectancy for the first time in recent history due to numerous co-morbid disorders [31] and it is a risk factor for many human diseases [34]. Obesity is associated with an increased risk of developing IR and T2DM [34, 35]. The primary defects in obese individuals are the dysfunction of adipocyte and adipose tissue [34].

IR in obese subjects is determined by the release of high amounts of non-esterified FA, glycerol, hormones, pro-inflammatory cytokines and many other factors from adipose or fat tissue. This is followed by dysfunction of pancreatic β- cells and failure to secret insulin to control blood glucose levels. These metabolic and inflammatory changes are critical in defining the risk and the development of T2DM. [35]. There is a clear hyperbolic relationship between IS and insulin secretion by the β-cells of the pancreas. This demonstrates the concept of a feedback loop governs the interaction between the β-cells function and IS tissues. This helpful in explain that patients or subjects with IR have significant increase in insulin response compared with low responses in IS group [11, 36].

IR is a characteristic feature of T2DM and obesity, and the majority of patients with T2DM are obese. Obesity has a major impact to cause IR in subjects without DM. IR is the primary defect in obese elderly and middle aged patients with T2DM despite, adequate circulating insulin. But, in the second group the impairment of insulin release and the alteration of hepatic glucose output are other defects contributing to the development of the disease [37, 38, 39]. The intra-abdominal fat is a major determinant of IR among other distributed fat in the body while the dysfunction of the β- cells is correlated with reduction of β-cells mass and subsequently reduction in IS. The genetic and the molecular basis of these pathological abnormalities are there. But, not fully understood. As mentioned, the progressive declining or failure of the β-cells function and IS are associated with development of T2DM. Prior to the onset of T2DM, there are stages from normal glucose concentration to dysglycemia (IFG, IGT) emphasizing in number of ethnic group the OGTT response is a major determinant of β-cells function [25, 36]. The elevations in plasma FFA concentrations in obese subjects and in patients with T2DM inhibit insulin stimulated peripheral glucose uptake (fat and skeletal muscle) and glycogen synthesis [40, 41].

The impairment of adipose tissue functions in obese subjects caused by interaction of genetic and environmental factors and subsequently leads to obesity medical co-morbidities. However, not all obese patients develop the same complications. The adipocyte dysfunctions or impairment occur in form of ectopic fat deposition, adipocyte hypertrophy, hypoxia, changes in the cellular composition with a variety of stresses and inflammatory processes in the fat tissue (release a proinflammatory, atherogenic, and diabetogenic adipokine pattern), increased lipid storage and impaired IS [33]. Obese individuals have large or expanded fat mass and have high or elevated plasma concentration fatty acids [42, 43, 44].

Glucose uptake rather than intracellular glucose metabolism has been implicated as the rate-limiting step for FA-induced IR [45].

In adipose tissue, the glucocorticoids can be produced locally from inactive 11-keto forms through the enzyme 11beta hydroxysteroid dehydrogenase type 1 (11beta HSD-1). In obese human, the glucocorticoids are normal. However, the excess of glucocorticoids produce visceral obesity, IR and DM. In mice, the transgenic mice overexpressing 11beta HSD-1 selectively in adipose tissue was exaggerated by high fat diet showed an increase in the level of corticosterone in adipose tissue by increased adipocyte 11beta HSD-1 activity. This could have the same effect in human[46] suggesting that increases in endogenous 11β-HSD1 in the adipose tissue of obese humans and rodents [47,48] contribute to obesity-associated IR, in part due to increased delivery of glucocorticoids to the liver via the portal vein. The c-Jun amino-terminal kinases (JNKs) interfere with insulin action and it is crucial mediator of obesity and IR. In obese mouse, the JNK activity is abnormally elevated and the absence of JNK1 results in decreased adiposity and improved IS. Therefore, it is a potential target for therapeutics [49].

The activation of JNK1 leads to serine phosphorylation of IRS-1 that impairs insulin action [50, 51]. In addition, IKK-β is a mediator of TNF-induced IR [52, 53, 54, 55] demonstrated the TLR4 (Lipopolysaccharide receptor) activation by FFA, plays a critical role in innate immunity and IR in obese human and animals through activation of inflammatory pathways. In mice the lack of TLR4 will protect insulin suppression signaling and reduce insulin mediated changes in systemic glucose metabolism by lipid infusion. This indicates the effect of nutrition as environmental factor on TLR4 and subsequently on IR. The Apoptosis signal-regulating kinase 1 (ASK1) is an evolutionarily conserved mitogen-activated protein 3-kinase that activates both Jnk and p38 mitogen-activated protein kinases. The reactive oxygen species-dependent TRAF6-ASK1-p38 axis is crucial for TLR4-mediated mammalian innate immunity [53, 54]. This finding may provide an additional link between innate immunity, cellular stress, and IR. The protein tyrosine phosphatase receptor T (PTPRT) knockout mice are resistant to high-fat diet-induced obesity. The PTPRT-modulated STAT3 signaling in the regulation of high-fat diet-induced obesity [34]. Figures 3 and 4 with Table 1.

Adipokine	Distribution	Function	Effect in obesity
Leptin	Secreted predominantly by WAT, to lesser degree, in ypothalamus, gastric epithelium, placenta & gonads.	Regulates energy intake, expenditure & feeding behavior. Also regulates storage of fat & insulin signaling.	↑ in mouse models of obesity. ↑ in human obesity & correlated with BMI & ↓ in weight loss.
Adiponcktin	Secreted exclusively by adipocytes. mRNA & protein in Sc AT > Omental AT.	Improves energy homeostasis, IS & Glucose uptake. Anti-Inflammatory properties.	↓ in mouse models of obesity and IR (ob/ob and db/db).

http://dx.doi.org/10.5772/59183

Adipokine	Distribution	Function	Effect in obesity
	2–3 times greater secretion in females.		↓ in human obesity & T2DM patients. ↑ after weight loss
Resistin	In rodents, secreted by adipocytes. In humans, secreted predominantly by circulating macrophages & monocytes, to a lesser degree, by WAT.	Implicated in glucose metabolism, in the regulation of gluconeogenesis & IR in rodents. More roinflammatory role in humans.	↑ circulating concentrations in mouse models of obesity. ↑ in human obesity & correlated with IR in T2DM patients.
TNF-α	Expressed by macrophages & adipocytes (visceral WAT > subcutaneous WAT).	Affects insulin & glucose metabolism. Provokes IR & stimulates lipolysis.	↑ in mouse models of obesity. ↑ in human obesity & correlated with BMI
IL-6	One-third of total circulating levels are expressed predominantly by adipocytes. Also expressed in macrophages, skeletal muscle, endothelial cells & fibroblasts.	Controversial role in the development of IR. Affects glucose metabolism	↑ circulating levels in human obese subjects & correlated with adiposity& reduced with weight loss. ↑ in plasma of T2DM patients.
IL-7	Secreted by stromal & vascular endothelial cells.	Homeostatic immune cytokine. Also regulates body weight, AT mass & function, and insulin signaling.	↑ in morbidly obese subjects.
IL-8	Secreted by adipocytes (visceral WAT > SC WAT) & macrophages.	Neutrophil chemotaxis.	↑ in obese subjects & related to fat mass & TNF-α levels.
IL-1	Secreted mainly by adipocytes & macrophages.	Role in macrophages chemotaxis & thermogenesis	↑ in obese mice. ↑ in human obesity & predictive of T2DM.
IL-10	Secreted by monocytes, macrophages, dendritic cells, B & T cells.	Improves IS & glucose transport.	Attenuated in T2DM patients & ↑ with weight loss
RBP4	Secreted by adipocytes, macrophages & hepatocytes.	Affects IS, hepatic glucose output & muscle insulin signaling.	↑ circulating levels in obese subjects & correlated with BMI & IR.
MCP-1	Secreted by AT.	Affects IS & ↑ macrophage recruitment in AT and inflammation.	↑ in mouse models of obesity. ↑ in T2DM subjects.
PAI-1	Expressed by WAT.	Potent inhibitor of fibrinolytic pathway.	↑ in human obesity and T2DM subjects.

Adipokine	Distribution	Function	Effect in obesity
CXCL5	Secreted by macrophages within the stromal vascular fraction.	Interferes with insulin signaling in muscle.	Circulating levels are higher in obese IR individuals than in obese IS & ↓ after a 4-weeks period on low-calorie diet.
Visfatin	Expressed in liver, muscle, WAT, bone marrow & lymphocytes	Role in IS, insulin secretion & inflammatory properties.	↑ in obesity & correlates with visceral adiposity in humans.
Chemerin	In rodents & humans, expressed in placenta & WAT.	Regulates adipocyte development & metabolic function.	↑ circulating levels in obese & T2DM patients and correlated with body fat, glucose & lipid metabolism.
Vaspin	Secreted by WAT, hypothalamus, pancreatic islets & skin.	Improves IS.	↑ in obesity & T2DM patients
Omentin	Secreted by omental AT.	↑ IS	↓ in obesity.
Apelin	Produced in a wide range of tissues.	Improves IS mainly acting in skeletal muscle & adipocytes in mice.	↑ in obesity, IGT & T2DM patients. ↓ after weight loss following diet & bariatric surgery.
Nesfatin	Secreted in brain tissue, B cells and AT.	Central action to ↓ Appetite.	↓ in obesity.
TGFβ	Multifunctional, produced By variety of cells. Inhibitor of differentiation.	Varied role in proliferation, differentiation, apoptosis and development.	↑ ob/ob and db/db mice. ↑ preadipocyte cell proliferation as with TNFα. ↑ in obesity, T2DM patients & CVD.
Rantes	Pro -inflammatory secreted by T cells, monocytes & to lesser degree in WAT.	↑ gene expression in AT.	No correlation of serum level with obesity.
Preptin	It is a novel hormone that is co-secreted with insulin and amylin from pancreatic β-cells [60].	Synthetic prepin ↑ insulin secretion from glucose stimulated β TC6-F7 in a concentration- dependent and saturable manner [61].	Plasma preptin level ↑ with higher BMI [62]. It is ↑ in patients with T2DM compared with patients with IGT and normal subjects [61].
Uncoupling protein 2	It is expressed in AT, skeletal muscle and tissue of immune system [63].	It protects cell function from damage and it impairs insulin secretion from β-cells [64].	Anti-oxidant in pancreatic β-cells [65]. The level and activity has impact on glucose stimulated insulin secretion [66].

Table 1. Adipokines increased in obesity and/or diabetes [58, 59].

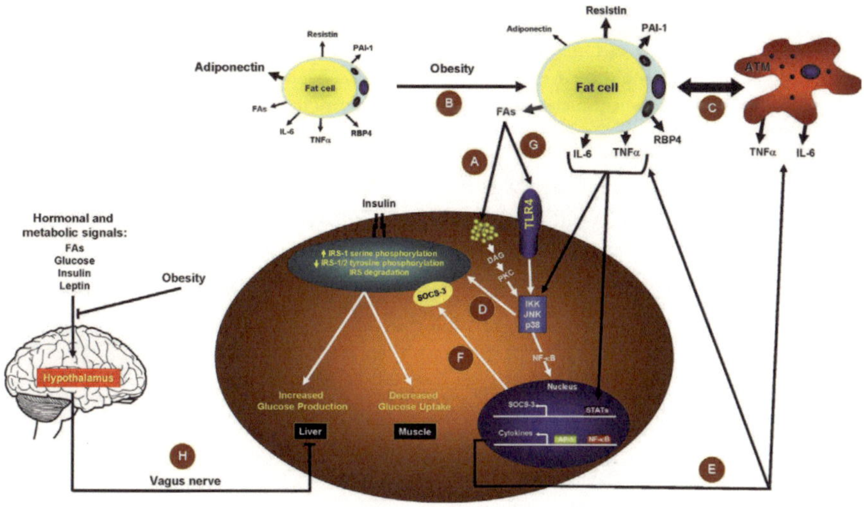

Figure 3. The molecular linked pathway between obesity and IR. (*A*) IR triggered by the increase in FAs through intracellular metabolites that activate PKC, leading to inhibit insulin signaling by activation of serine/threonine kinases. (*B*) Insulin signaling modulated by changes in adipokines secretion. (*C*) In the adipose tissue; the increased in the ATMs mediated the increase of the inflammatory cytokines that inhibit insulin signaling. (*D*) Insulin signaling inhibited by mediators (Endocrine and Inflammatory) converging on serine/threonine kinases. (*E*) IR exacerbated by activation of NF-κB heightens inflammatory responses. (*F*) Adipokines induced SOCS family proteins interfering with IRS-1 and IRS-2 tyrosine phosphorylation or by targeting IRS-1 and IRS-2 for proteosomal degradation inducing IR. (*G*) IR triggered by activation TLR4 and innate immune response by FAs. (*H*) Alteration in peripheral IS is related to the central response to hormonal and nutrient signals [57].

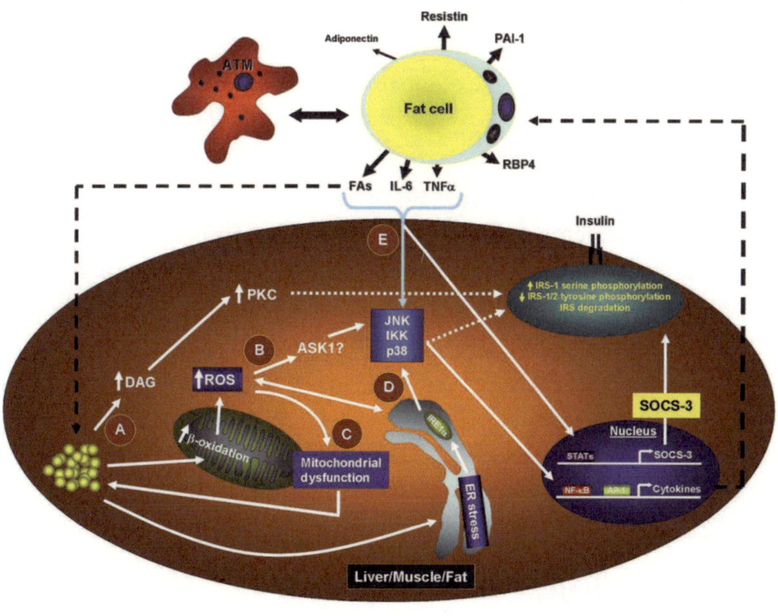

Figure 4. There are several cell-intrinsic mediators and pathways dysregulation in obesity with negative impact on IR. (*A*) Activation of PKC in the liver and muscles inhibits insulin signaling by increasing FA from ectopic adipose tissue. (*B*) Direct inhibition of insulin signaling through IRS-1 or IRS-2 serine phosphorylation or indirectly through a series of

transcriptional events mediated by NF-κB. Inhibition occurs due to activation of several serine/threoning kinases (JNK, IKK, and p38 MAPK) by excess in ROS. The later generation increased by mitochondrial β- oxidation triggered by excess fat accumulation. (*C*) IR exacerbated by mitochondrial dysfunction through increasing intracellular lipid accumulation. (*D*) Insulin signaling suppressed by activation of JNK or through a potential increase in ROS production and both activated by cellular ER stresses responses. (*E*) The cell-extrinsic modulators such as endocrine and inflammatory signals can intensified IR [57].

WAT: White adipose tissue, AT: adipose tissue, T2DM: type 2 diabetes mellitus, IR: insulin resistance, IS: insulin sensitivity, IGT: impaired glucose tolerance, TNF-α: tumor necrosis alpha, IL: interleukin, RBP4: Retinol binding protein, SC: subcutaneous, MCP-1: monocyte chemotactic protein 1, PAI: plasminogen activator inhibitor, CXCL5: chemokines molecules (CXCL5 ligand 5), TGFβ: transforming growth factor β.

6. Others

6.1. Glucose transporters

Glucose transporters (GLUT) are integral membrane proteins that mediate the transport of glucose and structurally-related substances across the cellular membranes [67].

Sugar transport catalyzed by 11 out of 14 members of the human GLUT family. There are specific characteristics of each isotypes. They are different in expression profile, substrate specificity and kinetic characteristics. Therefore, the tissue adaptation of the glucose uptake will be determined and regulated by specific tissue gene expression. GLUT4 malfunction in expression or regulation contributes to IR while GLU2 plays a role in hormonal and neuronal control by acting a glucose sensor in β-cells of the pancreas and neuronal cells [68]. GLUT1 is ubiquitously expressed with particularly high levels in human erythrocytes and in the endothelial cells lining the blood vessels of the brain. GLUT3 is expressed primarily in neurons and, together, GLUT1 and GLUT3 allow glucose to cross the blood-brain barrier and enter neurons [69].

The GLUTI, GLUT2, and GLUU3 are the major glucose transporters isoforms present in these cells and they are constitutively localized to the plasma membrane. The glucose flux across the membrane is largely dependent upon the circulating blood glucose level or concentration. In acute state, the glucose regulated the transport system in the muscles and fat cells responded within minutes to insulin [70].

GLUT4 is the primary hormonally-responsive transporter and it is the major insulin-responsive transporter [69]. GLUT4 expression is also reduced by low insulin states, such as in muscle during fasting, and in IR adipose tissue [71]. The malfunction of glucose transporter expression or regulation (GLUT4) appears to contribute to the IR syndrome [68].

7. Genes in type 2 Diabetes Mellitus

T2DM is a complex diseases arise from interactions of multiple genes with environmental factors. These genes are variables in strength, site of interaction and are different in general

http://dx.doi.org/10.5772/59183

population according to race and ethnicity. The diabetes genes are involved in insulin signaling, insulin secretion, IR, glucose metabolism and obesity. In addition, T2DM could be a component of many syndromes of identified inherited genes [72]. The genetic risk for T2DM changes as humans first began migrating around the world, implying a strong environmental component has affected the genetic-basis of the disease [73, 74]. Immigrants to Western developed countries, for instance, may be more prone to diabetes as compared to its lower incidence in their countries of origins [75]. In meta-analysis of different ethnicities was included in a cross–sectional data from 16 cohorts from the DECODA (Diabetes Epidemiology: Collaborative Analysis of Diagnostic Criteria in Asia) demonstrated; the waist-to-stature ratio in Asian was stronger than BMI is associated with DM in adjusted age group in both genders [76]. In Japanese-American the prevalence of DM was reduced among the men who had retained a more Japanese lifestyle through higher levels of physical activity and consumed more carbohydrates with less fat and animal protein in their diet. An inverse association between DM and being bom in Japan was observed independent of age, body mass index, physical activity, and percentages of calories from fat or carbohydrates [77]. In Fiji population the disease pattern is determined by the modern lifestyle as in many industrial counties. The increase in mortality in this population was contributing to 6% and 30% due to DM and CVD respectively [78]. In USA, the large burden of T2DM in relative to non-Latino Whites, Latinos —those of Mexican origin in particular is related to mixed acculturation to US lifestyles and with greater time living in the States [79]. This was supported by other two studies. The first showed IR, hyperinsulineamia and T2DM with secondary lipid disturbances are the possible mechanism of higher morbidity and mortality from CHD in UK immigrants from the Indian subcontinent (South Asian) than other general population independently of the dietary fat intakes, smoking, blood pressure, or plasma lipids [80]. The second study also observed IR is the common pathogenic mechanism and is a risk factor of increasing the prevalence of CHD, T2DM, low HDL and hypertriglyceridemia in first generation immigrant Asian Indian to the USA compared with native Caucasian population [81]. The two major environmental risk factors for T2DM are obesity (≥ 120% ideal body weight or a body mass index > 30 k/m^2) and the sedentary lifestyle [82, 83]. Thus, the tremendous increase in the rates of T2DM in recent years has been attributed, primarily, to the dramatic rise in obesity worldwide [84]. Obesity is a progressive disease and up to 80% of patients with T2DM and PCOS patients can be attributed to obesity. It is a progressive condition leads to medical co-morbidities which are more prevalent with age and higher BMI, particularly in those with a central obesity [85]. In Pima Indians adolescents, the prevalence of T2DM was 50.9 per 1000 in 1967-1976 increased to 6 folds in 1987-1996. In American Indian and first nation youth, T2DM was more prevalent in 10-19 years old young group. Mainly in obese subjects with acanthosis nigiricans and had family history of the disease [86]. Sinha R, reported 25% of obese children (4 to 10 years of age) and 21%t of obese adolescents (11 to 18 years of age) had IGT and 4% of the obese adolescent has silent T2DM [87]. The increase in physical activity plays an important role in reducing risk of obesity and T2DM. The prolonged TV watching is associated with a significantly increased risk of obesity and T2DM, independent of diet and exercise. Men watching TV more than 40 hours per week have threefold of increase risk of developing T2DM compared with those less than I hour TV watching. Therefore, the public health campaign of decrease sedentary life should accompany the increase in physical activity [88].

Physical activity has also been inversely related to body mass index and IGT. Interventional studies in China, Finland and the US demonstrated the decrease in the risk of incidence and in the progression from pre-diabetes stage (IGT) to T2DM by intensive lifestyle interventions targeting diet and exercise. The Finnish Diabetes Prevention Study showed a reduction by 58% and in the china study was 31% with diet and 42% with diet and exercise. This was supported by USA study showed the same risk reduction with intensive lifestyle as in the Finnish study and also a reduction of 31% with metformin indicating that lifestyle intervention is better than drugs in T2DM prevention [89, 90, 91].

Xue Sun [92] reviewed a large-scale of association studies, and the genome-wide association studies (GWAS). Both have successfully identified multiple genes that contribute to T2DM susceptibility. Linkage analysis, candidate gene approach, large-scale association studies, and GWAS have identified approximately 70 loci conferring susceptibility to T2DM. Among them, 45 loci were identified in European populations, and the other 29 loci were identified in Asian populations, especially in East and South Asians. The immediate benefit derived from these findings was the better understanding of the pathophysiology of T2DM. A great number of studies have suggested that genetic variants in or near KCNJ11, TCF7L2, WFS1, HNF1B, IGF2BP2, CDKN2ACDKN2B, CDKAL1, SLC30A8, HHEX/IDE, KCNQ1, THADA, TSPAN8/LGR5, DC123/CAMK1D, JAZF1, MTNR1B, DGKB/TMEM195, GCK, PROX1, ADCY5, SRR, CENTD2, ST6GAL1, HNF4A, KCNK16, FITM2-R3HDML-HNF4A, GLIS3, GRB14, ANK1, BCAR1, RASGRP1, and TMEM163 may confer T2DM risk through impaired -β-cell function [93-97] whereas PPARγ, ADAMTS9, IRS1, GCKR, RBMS1/ITGB6, PTPRD, DUSP9, HMGA2, KLF14, GRB14, ANKRD55, and GRK5 have an impact on insulin action [94,98-100]. FTO and MC4R, previously identified genes associated with obesity, appear to confer T2DM risk through their primary effects on BMI, but recent GWAS have shown that their effects on T2DM were independent of BMI, though FTO may have a small but detectable influence on T2DM risk through insulin action [101,102].

Barnet AH; concluded the higher concordance rate in identical twins than in non-identical twins regardless the age of the onset of the disease and in identical twins, the concordant for DM is usually in older age group compared with the younger [103]. In Japan, The Concordance between monozygotic twins was 83% for T2DM and was 40% between dizygotic twins for T2DM. This concordance was significantly greater in monozygotic than in dizygotic twins and among twins with later onset of DM (after the age of 20) than early onset. It was also observed, the loss of the early-phase insulin response for OGTT in T2DM co-twins [104]. The role of obesity or BMI in twins as a risk of DM varies in heterogeneous genetic background. The index twins of concordant pairs had been less obese than discordant pairs. This is suggestive obesity has a role in pathogenesis of DM in those with weaker genetic susceptibility for the disease [5].

Nonetheless, non diabetes first-degree relatives of T2DM patients have an almost three fold increased lifetime risk of T2DM in comparison to the background population [106]. In other study 40% of first-degree relatives of T2DM patients develop diabetes as compared to 6% in the general population [106]. IR is an early metabolic feature of nondiabetic first-degree relatives of T2DM patients [107,108] and also shows familial clustering in keeping with an underlying genetic predisposition [109,110]. The defects of insulin action are retained in cultured skeletal

http://dx.doi.org/10.5772/59183

muscle cells from IR subjects and T2DM patients [111,112] suggesting that genetic variation contributes to decreased insulin action. While IR is a common feature of T2DM, the severity and clinical importance varies considerably across the T2DM population [113].

7.1. Inherited DM: Maturity onset diabetes of the young or MODY

The transcription factor genes play a crucial role in the normal development and function of the β-cell. MODY is a distinct type of heterogeneous group of disorders caused by mutations in β-cell transcription factors. MODY is an autosomal dominant mode of inheritance β- cell dysfunction in young age group (usually before 25 years). It is difficult to distinguish between MODY and other forms of DM because of primary defect is pancreatic β-cell dysfunction in patients with MODY. There are at least nine mutations of different gens that result in MODY phenotypes which account in about 1-2% or 2-5% of patients diagnosed with DM (approximately 20000 in UK). The transcription factors hepatocyte nuclear factor HNF - α1, HNF-4α, insulin promoter factor (IPF)-1, HNF-1β, and NeuroD1 are the main identified genes in MODY. The Glucokinase (GCK) is an enzyme responsible for glucose phosphorylation, whereas HNF-1α, HNF-4α, IPF1, HNF-1β, and NEUROD1 are all transcription factors that modulate the expression of several genes involved in differentiation and function of β-cells. This enzyme is a key in blood glucose homeostasis and the defective in kinase gene metabolism implicated in the pathogenesis of DM. There is a linkage between the GCK locus on chromosome 7p and diabetes in 16 French families with MODY and the same linkage was demonstrated in a large 5-generation pedigree (BX) with 15 members with DM. Mutations in the GCK gene cause a mild, asymptomatic and non-progressive fasting hyperglycaemia from birth usually requiring no treatment. The gene on chromosome 7 (MODY2) encodes the glycolytic enzyme glucokinases plays a key role in generating the metabolic signal for insulin secretion and in integrating hepatic glucose uptake. Other linkage studies have localized other genes mutation in MODY on human chromosomes 20 (MODY1) and 12 (MODY3), with MODY2 and MODY3 being allelic with the genes encoding glucokinase. MODY1 is an encoding (hepatocyte nuclear factor) HNF-4α (gene symbol, TCF14), a member of the steroid/thyroid hormone receptor superfamily and an upstream regulator of HNF-1 α expression. This is a transcription factor involved in tissue-specific regulation of liver genes but also expressed in pancreatic islets, insulinoma cells and other tissues. Mutations in the GCK and HNF1- α/4-α genes account for up to 80% of all MODY cases, these mutations appear in different transcription factor genes result in different clinical presentations. Mutations in the genes encoding the transcription factors HNF-1α and HNF-4α cause a progressive insulin secretory defect and hyperglycemia while mutations in the GCK gene cause a mild and non-progressive disease. MODY3 form has also mutations in the gene encoding hepatocyte nuclear factor-1 α (HNF-1α, which is encoded by the gene TCF1). Mutations in HNF-1α are highly penetrant with 63%of mutation carriers having diabetes by the age of 25 years, 78.6% by 35 years, and 95.5% by 55 years resulted in progressive β- cell dysfunction with increasing treatment requirements, greater risk of complications with age and appear to be renal dysfunction, which is often diagnosed before diabetes. Mutations in HNF-4α result in same mode of β- cell deterioration in β-cells function but the diagnosis in the later age. Mutations in IPF-1 (PDX-1) are not a common cause of MODY. MODY1 form has mutations in the gene encoding hepatonuclear factor HNF-4 α (gene symbol, TCF14) is a member of the steroid/thyroid hormone receptor superfamily and an upstream regulator of HNF-1α expression. The deficient binding of NEUROD1 or binding of a transcriptionally inactive NEUROD1 polypeptide to target promoters in pancreatic islets leads to the development of T2DM in humans. In mice, two mutations in NEUROD1 in the heterozygous state were described in development of T2DM. The truncated polypeptide lacking the carboxy-terminal trans-activation domain, a region that associates with the co-activators CBP and p300 is more severe clinically than mutation at Arg 111 in the DNA-binding domain, abolishes E-box binding activity of NEUROD1 [114-125]. Other rare forms of MODY are CEL-MODY, ABCC8, KCNJ11 and UPD6 [126]. There are many factors determined the clinical presentation of various subtype of MODY including, the severity, the course of insulin secretion defect, the risk of microvascular complications and the presence of other abnormalities or defects in diabetes patients [127].

7.2. Mitochondrial diabetes: A monogenic Diabetes Mellitus

Maternally inherited diabetes and deafness (MIDD) is a new sub-type of diabetes with mutation in mitochondrial DNA. The mitochondrial genome is passed and inherited exclusively by maternal line. In patients with T2DM there could be increase in transmission of inherited diseases by maternal line more than paternal. However, only 0.5-2.8% of patients with DM demonstrated the frequency of adenine to guanine mutation. The adenine to guanine transition mutation at position 3243 in the dihydrouridine loop of mitochondrial $tRNA^{Leu(UUR)}$ gene is specific to patients with a neurological syndrome MELAS (myopathy, encephalopathy, lactic acidosis and stroke like disease). There is also 3243 mutation is associated with the phenotypical distinct of MIDD sub-type. In a study of the genotype of patients with T2DM of North European extraction with one or more features of MIDD and/or MELAS, Two patients were identified with the mutation giving a prevalence rate of 0.13% for the whole study population, and 0.45% for the sample with phenotypic features of MIDD. Other mitochondrial gene defects and mutation of 3234 are linked to the development of T2DM [128-133].

8. The monogenic forms of Insulin Resistance (IR)

A clear genotype-phenotype association is emerging following description of more than 60 mutations in insulin receptor gene which subsequently causing IR and tend to genera extreme and severe forms of IR patients. The most abundant mutations are heterozygous leading to decreased tyrosine phosphorylation of the β-subunit of the insulin receptor.

- Type A insulin resistance syndrome, it is a heterozygous mutations in the tyrosine kinase domain of the insulin receptor gene and it is the most common phenotype. It is characterized by acanthosis nigricans and hyperandrogenism without obesity or lipoatrophy.
- Homozygous or compound heterozygous mutations lead to the Rabson–Mendelhall syndrome with severe impairment of insulin receptor function.

http://dx.doi.org/10.5772/59183

- Donohue syndrome (Leprechaunism) is the most extreme form of IR in humans in whom mutations resulting in complete or near-complete absence of functional insulin receptors. [134,135,136]

- Dunnigan-type familial partial lipodystrophy (FPLD) is a rare autosomal dominant form of monogenic IR. FPLD patients are born with normal fat distribution but after the onset of puberty, they lose fat from their extremities and gluteal region. The mutation of LMNA, which encodes nuclear lamin A and C on chromosome 1q21, underlies FPLD. These patients have low leptin levels and FPDL is linked to early coronary heart disease. The LMNA codon 482 missense mutation was observed to strongly associated with hyperinsulinemia, dyslipidemia, hypertension, and T2DM [137,138,139].

- The PPARγ gene, encoding the receptor through which the insulin-sensitizing drugs, the thiazolidinediones, mediate their effects the peroxisome proliferator-activated receptor gamma (PPARγ) has become a prime candidate in the search for mutations causing IR [140]. The new missense mutations in the ligand-binding domain of PPARγ were found in family (mother and her son) was heterozygous for a single nucleotide substitution with mutation at codon P467L. The mother had history of irregular period, infertility disorder, Gestational DM followed by frank DM requiring high doses of insulin (severe IR). Her son had history of early onset T2DM and hypertension. The third subject was a young female from another family presented with primary amenorrhoea, hirsutism, acanthosis nigricans and hypertension. She was heterozygous from different mutation at codon V290 of a single nucleotide substitution. These new subtypes of dominantly inherited T2DM due to defective transcription factor function resulting in impaired insulin action rather than secretion [141]. Studies to determine if mutations in the PPARγ gene predispose to diabetes in the general population show a complex relationship.

8.1. Insulin gene

Several phenotypes, including T2DM, polycystic ovary syndrome, and birth weight are associated with tandem repeat (VNTR) minisatellite 5' of the insulin gene (INS). A study analyzed this insulin gene class III VNTR minisatellite in 155 European T2DM parent-offspring trios from the British Diabetes Association demonstrated that variation within the TH-INS-IGF2 locus, most plausibly at the VNTR itself at this regulatory element is a significant determinant of T2DM susceptibility. This susceptibility is exclusively mediated by paternally derived alleles [142].

8.1.1. SUR-1gene

In Dutch population, the exon 16-3t allele of the single nucleotide polymorphisms in the sulphonylurea receptor gene (SUR1) has been reported to be associated with T2DM patients compared with the control group. But there was no association between T2DM patients and the variant in exon 18 or the combination of both variants. Other studies in Caucasian population, strong linkage disequilibrium between the exon 16 and exon 18 variants was demonstrated in patients with T2DM but was not shown in the control group [143].

8.1.2. IRS-1gene

The utilization of insulin receptor substrate (IRS)-proteins (IRS-1 and IRS-2) emerged many interactive proteins in the insulin signaling system. This can be amplified or attenuated independently insulin binding and tyrosine kinase activity, providing an extensible mechanism for signal transmission in multiple cellular backgrounds [144]. Patient with T2DM with IRS-1 variants did not differ in their degree of IR compared with patients without known IRS-1 polymorphisms. However, carriers of the codon 972 variant had significantly lower plasma levels of fasting insulin and C-peptide [145, 146]. Many other studies demonstrated several polymorphisms in the IRS-1 gene variant, a Gly-->Arg change at the codon 972 may contribute in impairment of insulin secretion and increased in prevalence among patients with T2DM [146].

8.1.3. PC-1gene

In Swedish and Finnish people, the Q allele of the human glycoprotein PC-1 gene is associated with surrogate measures of IR, but it may not be enough to increase the susceptibility to T2DM. An observation showed there was no difference in the Q allele frequency between the patients with T2DM and control group. There were higher fasting plasma glucose and 2 hours in QK genotype siblings with diabetes compared with carrier of KK genotype. While in sibling with QK genotype and without diabetes have higher fasting plasma glucose and insulin than KK genotype carrier [147].

8.2. Glycogen synthase gene

An Xbal polymorphism has been described in the glycogen synthase gene associated with IR [148]. More features of metabolic syndrome and increased susceptibility to T2DM were described in sibling with rare A2 allele of discordant sib-pair analysis [149]. A set of polymorphic microsatellite markers that span the genome was implemented in genotyping of families with this condition to essence this approach [150].

8.2.1. Calpain 10 (CAPN10) gene

Calpain gene is cytoplasmic cystiene protease requiring calcium ions for activity. CAPN10 gene was proposed as susceptibility locus of T2DM based on the initial report of association between the T2DM and CAPN10 gene [151]. It has been reported of association with T2DM in Pima Indians [152], in African Americans [153] in Mexican Americans [154], in the Botnia area of Finland, German patients [155] and in South Indians [156].

8.2.2. Foxo 1 gene

Insulin signalling downstream of the phosphatidylinositol 3-kinase (PI3K)/Akt pathway is at least in part controls glucose on β-cells mass and function. The activation of Akt is negatively affected the proliferation and metabolism of Foxo transcription factors. The changes in Foxo 1 transcriptional activity are associated with nutritional alteration of β-cells. Glucose-stimulated insulin secretion acts through its own receptor as the predominant mediator of these changes in β-cells [157]. Ghrelin increases pancreatic β-cell proliferation and survival via sequential activation of phosphatidylinositol-3 kinase (PI3K) and Akt ghrelin. It protects pancreatic β-cells from lipotoxicity by inhibiting the nuclear translocation of Foxo1 [158].

8.3. Beta 3-adrenergic receptor gene

The energy balance by increasing in lipolysis and thermogenesis could be regulated by the beta 3-adrenergic receptor (beta 3-AR) gene. The ability to gain weight and the early onset of T2DM are associated with mutation in the beta 3-AR gene (Trp64Arg). But this is not in Dutch population [159]. Many studies in different ethnic groups showed an association of beta3-AR gene polymorphism with IR, obesity and its metabolic disorders such as T2DM, coronary heart disease and hypertension [160].

8.3.1. TCF7L2

The risk alleles of TCF7L2 were associated with enhanced expression of this gene in human islets as well as impaired insulin secretion both in vitro and in vivo. TCF7L2 has also been linked to altered pancreatic islet morphology as exemplified by increased individual islet size and altered α and β cell ratio/distribution within human islets [161]. TCF7L2 encodes the transcription factor TCF4 which is related to Wnt signaling pathway and which plays a critical role in the pathogenesis of T2DM. The risks of alleles in TCF7L2 were associated with hepatic but not peripheral IR and enhanced the rate of hepatic glucose production in human [162]. This is indirectly disturbing beta cells function of the pancreas.

8.3.2. SCL30A8

SCL30A8 encodes the islet specific zinc transporter ZnT-8, which delivers zinc ions from cytoplasm into intracellular insulin-containing granules and is implicated in insulin maturation and/or storage processes in β-cells [163]. The expression level of ZnT-8 was remarkably down regulated in the pancreas of db/db and Akitamice in the early stage of diabetes. Global SCL30A8 knockout mice demonstrated reduced plasma insulin, impaired glucose –stimulated insulin secretion, and markedly reduced islet zinc content [164].

8.4. Others genetic syndromes associated with diabetes

Down syndrome, Klinefelter syndrome, Turner syndrome, Wolfram syndrome, Friedreichataxia, Huntington chorea, Laurence-Moon-Biedlsyndrome, Myotonicdystrophy, Porphyria and Prader-Willi syndrome.

9. Drugs induced hyperglycemia and DM

Many pharmacologic and chemical agents can predispose, induce or precipitate hyperglycemia in normal subjects with high risk of T2DM or patients with IGT and DM. The individual effect of each agent could be weak or strong and subsequently the new glycemic state will be variable from transient to permanent. There are many mechanisms to induce diabetes by interfere with insulin production or secretion (e.g. Beta- Blockers), block insulin action (e.g. Steroids), interfere with both insulin secretion and action (e.g. Thiazides), and finally increase blood glucose using mechanisms independent of insulin's actions (e.g. Nicotinic acid) [165].

Table 2 shows the most common drugs that used in clinical practice with the mechanism of each drug or group.

Drugs	Mechanisms	Notes
Thiazide and thiazide like drugs. Chlorothiazide Chlorothalidone Hydrocholorthiazide Idapamide Methyclothiazide Metolazone	Decreases insulin release by hypokalemia [167,168] and down regulation of PPARγ Receptor.	Avoided in patients with DM and patients at risk of hyperglycemia. Use small dose if requires [167, 168].
*Spironolactone does not cause IGT even at high dosage [167].	In hypertensive elderly on Thiazide but without DM, each 0.5meq/L reduction in serum potassium was associated with 45% higher risk of new DM [169].	Indapamide does not interfere with blood sugar control in T2DM but higher doses that cause potassium loss may cause deterioration.
	Increases aldosterone release and IR [170,171].	Loop diuretics have been reported to reduce glucose control to a lesser extent than Thiazides [168].
Atypical antipsychotics **High risk** Clozapine Olanzapine	Wight gain [172, 173] and adiposity [174]	Risk of hyperglycemia is more in patients with obesity, age, ethnic status, and certain neuropsychiatric conditions [173].
Intermediate risk Paliperidone Quietiapine Resperidone	Sympathetic stimulation [175].	
Low risk Aripiprazole Ziprasidone	Decrease insulin action [173] and increase IR [176].	
Unknown Iloperidone	Potential Individual Polymorphisms in the leptin gene and leptin receptor gene to antipsychotic induced obesity [177].	
B- blockers Atenolol Metoprolol Propranolol	Increase fasting glucose [178].	The risk of hyperglycemia is increased in patient on B-blocker and thiazide diuretics [180].

Drugs	Mechanisms	Notes
*Carvidolol and nebivolol are not associated with hyperglycemia.	Impair insulin secretion [179]	
Corticosteroids Betamethasone acetate Cortisone Methylprednisolone Hydrocortisone Fludrocortisone Hydrocortisone Triamcinolone Prednisolone Dexamethasone	Decrease in both hepatic and extrahepatic sensitivity to insulin [182].	Identify high risk patient of hyperglycemia.
Oral contraceptive pills	Increase IR [182,183].	Risk of hyperglycemia is increased with higher doses and longer duration therapy.
Megasterol acetate [181].		Monitor the blood glucose to optimize the diabetes therapy by tablets or insulin to avoid short and long term complications of hyperglycemia.
Growth Hormone	Accelerated lipolysis resulting in increased circulating non-esterified fatty acids levels [184,185]. This may contribute to IR, hyperinsulinemia and defective glycogen synthesis [186].	Used as replacement therapy in patients with GH deficiency.
Protease inhibitors Atazanavir, Darunavir Fosamprenavir Indinavir Nelfinavir Ritonivir Saquinavir Tipranivir. Etravirine Maraviroc Raltegravir	Inhibition of GLUT4 Transporter contributes to decrease peripheral insulin sensitivity and induce IR. [187].	Lipodystrophy and Dyslipidaemia are major side effects of this group [188].
Didanosine Nucleoside reverse transcriptase inhibitor	Causes β-cell injury by pancreatitis [189].	Used in treatment of HIV infection. The risk is increased with high dose and in combination with tenofovir [190].
Antibiotics **(Quinolone group)**		

Drugs	Mechanisms	Notes
Gatifloxacin Temafloxacin Levofloxacin	Stimulation of insulin secretion by inhibition of pancreatic beta-cell K(ATP) channels causes hypoglycemia [192]. It may also cause hyperglycemia. [193].	Gatifloxacin was withdrawn from the market because of this effect [193]. Levofloxacin has a small effect. [192].
Rifampicin [191].	Possibly by augmenting intestinal absorption of glucose.	It is an early phase of hyperglycemia and disappeared after few days of treatment. This effect in rat [194].
Tetracyclines Tetracycline chlortetracycline	Causes hyperglycemia.	
\Calcineurin inhibitors Cyclosporine	Impair the function β-cells by impairing insulin gene expression [195-197].	The incidence of new onset DM was 14 to 16% augmented in the first post-transplantation year, declining thereafter to an annual incidence of 4 to 6%, similar to the pre-transplantation baseline rate [205, 206].
Sirolimus Tacrolimus Cyclosporine	Direct β-cells toxicity [198-200]. Decreases in IS [201].	The cumulative incidence of new onset DM was 24% at 3 yr after transplantation [205].
	Impair insulin-mediated suppression of hepatic glucose production [202]. May cause ectopic triglyceride deposition, leading to IR [203, 204].	There is a synergetic effect of cyclosporine to induce DM if given with other diabetogenic drug [207].
	The above aggravated by many modifiable and non-modifiable risk factors [201].	
Thalidomide [208].	Decreases insulin-stimulated peripheral glucose uptake by 31% (increased insulin resistance)	Thalidomide, withdrawn for teratogenicity and was reintroduced in 1997 as an immunomodulator to treat erythema nodosum leprosum.
	Decreases glycogen synthesis by 48%.	
Fish oil or Omega -3 polyunsaturated fatty acids (PUFAs).	PUFAs may affect glucose metabolism through increased IS, but studies to date have been inconclusive [209].	Among all adults who use natural products, more than 37% report taking fish oil or omega-3s. [210].
Interferon α [211].	Risk of hyperglycemia only in patient with chronic hepatitis C infection.	Sustained virological responses reduce the risk of developing glucose abnormalities, especially in patients with normal glucose baseline.

Drugs	Mechanisms	Notes
Ritodrine [212].	Ritodrine induced hypokalemia.	It is selective β2- adrenergic agonist used for premature labour.
Pentamidine [213].	Inappropriate insulin release and toxicity to the islet β-cells. It may cause hypoglycemia, IGT and DM.	It is anti-protozoa agent. These effects worsening with higher doses prolong course and renal impairment.
Statins [214].	Impairing β-cell function and decreasing peripheral insulin sensitivity.	Elderly women and Asians are at particular risk.
Nicotinamide [215].	Enhanced gluconeogenesis.	Hyperglycemia may occur in both normal subjects and in patients with DM.
Diazoxide [216].	Inhibits insulin secretion	Used in treatment of insulinoma.
diphenylhydantoin [217].	Inhibiting apoptosis, increases islet insulin content, accompanied with ameliorated glucose tolerance.	It may be useful in treatment and prevention of DM.
	Inhibits insulin secretion.	Hyperglycemia is more likely to develop in subjects with other risk factors for DM.
L-Asparaginase	Non injury to β-cells [218]. In Rabbits, the anti-tumor enzyme, L-asparaginase, is produced at least in part by the suppression of insulin release [219].	It is transient hyperglycemia that ends following stop the drug.
Vacor Rodenticide poisoning [220].	It has antineoplastic activity and cause pancreatic β-cell damage.	Accidental ingestion by subjects causes severe form of diabetes Ketoacidosis.
Total Parenteral Nutrition	These patients are often critically ill and are administered preparations with high glucose content [221].	It is associated with poor outcome in severely ill patients [221,222].

Table 2. A modified and updated table of mechanisms of drugs induced hyperglycemia [166].

10. Gestational Diabetes Mellitus

Gestational diabetes mellitus (GDM) is a heterogeneous pathogenic condition affecting 2-5% of all pregnant women during pregnancy [223, 224] in other data is 5-6% [225]. GDM and T2DM share a common pathophysiological background, including β-cell dysfunction and IR [226, 227]. In addition, women with GDM are at increased risk of developing T2DM later in life [226]. The pancreatic β- cells failure and impairment is the primary characteristic of GDM. In this group of patients with diabetes, there is a genetic predisposition triggered by increased IR during pregnancy leading to malfunction of the pancreatic β-cells [224]. The clustering of the GDM within family members suggestive of genetic predisposition to the development of this disease. Furthermore, women with MODY gene mutations are reported to have GDM more often [223,224]. In addition, the mutations in other genes include glucokinase (GCK), HLA antigens, insulin receptor (INSR), insulin-like growth factor-2 (IGF2), HNF4A, insulin gene (INS-VNTR), plasminogen activator inhibitor 1 (PAI-1), potassium inwardly rectifying channel subfamily J, member 11 (KCNJ11), hepatocyte nuclear factor-4a (HNF4A) and 1α (HNF1A) [224] suggest the susceptibility to increase the risk of GDM in certain patients.

The stimulators or the inducers of IR and phosphorylate insulin receptor substrate (IRS) proteins are activated in uncontrollable method several kinases, including inhibitor of nuclear factor κB kinase β (IKK β), c-Jun N-terminal kinase (JNK), mammalian target of rapamycin (mTOR), protein kinase C (PKC) and ribosomal S6 protein kinase (S6K). Substance P is a potent cytokine and is considered one of the crucial activators that contribute in the development of IR by impairment of insulin signaling [225]. The genetic variants in TCF7L2 is the strongest gene associated with GDM risk among other minor alleles of rs7903146 (TCF7L2), rs1225 5372 (TCF7L2), rs1799884 (-30G/A, GCK), rs5219 (E23K, KCNJ11), rs7754840 (CDKAL1), rs4402960 (IGF2BP2), rs10830963 (MTNR1B), rs1387153 (MTNR1B) and rs1801278 (Gly972Arg, IRS1) significantly associated with a higher risk of GDM. There are 12 SNPs from 10 genes are associated GDM [228].

The E23K polymorphism of KCNJ11 seems to predispose to GDM in Scandinavian women [226] and the polymorphism of TCF7L2 (rs7903146 C/T) gene, and the G972R polymorphism of the IRS1 gene, seems to predispose to GDM in Greek women [227]. In women of Han nationality in north China, The defect in sulfonylurea receptor-1 (SUR1) gene (cc and AA) may contribute to insulin hypersecretion, which might be the cause of increased body weight and decreased IS and genotype cc of SUR1 is connected with severe type of GDM [229].

In animals but not in human, Galanin inhibits glucose-stimulated insulin release [230]. In the human, the initial postprandial rise of glucose and insulin are suppressed by galanin administration [231]. Galanin and IL-6 were found to be significantly associated with IR markers in GDM, thus may play important roles in the regulation of glucose hemostasis [232].The higher level of plasma galanin is a novel biomarker for the prediction of GDM [233].

In late pregnancy the relative proinsulin secretion is mainly related to IR and does not necessarily reflect β-cell function. T2DM is not independently associated with hyperproinsulinemia as measured by the proinsulin-to-C-peptide ratio. While, in pregnant women, the increased in IR is associated with decreased proinsulin to C-peptide ratio, independently of glucose tolerance status [234].

The islet amyloid pancreatic polypeptid hypersecretion is characteristic for pregnancy and might partially decrease hyperinsulinemia in pregnancy by inhibiting insulin secretion [235].

The β- cells dysfunction and IR are the core in the pathogenesis of T2DM and both are mediated by Adiponectin. Therefore, in late pregnancy the Adiponectin is an independent factor correlated with β- cells dysfunction [236].

In pregnancy IR and GDM caused by the placental hormones and cytokines such as tumor necrosis factor alpha (TNFα), resisten and leptin. All of these are secreted by placenta independently. The human chorionic somatomammotropin (HCS), cortisol, estrogen, progesterone, and human placental growth hormone (hPGH) are important placental hormones. Severe IR produced by overexpression of hPGH and the increase of the HCS throughout pregnancy stimulates maternal pancreatic insulin release [237].

The fall of IS during pregnancy is counteracted by increase maternal insulin secretion to maintain glucose control [238]. The insufficient insulin secretion to counteract the pregnancy-related decrease in IS is contributing in development of DM [239]. Women at high risk of GDM should have a prior conception plan to prevent DM by normalize body weight, regular physical exercise, reducing excess intake of animal protein and soft drinks, planning of pregnancy in younger ages, avoiding pollutant exposition and smoking cessation [240].

11. Uncommon diseases cause hyperglycemia and DM

11.1. Endocrine diseases

Acromegaly and hypercortisolism are frequently associated with IGT and T2DM. It is a recognized finding of occurrence of secondary T2DM with many hormonal diseases (pituitary, adrenal/or thyroid disease). Patients with Acromegaly have IR, both in the liver and in the periphery displaying hyperinsulinemia and increased glucose turnover in the basal post-absorptive states. There is increase in blood glucose level and free fatty acids due to stimulation of gluconeogenesis and lipolysis. Although, insulin growth factor-1(IGF-1) level is increased but it is unable to counteract IR induced by abnormal excess GH level. On the other hand, IS primarily enhanced in the skeletal muscles by increased IGF-1. The excess of the GH and IGF-1 in patients with Acromegaly could be controlled by somatostatin analogues (SSAs) therapy in most of the patients. On the contrast, the overall glucose tolerance might be complicated by the inhibitory effect of SSAs on pancreatic insulin secretion.

The visceral obesity and IR are induced by hypercortisolemia. It also leads to hyperglycemia and reduced glucose tolerance, determines IR and stimulates hepatic gluconeogenesis and glycogenolysis. The hyperglycemia is due to decreased insulin secretion in patients with neuroendocrine tumors (NETs), patients with pancreatic surgery and in those with pheochromocytoma. While in somatostatinoma or gluconoma the hyperglycemia is related to alteration in the counterbalance between these hormones. In the symptomatic treatment of NETs, the SSAs represent a valid therapeutic choice and it may have a significant impact on the prevalence of glucose metabolism imbalance.

Hyperthyroidism is the principally cause of hyperglycemia among thyroid disorders [241]. IR is associated positively with abnormal increase in the thyroid hormone levels [242]. The uncontrolled diabetes in patient with diabetes developing thyrotoxicosis is related to the stimulation of hepatic glucose production by thyroid hormones acting via a sympathetic pathway from the hypothalamus and FT3 influenced the transcriptional regulators of metabolic and mitochondrial genes may contribute to the development of IR. In contrast, hypothyroidism is linked to decreased IS. The thyroid hormones have insulin antagonistic effects at the liver that lead to an increase in glucose hepatic output, via an enhanced rate of gluconeogenesis and glycogenolysis. Lipid metabolism (lipogenesis and lipolysis) are stimulated by FT3 further aggravating the dysregulation of liver glucose and lipid metabolism predispose to IR There are several genes are involved in gluconeogenesis, glycogen metabolism, insulin signaling and many hepatic glucogenic enzymes are regulated by thyroid hormones. The thyroid hormones also could cause an increase in hepatic glucose output, through increased hepatic expression of the glucose transporter GLUT2 [243].

11.2. Polycystic ovary syndrome

The features of PCOS are hyperinsulinemia, IR and hyperandrogenesim. The later presented in those patients with hirsutism, acne, irregular periods and reproductive disorders. These features are more marked and severe in obese females and the combination of both (these features with obesity) have a synergistic effect on increased insulin secretion by β-cells and development of compensatory hyperinsulinemia. Subsequently, with the decline of the β-cell compensatory response a relative or absolute insulin secretion and production insufficiency develops which may lead to dysglycemia (IFG, IGT and T2DM). Therefore, it is well-known that PCOS and IR are considered risk factors for GDM [244]. This risk is increased in obese females, presence of family history of T2DM and to the severity of high androgenic activity. Therefore, the dysglycemia could occur in earlier age group than normal population. It could be in the 3rd or 4th decade of life and it is approximately 5 to 10 folds higher than normal population. No doubt, it is higher compared with age and weight matched control age group [245].

11.3. Pancreatic damage or β-cell damage of the pancreas

Chronic alcoholism and tropical calcified pancreatitis are most commonly associated with diabetes [247]. Pancreatic exocrine disease associated with hyperglycemia or DM has a unique clinical and metabolic form. It is painless occasionally and malabsorption occurs after clinical hyperglycemia or DM following failure or impairment of endocrine and exocrine pancreatic function of both α and β cells [246]

11.4. Hereditary hemochromatosis

Iron overload and excessive tissues deposition of iron including the pancreas. It is an autosomal recessive genetic disorder caused by a mutation in the HFE gene located on the short arm of chromosome 6. Approximately 50% of patients diagnosed with hemochromatosis will have either type 1 or T2DM [248].

11.5. Cystic fibrosis

Diabetes Mellitus is the most common morbidity in patients with cystic fibrosis (CF). It occurs in about 20% of adolescent and 40-50% of adults with this disease. CF primarily caused by insulin insufficiency. However, there is a role for IR in acute and chronic stages of this disease due to fluctuation level of insulin. DM has a unique distinct entity in patient with CF because it has mixed features of TIDM and T2DM [249].

Other causes of damage of the pancreas are toxins like alcohol, surgical resection of the pancreas and pancreatic cancer.

11.6. Smoking

There are several studies suggestive of smoking is a risk factor for T2DM, it is an independent and modifiable risk. The early weight gain following smoking cessation is far more beneficial compared with the long term effect of smoking. This weight gain could increase the risk of diabetes [250-252]. Smoking deteriorates glucose metabolism and it is considered a possible a risk factor for development of IR and subsequently T2DM [253]. Smoking is also through a body mass index independent mechanism increasing the risk of T2DM [254, 255]. Pancreatic damage by toxic agents cause insufficient insulin secretion and development of the disease. Tobacco is one of the toxic agent to the human body and organ damage; on the pancreas it is also considered a risk factor of pancreatic cancer and chronic pancreatitis [256].

11.7. Prematurity and birth weight

Hofman PL in 2004 reported an association between low birth weight, commonly a reflection of an adverse in utero environment, and the subsequent development of diseases such as T2DM and hypertension in later life is now generally accepted as is an association between an adverse perinatal environment and a permanent reduction in IS [257, 258].This concept was changed in other report by the evidence has accumulated that small for gestational age children have long-term adult health consequences including obesity, T2DM, hypertension, coronary artery disease and stroke. This increased risk of later adult disease is likely a consequence of an early, persistent reduction in IS [259]. Reduced fetal growth is associated with increased risk of diabetes and suggested a specific association with thinness at birth [260]. Prevalence of T2DM and IGT depended on the synergic effect of thin body size at birth and obesity during adulthood [261]. IGT and T2DM are early signs and indications of growth retardation in early life. The raise in plasma levels of 32-33 split proinsulin is closely related to growth retardation and reflects the β-cells dysfunction [262]. A review and analysis of 14 studies low birth weight (<2,500 g), as compared with a birth weight of >/=2,500 g, was associated with increased risk of T2DM. The risk is the same in high birth weight (>4,000 g), as compared with a birth weight of (</=4,000 g) [263]. The two strongest predictor factors for development of T2DM in adult life are low birth weight and abdominal obesity. The risk of T2DM in Chinese adults is inversely correlated to birth weight. Subjects with high risk of developing hypertension and abdominal obesity are those with the lowest or highest birth weight [264].

12. Conclusion

The evolution of T2DM requires the presence of defects in both insulin secretion and insulin action, and both of these defects can have a genetic and an acquired component. There are many discovered complex alterations in adipose tissue secretion of cytokines, adipokines, and chemokines and immune cell composition observed in adipose tissue-related pathologies such as obesity and IR. The later is a nearly universal finding in patients with established disease. There are many recognized genes involved in β-cell development, function and regulation. These could lead to disorders in insulin secretion, IR and glucose sensing. Physicians should be aware about the potential drugs contribute to the development of hyperglycemia and diabetes. Ladies at high risk of GDM should be identified and screened for diabetes before conception and to be followed after delivery. Early identification and diagnosis of many medical conditions and other risk factors could induce hyperglycemia or precipitate a pre-existing condition of DM.

The above demonstrated a wide range of research in this area that should be encouraged to improve our understanding of the disease. T2DM is a complex interaction between genetics, cytokines, immune cells and tissues during inflammatory responses with obesity, insulin function, IR and β-cells failure. Subsequently this could help in discovery new drugs to treat T2DM that could interfere or stop any stage of these mechanisms at molecular or genetic level.

Author details

Fuad AlSaraj*

Address all correspondence to: fuad.alsaraj@mediclinic.ae

Mediclinic Welcare Hospital, Dubai, UAE

References

[1] Defronzo RA. Banting Lecture. From the triumvirate to the ominous octet: a new paradigm for the treatment of type 2 diabetes mellitus. Diabetes 2009; 58 (4):773–795.

[2] Consoli A. Predominant role of gluconeogenesis in increased hepatic glucose production in NIDDM. Diabetes 1989 ;38 (5):550-557.

[3] Consoli A. Role of liver in pathophysiology of NIDDM. Diabetes Care 1992; 15(3): 430-441.

[4] Ramnanan CJ. Physiologic action of glucagon on liver glucose metabolism. Diabetes Obes Metab 2011 ;13 Suppl 1:118-125.

[5] Gerich JE. Control of glycaemia. Baillieres Best Pract Res Clin Endocrinol Metab 1993; 7 (3):551–586.

[6] Porte D Jr, Kahn SE. The key role of islet dysfunction in type II diabetes mellitus. Clin Invest Med 1995; 18 (4):247-254.

[7] Kahn SE, Porte D Jr. Islet dysfunction in non-insulin-dependent diabetes mellitus. Am J Med. 1988; 85 (5A):4-8.

[8] Porte D Jr. Banting lecture 1990. Beta-cells in type II diabetes mellitus. Diabetes 1991; 40 (2):166-180.

[9] Mitrakou A. Contribution of abnormal muscle and liver glucose metabolism to postprandial hyperglycemia in NIDDM. Diabetes 1990; 39 (11):1381-1390.

[10] Tappy L. Regulation of hepatic glucose production in healthy subjects and patients with non-insulin-dependent diabetes mellitus. Diabete Metab 1995; 21(4):233-240.

[11] Halter JB. Glucose regulation in non-insulin-dependent diabetes mellitus. Interaction between pancreatic islets and the liver. Am J Med 1985; 79 (2B):6-12.

[12] Porte D. β-Cell Dysfunction and Failure in Type 2 Diabetes Potential Mechanisms. Diabetes 2001; 50 (1): S160-S163.

[13] Arthur C. Chapter 78: Insulin, Glucagon, and Diabetes Mellitus. Textbook of Medical Physiology (11th ed.). Philadelphia: Elsevier Saunders 2006. P 963–P968.

[14] Vinay K. Chapter 24: The Endocrine System. Robbins and Cotran Pathologic Basis of Disease (7th ed.). Philadelphia: Elsevier Saunders 2005. P1191–1193.

[15] Cheng K. First phase insulin secretion and type 2 diabetes. Curr Mol Med 2013; 13 (1):126-139.

[16] Byrne MM.Elevated plasma glucose 2 h post challenge predicts defects in β-cell function. Am J Physiol 1996; 270 (4 pt 1): E572-E579.

[17] Gerich JE. Is reduced first-phase insulin release the earliest detectable abnormality in individuals destined to develop type 2 diabetes? Diabetes 2002; 51 (Suppl 1):S117-S121.

[18] Del Prato S. Phasic insulin release and metabolic regulation in type 2 diabetes. Diabetes. 2002 ;51 Suppl 1:S109-S116.

[19] Barg S. A subset of 50 secretory granules in close contact with L-type Ca2+ channels accounts for first-phase insulin secretion in mouse beta-cells. Diabetes 2002; 51 (Suppl 1):S74-S82.

[20] Kühl C. Etiology and pathogenesis of gestational diabetes. Diabetes Care 1998 ;21 Suppl 2:B19-B26.

[21] Nijpels G. Determinants for the progression from impaired glucose tolerance to non-insulin-dependent diabetes mellitus. Eur J Clin Invest 1998 ;28 Suppl 2:8-13.

[22] Abdul-Ghani MA. Contributions of beta-cell dysfunction and insulin resistance to the pathogenesis of impaired glucose tolerance and impaired fasting glucose. Diabetes Care. 2006 ; 29(5):1130-1139.

[23] Magnusson I. Increased rate of gluconeogenesis in type II diabetes mellitus. A ^{13}C nuclear magnetic resonance study. J Clin Invest 1992; 90 (4):1323–1327.

[24] Sesti G. Pathophysiology of insulin resistance. Best Pract Res Clin Endocrinol Metab 2006; 20 (4):665-679.

[25] Ahrén B. Islet adaptation to insulin resistance: mechanisms and implications for intervention. Diabetes Obes Metab 2005; 7 (1):2-8.

[26] Brancati FL. Body weight patterns from 20 to 49 years of age and subsequent risk for diabetes mellitus: the Johns Hopkins Precursors Study. Arch Intern Med 1999; 159 (91):957–963.

[27] Roberts CK. Metabolic Syndrome and Insulin Resistance: Underlying Causes and Modification by Exercise Training. Compr Physio. 2013; 3 (1):1-58.

[28] Petersen KF. Pathogenesis of skeletal muscle insulin resistance in type 2 diabetes mellitus. Am J Cardiol 2002; 90 (5A):11G-18G.

[29] Moller DE. Prevalence of mutations in the insulin receptor gene in subjects with features of the type A syndrome of insulin resistance. Diabetes 1994; 43(2):247-255.

[30] Taylor SI. Insulin resistance associated with androgen excess in women with autoantibodies to the insulin receptor. Ann Intern Med 1982; 97 (6):851-855.

[31] Olshansky SJ. A potential decline in life expectancy in the United States in the 21st century. N Engl J Med 2005; 352 (11): 1138-1145.

[32] Smyth S. Diabetes and obesity: the twin epidemics. Nat Med 2006; 12 (1): 75–80.

[33] Blüher M. Adipose tissue dysfunction in obesity. Exp Clin Endocrinol Diabetes 2009; 117 (6):241-250.

[34] Feng X. PTPRT Regulates High-Fat Diet-Induced Obesity and Insulin Resistance. PLoS One 2014 ;9 (6): e 1100783.

[35] Kahn SE. Mechanisms linking obesity to insulin resistance and type 2 diabetes. Nature 2006; 444(7121):840-846.

[36] Kahn SE. The relative contributions of insulin resistance and beta-cell dysfunction to the pathophysiology of Type 2 diabetes. Diabetologia 2003; 46 (1):3-19.

[37] Meneilly GS. NIDDM in the elderly. Diabetes Care 1996; 19 (12):1320-1325.

[38] Meneilly GS. Metabolic alterations in middle-aged and elderly obese patients with type 2 diabetes. Diabetes Care 1999; 22 (1):112-118.

[39] Ludvik B. Effect of obesity on insulin resistance in normal subjects and patients with NIDDM. Diabetes 1995 ;44 (9):1121-1125.

[40] Boden G. Role of fatty acids in the pathogenesis of insulin resistance and NIDDM. Diabetes. 1997; 46 (1):3-10

[41] Boden G. Effects of free fatty acids (FFA) on glucose metabolism: significance for insulin resistance and type 2 diabetes. Exp Clin Endocrinol Diabetes. 2003; 111 (3): 121-124.

[42] Boden G. Free fatty acids (FFA), a link between obesity and insulin resistance. Front Biosci 1998 15; 3:d169-175.

[43] Boden G. Obesity and Free Fatty Acids (FFA). Endocrinol Metab Clin North Am 2 008; 37 (3): 635–646.

[44] Boden G. Fatty acid-induced inflammation and insulin resistance in skeletal muscle and liver. Curr Diab Rep. 2006; 6(3):177-81.

[45] Shulman G. Cellular mechanisms of insulin resistance. J Clin Invest 2000; 106 (2): 171–176.

[46] Masuzaki H. A transgenic model of visceral obesity and the metabolic syndrome. Science 2001; 294 (5549): 2166–2170.

[47] Rask E. Tissue-specific dysregulation of cortisol metabolism in human obesity. J Clin Endocrinol Metab 2001; 86 (3): 1418–1421.

[48] Paulmyer-Lacroix O. Expression of the mRNA coding for 11β hydroxysteroid dehydrogenase type 1 in adipose tissue from obese patients: An in situ hybridization study. J Clin Endocrinol Metab 2002; 87 (6): 2701–2705.

[49] Hirosumi J. A central role for JNK in obesity and insulin resistance. Nature 2002; 420 (6913): 333–336.

[50] Aguirre V. The c-Jun NH(2)-terminal kinase promotes insulin resistance during association with insulin receptor substrate-1 and phosphorylation of Ser(307). J Biol Chem 2000; 275 (12): 9047– 9054.

[51] Gao Z. Inhibition of insulin sensitivity by free fatty acids requires activation of multiple serine kinases in 3T3-L1 adipocytes. Mol Endocrinol 2004; 18 (8): 2024–2034.

[52] Yuan M. Reversal of obesity- and diet-induced insulin resistance with salicylates or targeted disruption of Ikkbeta. Science 2001; (5539); 293:1673–1677.

[53] Matsuzawa A. ROS-dependent activation of the TRAF6–ASK1–p38 pathway is selectively required for TLR4- mediated innate immunity. Nat Immunol 2005; 6 (6): 587–592.

[54] Shi H. TLR4 links innate immunity and fatty acidinduced insulin resistance. J Clin Invest 2006; 116 (11): 3015–3025.

[55] Suganami T. Role of the Toll-like receptor 4/NF- κB pathway in saturated fatty acid-induced inflammatory changes in the interaction between adipocytes and macrophages. Arterioscler Thromb Vasc Biol 2007; 27 (11): 84 91.

[56] Tobiume K ASK1 is required for sustained activations of JNK/p38 MAP kinases and apoptosis. EMBO Rep 2001; 2 (3): 222–228.

[57] Qatanani M. Mechanisms of obesity-associated insulin resistance: many choices on the menu. Genes Dev 2007; 21 (12): 1443-1455.

[58] Kassem M. Adipose Tissue in Obesity-Related Inflammation and Insulin Resistance: Cells, Cytokines, and Chemokines. ISRN Inflammation 2013; 2013: 139239:1-12.

[59] Piya M. Adipokine inflammation and insulin resistance: the role of glucose, lipids and endotoxin. Journal of Endocrinology 2013; 216 (1): T1–T15.

[60] Cheng KC. Characterization of preptin-induced insulin secretion in pancreatic β-cells. J Endocrinol 2012; 215 (1):43-49.

[61] Buchanan CM. Preptin derived from proinsulin-like growth factor II (proIGF-II) is secreted from pancreatic islet beta-cells and enhances insulin secretion. Biochem J 2001; 360 (pt2):431-439.

[62] Ozkan Y. Acylated and desacylated ghrelin, preptin, leptin, and nesfatin-1 Peptide changes related to the body mass index. Int J Endocrinol 2013; 2013 (236085): 1-7.

[63] Schrauwen P. UCP2 and UCP3 in muscle controlling body metabolism. J Exp Biol. 2002; 205 (pt15):2275-2285.

[64] Zaninovich AA. Role of uncoupling proteins UCP1, UCP2 and UCP3 in energy balance, type 2 diabetes and obesity. Synergism with the thyroid. Medicina (B Aires) 2005; 65 (2):163-169.

[65] Ježek P. Antioxidant and regulatory role of mitochondrial uncoupling protein UCP2 in pancreatic beta-cells. Physiol Res 2014; 63 (Suppl 1):S73-S91.

[66] Pi J. Reactive oxygen species and uncoupling protein 2 in pancreatic β-cell function. Diabetes Obes Metab 2010; 12 (Suppl 2):141-148.

[67] Takata K. Glucose transporters in the transepithelial transport of glucose. J Electron Microsc 1996; 45 (4):275-284.

[68] Scheepers A. The glucose transporter families SGLT and GLUT: molecular basis of normal and aberrant function. JPEN J Parenter Enteral Nutr 2004; 28 (5):364-371.

[69] Watson RT. Intracellular organization of insulin signaling and GLUT4 translocation. Recent Prog Horm Res 2001; 56:175-193.

[70] Haney PM. Intracellular targeting of the insulin-regulatable glucose transporter (GLUT4) is isoform specific and independent of cell type. J Cell Biol 1991;114 (4): 689-699.

[71] Sabino-Silva R. The Na (+)/glucose cotransporters: from genes to therapy. Braz J Med Biol Res 2010; 43(11):1019-1026.

[72] McIntyre EA. Genetics of type 2 diabetes and insulin resistance: knowledge from human studies. Clin Endocrinol (Oxf) 2002; 57 (3):303-311.

[73] Bastian W. Genes with linkage or association with type 2 diabetes mellitus. J Pediatr Endocrinol Metab 2002; 15 (Suppl 1):471-484.

[74] Gibbons Ann. 12th International Congress of Human Genetics. Diabetes Genes Decline Out of Africa. Science 2011; 334 (6056): 583.

[75] Levine JA. Poverty and Obesity in the U.S. Diabetes 2011, 60: 2667-2668.

[76] Nyamdorj R. BMI compared with central obesity indicators in relation to diabetes and hypertension in Asians. Obesity 2008; 16 (7): 1622-1635.

[77] Boji Huang. Acculturation and Prevalence of Diabetes among Japanese-American Men in Hawaii. Am J Epidemiol 1996; 144:674- 681.

[78] Tuomilehto J. Cardiovascular diseases and diabetes mellitus in Fiji: analysis of mortality, morbidity and risk factors. Bull World Health Organ 1984; 62 (1):133-143.

[79] Afable-Munsuz A. Immigrant generation and diabetes risk among Mexican Americans: the Sacramento area Latino study on aging. Am J Public Health 2014; 104 Suppl 2:S234-S250.

[80] McKeigue PM. Diabetes, hyperinsulinaemia, and coronary risk factors in Bangladeshis in east London. Br Heart J 1988; 60 (5): 390-396.

[81] Enas EA. Coronary heart disease and its risk factors in first-generation immigrant Asian Indians to the United States of America. Indian Heart J 1996; 48 (4): 343-353.

[82] Van Dam RM. The epidemiology of lifestyle and risk for type 2 diabetes. Eur J Epidemiol 2003; 18 (12): 1115-1125.

[83] Shaw J. Epidemiology and prevention of type 2 diabetes and the metabolic syndrome. MJA 2003; 179 (7): 379-383.

[84] Zimmett P. Global and societal implication of the diabetes epidemic. Nature 2001; 414 (6865): 782-787.

[85] Lean ME. Obesity: burdens of illness and strategies for prevention or management. Drugs Today (Barc) 2000; 36 (11): 773-784.

[86] Fagot-Campagna A. Type 2 diabetes among North American children and adolescents: an epidemiologic review and a public health perspective. J Pediatr 2000; 136 (5): 664-672.

[87] Sinha R. Prevalence of impaired glucose tolerance among children and adolescents with marked obesity. N Engl J Med 2002;346 (11): 802-810.

[88] Hu FB. Sedentary lifestyle and risk of obesity and type 2 diabetes. Lipids 2003; 38 (2): 103-108.

[89] Pan XR. Effects of diet and exercise in preventing NIDDM in people with impaired glucose tolerance. The Da Qing IGT and Diabetes Study. Diabetes Care 1997; 20 (4): 537-544.

[90] Tuomilehto J. Prevention of type 2 diabetes mellitus by changes in lifestyle among subjects with impaired glucose tolerance. N Engl J Med 2001; 344 (18): 1343-1350.

[91] Knowler WC. Reduction in the Incidence of Type 2 Diabetes with Lifestyle Intervention or Metformin. N Engl J Med 2002; 346 (6):393-403.

[92] Xue Sun. Genetics of Type 2 Diabetes: Insights into the Pathogenesis and Its Clinical Application. BioMed Research International 2014; 2014 (926713): 1-15.

[93] Steinthorsdottir V. A variant in CDKAL1 influences insulin response and risk of type 2 diabetes. Nature Genetics 2007; 39 (6): 770-775.

[94] Voight BF. Twelve type 2 diabetes susceptibility loci identified through large-scale association analysis. Nature Genetics 2010; 42 (7): 579–589.

[95] Silander K. Genetic variation near the hepatocyte nuclear factor-4α gene predicts susceptibility to type 2 diabetes. Diabetes 2004; 53 (4): 1141–1149.

[96] Lyssenko V. Common variant in MTNR1B associated with increased risk of type 2 diabetes and impaired early insulin secretion. Nature 2009; 41(1): 82-88.

[97] Nielsen T. Type 2 diabetes risk allele near CENTD2 is associated with decreased glucose-stimulated insulin release. Diabetologia 2011; 54 (5):1052–1056.

[98] Boesgaard TW. Variant near ADAMTS9 known to associate with type 2 diabetes is related to insulin resistance in offspring of type 2 diabetes patients— EUGENE2 study. PLoS ONE 2009; 4: (9): e7236.

[99] Anand A. In vivo modulation of Hmgic reduces obesity. Nature Genetics 2000; 24 (4): 377–380.

[100] Rung J. Genetic variant near IRS1 is associated with type 2 diabetes, insulin resistance and hyperinsulinemia. Nature Genetics 2009; 41(10): 1110–1115.

[101] Binh T. Association of the common FTO-rs9939609 polymorphism with type 2 diabetes, independent of obesity-related traits in a Vietnamese population. Gene 2013; 513 (1): 31–35.

[102] Xi B. Common polymorphism near the MC4R gene is associated with type 2 diabetes: data fromameta-analysis of 123, 373 individuals. Diabetologia 2012; 55 (10): 2660–2666.

[103] Barnett AH. Diabetes in identical twins: A study of 200 pairs. Diabetologia 1981; 20 (2): 87–93.

[104] Committee on Diabetic Twins, Japan Diabetes Society. Diabetes mellitus in twins: a cooperative study in Japan. Committee on Diabetic Twins, Japan Diabetes Society. Diabetes Res Clin Pract 1988 14; 5 (4):271-280.

[105] Matsuda A. Relationship between obesity and concordance rate for type 2 (non-insulin-dependent) diabetes mellitus among twins. Diabetes Res Clin Pract 1994; 26 (2): 137-143.

[106] Kobberling J., Tillil H. Empirical risk figures for first-degree relatives of non-insulin dependent diabetics. In The Genetics of Diabetes Mellitus. (ed J. Kobberling, R Tattersall 1982. p201–p209.

[107] Eriksson J. Early metabolic defects in persons at increased risk for non- insulin-dependent diabetes mellitus. N Engl J Med 1989; 321 6): 337–343.

[108] Humphriss DB. Multiple metabolic abnormalities in normal glucose tolerant relatives of NIDDM families. Diabetologia 1997; 40 (10):1185–1190.

[109] Lillioja S. In vivo insulin action is familial characteristic in nondiabetic Pima Indians. Diabetes 1987; 36 (11):1329–1335.

[110] Martin BC. Familial clustering of insulin sensitivity. Diabetes 1992; 41 (7): 850–854.

[111] Henry RR. Insulin action and glucose metabolism in nondiabetic control and NIDDM subjects. Comparison using human skeletal muscle cell cultures. Diabetes 1995; 44 (8): 936–946.

[112] Jackson S. Decreased insulin responsiveness of glucose uptake in cultured human skeletal muscle cells from insulin-resistant nondiabetic relatives of type 2 diabetic families. Diabetes 2000; 49 (7):1169–1177.

[113] DeFronzo RA. Insulin resistance. A multifaceted syndrome responsible for NIDDM, obesity, hypertension, dyslipidemia, and atherosclerotic cardiovascular disease. Diabetes Care 1991; 14 (3):173–194.

[114] Frayling TM. Beta-cell genes and diabetes: molecular and clinical characterization of mutations in transcription factors. Diabetes 2001; 50 (Suppl 1):S94-S100.

[115] Gardner DS. Clinical features and treatment of maturity onset diabetes of the young (MODY). Diabetes Metab Syndr Obes 2012; 5: 101–108.

[116] Shepherd M. Predictive genetic testing in maturity-onset diabetes of the young (MODY) Diabet Med 2001; 18 (5):417–421.

[117] Froguel P. Close linkage of glucokinase locus on chromosome 7p to early-onset non-insulin-dependent diabetes mellitus. Nature 1992; 356 (6365):162 –164.

[118] Hattersley AT. Linkage of type 2 diabetes to the glucokinase gene. Lancet 1992; 339 (8805):1307–1310.

[119] Yamagata K. Mutations in the hepatocyte nuclear factor-4α gene in maturity-onset diabetes of the young (MODY1). Nature 1996; 384 (6608):458 –460.

[120] Yamagata K. Mutations in the hepatocyte nuclear factor-1α gene in maturity-onset diabetes of the young (MODY3). Nature 1996; 384 (6608):455–458.

[121] Alessandro D. Recent advances in the genetics of maturity onset diabetes of the young and other forms of autosomal dominant diabetes. Curr Opin Endocrinol & Diabetes 2000; 7 (4):203–210.

[122] McDonald TJ. Maturity onset diabetes of the young: identification and diagnosis. Ann Clin Biochem 2013; 50 (pt5):403-415.

[123] Stoffers DA. Early-onset type-II diabetes mellitus (MODY4) linked to IPF1. Nat Genet 1997; 17 (2):138-139.

[124] Horikawa Y. Mutation in hepatocyte nuclear factor-1 beta gene (TCF2) associated with MODY. Nat Genet 1997; 17 (4):384 –385.

[125] Malecki MT. Mutations in NEUROD1 are associated with the development of type 2 diabetes mellitus. Nat Genet 1999; 23 (3):323-328.

[126] Rochelle Naylor. Who should have genetic testing for maturity-onset diabetes of the young?. Clinical Endocrinology (Oxf) 2011; 75 (4): 422–426.

[127] Timsit J. Diagnosis and management of maturity-onset diabetes of the young. Treat Endocrinol 2005; 4 (1):9-18.

[128] GotoY. A mutation in the tRNA (Leu) (UUR) gene associated with the MELAS subgroup of mitochondrial encephalomyopathies. Nature1990; 348 (6302): 651–653.

[129] Vanden Ouweland JM. Mutation in mitochondrial tRNA (Leu) (UUR) gene in a large pedigree with maternally transmitted type II diabetes mellitus and deafness. Nat Genet 1992; 1 (5): 368–371.

[130] Maassen JA. Maternally inherited diabetes and deafness: a new diabetes subtype. Diabetologia 1996; 39 (4): 375–82.

[131] Vionnet N. Prevalence of mitochondrial gene mutations in families with diabetes mellitus. Lancet 1993; 342 (8884):1429–1430.

[132] Newkirk JE. Maternally inherited diabetes and deafness: prevalence in a hospital diabetic population. Diabet Med 1997; 14 (6): 457–460.

[133] Daly MJ. High resolution haplotype structure in the human genome. Nat Genet 2001; 29 (2):229-232.

[134] Krook A. Mutant insulin receptors in syndromes of insulin resistance. Clin Endocrinolo Metab 1996; 10 (1): 97–122.

[135] Whitehead JP. Molecular scanning of the insulin receptor substrate 1 gene in subjects with severe insulin resistance: detection and functional analysis of a naturally occurring mutation in a YMXM motif. Diabetes 1998; 47 (5): 837–838.

[136] Whitehead JP. Multiple molecular mechanisms of insulin receptor dysfunction in a patient with Donohue syndrome. Diabetes 1998; 47 (8):1362–1364.

[137] Hegele RA. Familial partial lipodystrophy: a monogenic form of the insulin resistance syndrome. Mole Genet Metab 2000; 71(4): 539–544.

[138] Shackleton S. LMNA, encoding lamin A/C, is mutated in partial lipodystrophy. Nat Genet 2000; 24 (2): 153–156.

[139] Hegele RA. Premature atherosclerosis associated with monogenic insulin resistancze. Circulation 2001; 103 (18): 2225–2229.

[140] Martin G. Coordinate regulation of the expression of the fatty acid transport protein and acyl-CoA synthetase genes by PPARalpha and PPARgamma activators. J Biol Chem 1997; 272(45):28210-28217.

[141] Barroso I. Dominant negative mutations in human PPARgamma associated with severe insulin resistance, diabetes mellitus and hypertension. Nature 1999; 402 (6764): 880–883.

[142] Huxtable SJ. Analysis of parent–offspring trios provides evidence for linkage and association between the insulin gene and type 2 diabetes mediated exclusively through paternally transmitted class III variable number tandem repeat alleles. Diabetes 2000; 49 (1): 126–130.

[143] Hart LM. Variants in the sulphonylurea receptor gene: association of the exon 16-3t variant with Type II diabetes mellitus in Dutch Caucasians. Diabetologia 1999; 42 (5): 617-620.

[144] White MF. The insulin signalling system and the IRS proteins. Dibetologia 1997; 40 (Suppl 2): S2-17.

[145] Almind K. Aminoacid polymorphisms of insulin receptor substrate-1 in non-insulin-dependent diabetes mellitus. Lancet 1993; 342 (8875): 828–832.

[146] Porzio O. The Gly972 → Arg amino acid polymorphism in IRS-1 impairs insulin secretion in pancreatic beta cells. J Clin Invest 1999; 104 (3): 357–364.

[147] Gu HF. Association between the human glycoprotein PC-1 gene and elevated glucose and insulin levels in a paired-sibling analysis. Diabetes 2000; 49 (9):1601–1603.

[148] Groop LC. Association between polymorphism of the glycogen synthase gene and non-insulin-dependent diabetes mellitus. N Eng J Med 1993; 328 (1):10–14.

[149] Orho-Melander M. A paired-sibling analysis of the XbaI polymorphism in the muscle glycogen synthase gene. Diabetologia 1999; 42 (9):1138–1145.

[150] McIntyre EA. Genetics of type 2 diabetes and insulin resistance: knowledge from human studies. Clin Endocrinol (Oxf) 2002; 57 (3):303-311.

[151] Horikawa Y. Genetic variation in the calapin 10 gene (CAPN10) is associated with type 2 diabetes mellitus. Nat Genet 2000; 26 (2): 163-175.

[152] Baier LJ. A calpain- 10 gene polymorphysim is associated with reduced muscle mRNA levels and insulin resistance. J Clin Invest 2000; 106 (7): R69-73.

[153] Garant MJ. SNP43 of CAPN10 and the risk of type 2 diabetes in African-Americans: the Atherosclerosis Risk in Communities Study. Diabetes 2002; 51(1):231–237.

[154] del Bosque-Plata L. Association of the calpain-10 gene with type 2 diabetes mellitus in a Mexican population. Mol Genet Metab 2004; 81(2):122-126.

[155] Fingerlin TE. Variation in three single nucleotide polymorphisms in the calpain-10 gene not associated with type 2 diabetes in a large Finnish cohort. Diabetes 2002; 51 (5):1644-1648.

[156] Cassell PG. Haplotype combinations of calpain 10 gene polymorphisms associate with increased risk of impaired glucose tolerance and type 2 diabetes in South Indians. Diabetes 2002; 51(5):1622–1628.

[157] Martinez SC. Glucose regulates Foxo1 through insulin receptor signaling in the pancreatic islet beta-cell. Diabetes 2006; 55 (6):1581-1591.

[158] Wang W. Inhibition of Foxo1 mediates protective effects of ghrelin against lipotoxicity in MIN6 pancreatic beta-cells. Peptides 2010; 31(1):307-314.

[159] Oeveren van-Dybicz AM. Beta 3-adrenergic receptor gene polymorphism and type 2 diabetes in a Caucasian population. Diabetes Obes and Metab 2001; 3 (1):47-51.

[160] Babol K. Beta3-adrenergic receptor. Postepy Biochem 2005; 51(1):80-87.

[161] Le Bacquer O. TCF7L2 rs7903146 impairs islet function and morphology in nondiabetic individuals. Diabetologia 2012; 55 (10): 2677–2681.

[162] Lyssenko V. Mechanisms by which common variants in the TCF7L2 gene increase risk of type 2 diabetes. The Journal of Clinical Investigation 2007; 117 (8):2155–2163.

[163] Chimienti F. ZnT-8, a pancreatic β-cell specific zinc transporter. Biometals 2005; 18 (4): 313–317.

[164] Pound LD. Deletion of the mouse Slc30a8 gene encoding zinc transporter-8 results in impaired insulin secretion. Biochemical Journal 2009; 421 (3): 371–376.

[165] Lohani Gaya. Drug- induced diabetes. Medicine Update 2010; 20 (72): 70-73.

[166] Abdur Rehman. Drug-Induced Glucose Alterations Part 2: Drug-Induced Hyperglycemia. Diabetes Spectrum 2011; 24 (4):234-238.

[167] Ramsay LE. Diabetes, impaired glucose tolerance and insulin resistance with diuretics. Eur Heart J 1992; 13 (Suppl G):68-71.

[168] O'Byrne S. Effects of drugs on glucose tolerance in non-insulin-dependent diabetics (Part I). Drugs 1990; 40 (1):6-18.

[169] Shafi T. Changes in serum potassium mediate thiazide-induced diabetes. Hypertension 2008; 52 (6):1022-1029.

[170] Carter B. Thiazide-induced dysglycemia: call for research from a working group from the National Heart, Lung, and Blood Institute. Hypertension 2008; 52 (1):30–36.

[171] Tham DM. Angtiotensin II is associated with activation of NF- kB-mediated genes and downregulation of PPARS. Physiol Genomics 2002; 11(1):21–30.

[172] Henderson DC. Clozapine, diabetes mellitus, weight gain, and lipid abnormalities: A five-year naturalistic study. Am J Psychiatry. 2000; 157 (6):975-981.

[173] Haupt DW. Hyperglycemia and antipsychotic medications. J Clin Psychiatry 2001; 62 (Suppl 27):15-26.

[174] Newcomer JW. Second-generation (atypical) antipsychotics and metabolic effects: a comprehensive literature review. CNS Drugs 2005; 19 (Suppl 1):1-93.

[175] Savoy YE. Differential effects of various typical and atypical antipsychotics on plasma glucose and insulin levels in the mouse: evidence for the involvement of sympathetic regulation. Schizophr Bull 2010; 36 (2):410–418.

[176] Leung JY. Cardiovascular side-effects of antipsychotic drugs: the role of the autonomic nervous system. Pharmacol Ther 2012; 135(2):113-122.

[177] Lee AK. Pharmacogenetics of leptin in antipsychotic-associated weight gain and obesity-related complications. Pharmacogenomics 2011; 12 (7):999-1016.

[178] Luna B. Drug-induced hyperglycemia. JAMA 2001; 286 (16):1945–1948.

[179] Greiss TW. Hypertension and antihypertensive therapy as risk factors for type 2 diabetes mellitus. N Engl J Med 2000; 342 (3) :905.

[180] Ferner RE. Drug-induced diabetes. Baillieres Clin Endocrinol Metab 1992;6 (4):849-66.

[181] Henry K. Diabetes mellitus induced by megestrol acetate in a patient with AIDS and cachexia. Ann Intern Med 1992 1; 116(1):53-54.

[182] Rizza RA. Cortisol-induced insulin resistance in man: impaired suppression of glucose production and stimulation of glucose utilization due to a postreceptor detect of insulin action. J Clin Endocrinol Metab 1982; 54 (1): 131-138.

[183] Paquot N. Effects of glucocorticoids and sympathomimetic agents on basal and insulin-stimulated glucose metabolism. Clin Physiol 1995; 15(3):231-240.

[184] Bak JF. Effects of growth hormone on fuel utilization and muscle glycogen synthase activity in normal humans. Am J Physiol 1991; 260 (5pt1):E736-E742.

[185] Sherwin RS. Effect of growth hormone on oral glucose tolerance and circulating metabolic fuels in man. Diabetologia 1983; 24 (3):155-161.

[186] Manthinda H. Growth Hormone-Induced Insulin Resistance and Its Relationship to Lipid Availability in the Rat. Diabetes 1996; 45 (4): 415-421.

[187] Joseph C. HIV Protease Inhibitors Acutely Impair Glucose-Stimulated Insulin Release. Diabetes 2003; 52 (7): 1695-1700.

[188] Calvo M. Update on metabolic issues in HIV patients. Curr Opin HIV AIDS 2014; 9 (4):332-339.

[189] Munshi M. Hyperosmolar nonketotic diabetic syndrome following treatment of human deficiency virus infection with didanosine. Diabetes Care 1994; 17(4): 316.

[190] Pecora F. Effect of tenofovir on didanosine absorption in patients with HIV. Ann Pharmacother 2003; 37 (9): 1325-1328.

[191] Takasu N. Rifampicin-induced early phase hyperglycemia in humans. Am Rev Respir Dis 1982; 125 (1):23-27.

[192] Saraya A. Effects of fluoroquinolones on insulin secretion and beta-cell ATP-sensitive K+ channels. Eur J Pharmacol 2004; 497 (1):111-117.

[193] Aspinall SL. Severe Dysglycemia with the Fluoroquinolones: A Class Effect? Clin Infect Dis 2009; 49 (3): 402-408.

[194] Storozhuk PG. Effect of certain antibiotics of tetracycline series on the level of blood sugar and the role of insulin in the mechanism of its regulation. Probl Endokrinol (Mosk) 1976 ;22 (6):106-110.

[195] Redmon JB. Effects of tacrolimus (FK506) on human insulin gene expression, insulin mRNA levels, and insulin secretion in HIT-T15 cells. J Clin Invest 1996; 98 (12): 2786–2793.

[196] Herold KC. Inhibition of glucose-stimulated insulin release from beta TC3 cells and rodent islets by an analog of FK506. Transplantation 1993; 55(1): 186–192.

[197] Hahn HJ.Reversibility of the acute toxic effect of cyclosporine A on pancreatic B cells of Wistar rats. Diabetologia 1986; 29(8): 489–494.

[198] Kwon G. Glucose-stimulated DNA synthesis through mammalian target of rapamycin (mTOR) is regulated by KATP channels: Effects on cell cycle progression in rodent islets. J Biol Chem 2006; 281(6): 3261–3267.

[199] Kwon G. Signaling elements involved in the metabolic regulation of mTOR by nutrients, incretins, and growth factors in islets. Diabetes 2004; 53(Suppl 3): S225–S232.

[200] Bussiere CT. The impact of the mTOR inhibitor sirolimus on the proliferation and function of pancreatic islets and ductal cells. Diabetologia 2006; 49 (10): 2341–2349.

[201] Micheal F. Transplant-Associated Hyperglycemia: A New Look at an old problem. Clin J Am Soc Nephrol 2007; 2(2):343-355.

[202] Kasiske BL. Diabetes mellitus after kidney transplantation in the United States. Am J Transplant 2003; 3 (2) 178–185.

[203] Woodward RS. Incidence and cost of new onset diabetes mellitus among US wait-listed and transplanted renal allograft recipients. Am J Transplant 2003; 3 (5): 590–598.

[204] Syed NA. Reciprocal regulation of glycogen phosphorylase and glycogen synthase by insulin involving phosphatidylinositol-3 kinase and protein phosphatase- 1 in HepG2 cells. Mol Cell Biochem 2000; 211(1-2): 123–136.

[205] Mittelman SD. Inhibition of lipolysis causes suppression of endogenous glucose production independent of changes in insulin. Am J Physiol Endocrinol Metab 2000; 279 (3): E630–E637.

[206] Lewis GF. Disordered fat storage and mobilization in the pathogenesis of insulin resistance and type 2 diabetes. Endocr Rev 2002; 23(2): 201–229.

[207] Ost L. impaired glucose tolerance in cyclosporine-prednisone treated renal graft recipients. Transplant 1988; 46 (3): 370-372.

[208] Wilson JS. Congenital deformities and insulin antagonism. Lancet 1996; 2 (7470): 940–941.

[209] Akinkuolie AO. Omega-3 polyunsaturated fatty acid and insulin sensitivity: a meta-analysis of randomized controlled trials. Clin Nutr 2011; 30 (6):702-707.

[210] Barnes PM. Complementary and alternative medicine use among adults and children: United States, 2007. Natl Health Stat Report 2008; 10 (12):1-23.

[211] Zhang W. Effects of interferon-alpha treatment on the incidence of hyperglycemia in chronic hepatitis C patients: a systematic review and meta-analysis. PLoS One 2012 (6); 7:e39272.

[212] Cano A. Metabolic disturbances during intravenous use of ritodrine: increased insulin levels and hypokalemia. Obstet Gynecol 1985; 65 (3):356-360.

[213] Roger A. Pentamidine-lnduced Derangements of Glucose Homeostasis. Diabetes Care 1995; 18 (1): 49-55.

[214] Goldstein MR. Do statins cause diabetes? Curr Diab Rep 2013; 13 (3):381-390.

[215] Henkin Y. Niacin revisited: clinical observations on an important but underutilized drug. Am J Med 1991; 91(3):239-246.

[216] Huang Q. Diazoxide prevents diabetes through inhibiting pancreatic beta-cells from apoptosis via Bcl-2/Bax rate and p38-beta mitogen-activated protein kinase. Endocrinology 2007; 148 (1): 81–91.

[217] Fariss BL. Diphenylhydantoin-induced hyperglycemia and impaired insulin release. Effect of dosage. Diabetes. 1971;20 (3):177-181.

[218] Gailau S. Diabetes in patients treated with asparaginase. Clin Pharmacol Ther 1971; 12(3): 487.

[219] Lavine RL. E.coli L-asparaginase and insulin release in vitro. Metabolism. 1982; 31(10):1009-1013.

[220] Leona VM. Diabetes Mellitus and Autonomic Dysfunction After Vacor Rodenticide Ingestion. Diabetes Care 1978; 1(2):73-76.

[221] Cheung NW. Hyperglycemia Is Associated With Adverse Outcomes in Patients Receiving Total Parenteral Nutrition. Diabetes Care 2005; 28 (10): 267-271.

[222] Francisco J. Hyperglycemia During Total Parenteral Nutrition An important marker of poor outcome and mortality in hospitalized patients. Diabetes Care 2010; 33 (4): 739–741.

[223] Shaat N. Genetics of gestational diabetes mellitus. Curr Med Chem 2007; 14 (5): 569-583.

[224] Lambrinoudaki I. Genetics in gestational diabetes mellitus: association with incidence, severity, pregnancy outcome and response to treatment. Curr Diabetes Rev 2010; 6 (6): 393-399.

[225] Patro-Malysza J. The Impact of Substance P on the Pathogenesis of Insulin Resistance Leading to Gestational Diabetes. Curr Pharm Biotechnol 2014; 15(1):32-37.

[226] Shaat N. Association of the E23K polymorphism in the KCNJ11 gene with gestational diabetes mellitus. Diabetologia 2005; 48 (12):2544-2551.

[227] Pappa KI. Gestational diabetes mellitus shares polymorphisms of genes associated with insulin resistance and type 2 diabetes in the Greek population. Gynecol Endocrinol 2011; 27 (4):267-272.

[228] Zhang C. Genetic variants and the risk of gestational diabetes mellitus: a systematic review. Hum Reprod Update 2013; 19 (4):376-390.

[229] Niu XM. Study on association between gestational diabetes mellitus and sulfonylurea receptor-1 gene polymorphism. Zhonghua Fu Chan Ke Za Zhi 2005; 40 (3):159-163.

[230] Holst JJ. On the effects of human galanin in man. Diabetologia 1993; 36 (7):653–657.

[231] Bauer FE. Inhibitory effect of galanin on postprandial gastrointestinal motility and gut hormone release in humans. Gastroenterology 1989; 97 (2):260–264.

[232] Nergiz S. Circulating galanin and IL-6 concentrations in gestational diabetes mellitus. Gynecol Endocrinol 2014; 30 (3):236-240.

[233] Zhang Z. Endogenous galanin as a novel biomarker to predict gestational diabetes mellitus. Peptides 2014; 54:186-189.

[234] Retnakaran R. The impact of insulin resistance on proinsulin secretion in pregnancy: hyperproinsulinemia is not feature of gestational diabetes. Diabetes Care 2005; 28 (11):2710-2715.

[235] Kautzky-Willer A. Elevated islet amyloid pancreatic polypeptide and proinsulin in lean gestational diabetes. Diabetes 1997; 46 (4):607-614.

[236] Retnakaran R. Adiponectin and beta cell dysfunction in gestational diabetes: pathophysiological implications. Diabetologia 2005; 48 (5):993-1001.

[237] Metzger BE. Summary and recommendations of the Fifth International Workshop-Conference on Gestational Diabetes Mellitus. Diabetes Care 2007; 30 (suppl 2):S251–S260.

[238] Sullivan B. Gestational diabetes. J Am Pharm Assoc 1998; 38 (3):364-371.

[239] Vambergue A. Pathophysiology of gestational diabetes. J Gynecol Obstet Biol Reprod (Paris) 2002; 31(6 suppl):4S3-4S10.

[240] Kleinwechter H. Predisposition and phenotypes of gestational diabetes. Dtsch Med Wochenschr 2014; 139 (21):1123-1126.

[241] Resmini E. Secondary diabetes associated with principal endocrinopathies: the impact of new treatment modalities. Acta Diabetol 2009; 46 (2):85-95.

[242] Lambadiari V. Thyroid hormones are positively associated with insulin resistance early in the development of type 2 diabetes. Endocrine 2011; 39 (1):28-32.

[243] Brenta G. Why Can Insulin Resistance Be a Natural Consequence of Thyroid Dysfunction? Journal of Thyroid Reserch 2011; 2011: 152850, 9 pages.

[244] De Leo V. Polycystic ovary syndrome and type 2 diabetes mellitus. Minerva Ginecol 2004; 56 (1): 53-62.

[245] Pelusi B. Type 2 diabetes and the polycystic ovary syndrome. Minerva Ginecol 2004; 56 (1):41-51.

[246] Sjoberg RJ. Pancreatic diabetes mellitus. Diabetes Care 1989; 12 (10):715-724.

[247] Choudhuri G. Pancreatic diabetes. Trop Gastroenterol 2009; 30 (2):71-75.

[248] Richard JS. Case Study: Screening and Treatment of Pre-Diabetes in Primary Care. Clinical Diabetes 2004; 22 (2): 98-104.

[249] Moran A. Clinical Care Guidelines for Cystic Fibrosis–Related Diabetes. A position statement of the American Diabetes Association and a clinical practice guideline of

the Cystic Fibrosis Foundation, endorsed by the Pediatric Endocrine Society. Diabetes Care 2010; 33 (12): 2697–2708.

[250] Yeh HC. Smoking cessation and risk for type 2 diabetes mellitus. A cohort study Annals of Internal Medicine 2010; 152(1): 10-17.

[251] Rimm EB. Prospective study of cigarette smoking, alcohol use, and the risk of diabetes in men. BMJ1995; 310 (6979): 555–559.

[252] Radzeviciene L. Smoking habits and the risk of type 2 diabetes: a case control study. Diabetes and Metabolism 2009; 35 (3):192-197.

[253] Fagard RH. Smoking and diabetes – the double health hazard. Primary Care Diabetes 2009; 3 (4): 205-209.

[254] Cullen MW. No interaction of body mass index and smoking on diabetes mellitus risk in elderly women. Preventative Medicine 2009; 48(1): 74-78.

[255] Nagaya T. Heavy smoking raises risk for type 2 diabetes milletus in obese men; but, light smoking reduces the risk in lean men: a follow up study in Japan. Annals of Epidemiology 2008; 18(2): 113-118.

[256] Lynch SM. Cigarette smoking and pancreatic cancer: a pooled analysis from the pancreatic cancer cohort consortium. American Journal of Epidemiology 2009; 170(4): 403-413.

[257] Hofman PL. Premature birth and later insulin resistance. N Engl J Med 2004; 351(21): 2179-2186.

[258] Hofman PL. The metabolic consequences of prematurity. Growth Horm IGF Res. 2004;14 (Suppl A):S136-S139.

[259] Hofman PL. Insulin sensitivity in people born pre-term, with low or very low birth weight and small for gestational age. J Endocrinol Invest 2006; 29 (1 Suppl):2-8.

[260] Lithell HO. Relation of size at birth to non-insulin dependent diabetes and insulin concentrations in men aged 50-60 years. BMJ 1996; 312 (7028):406-410.

[261] Mi J. Association of body size at birth with impaired glucose tolerance during their adulthood for men and women aged 41 to 47 years in Beijing of China. Zhonghua Yu Fang Yi Xue Za Zhi 1999; 33 (4):209-213.

[262] Hales CN. Fetal and infant growth and impaired glucose tolerance at age 64. BMJ. 1991; 303 (6809):1019-1022.

[263] Harder T. Birth weight and subsequent risk of type 2 diabetes: a meta-analysis. Am J Epidemiol 2007; 165 (8):849-857.

[264] Tian JY. Birth weight and risk of type 2 diabetes, abdominal obesity and hypertension among Chinese adults. Eur J Endocrinol 2006; 155(4):601-607.

Chapter 4

Can Adiponectin be a biomarker for Ethnic heterogeneity in Diabetes Mellitus?

Fatum Elshaari, F.A. Elshaari, D.S. Sheriff,
A.A. Alshaari and S. Omer Sheriff

Additional information is available at the end of the chapter

http://dx.doi.org/10.5772/59119

1. Introduction

There is considerable body of evidence to suggest that the effect of obesity as a major risk factor of chronic diseases differ due to variation in genetic predisposition and ethnic differences. This is due probably to the difference in body habitus and the distribution of adipose tissue. It is shown that Asians have a higher proportion of abdominal obesity compared to other ethnic groups and carry greater risk for diabetes, hypertension and coronary vascular diseases at a lower level of body mass index(BMI) compared to other populations. [1-3]. Japanese are reported to carry twice the risk of developing diabetes at all levels of BMI compared to Caucasians [4]. Therefore with a wide variety of studies reporting the importance of ethnicity playing an important role in the distribution of total body fat has created a need to identify a biomarker(s) or risk marker for ethnic heterogeneity in the development of chronic diseases.

In this regard adipocytokines adiponectin, leptin and resistin are considered as potential candidates to delineate the mechanisms involved in such ethnic differences related to chronic diseases. Adiponectin and leptin are reported to show reciprocal relationship with increasing adiposity. It is demonstrated that adiponectin levels reflect visceral adiposity and leptin the subcutaneous one. It is also reported that serum adiponectin levels are lower in Chinese, Malay, Japanese, Koreans, south Asians compared to Caucasians. [5]There is another adipocytokine which is related to adiposity. This adipocytokine was reported to resist the action of insulin and so it is named as Resistin. It is shown that Resistin is present more in visceral adipose tissue compared to other fat depots and a diet rich in fat induces greater secretion of resistin.[6] The adiponectin, leptin and resistin trio could be the biomarkers of ethnic heterogeneity.

Obesity is a major public health concern of Libya with higher prevalence of obesity related diseases hypertension, type 2 diabetes (T2DM) and coronary vascular disease.[7] Therefore, the present preliminary study was undertaken in Libyan subjects with their unique ethnicity, life style and cultural habits to demonstrate whether such differences occur in serum adiponectin, leptin and resistin levels in relation to adiposity particularly visceral adiposity. It was shown that BMI and Waist circumference could be taken as markers of subcutaneous obesity and abdominal obesity respectively. Along with these anthropometric measurements glycemic status, lipid profile were studied and correlated with adiponectin, leptin and resistin levels in obese and type 2 diabetes (T2DM) subjects.

2. Subjects taken for the study

The subjects included in the study were local Libyan subjects, Benghazi. Informed consent was taken from each participant and approval for the study taken from Institute Ethics Review Board(Faculty of Medicine, Benghazi University, Benghazi).

3. Anthropometric measurements

Height, weight, waist circumference, were measured. Their age, duration of diabetes and medicine usage as well as personal and family history were noted.The measurements and examinations were carried out by the same physician.

BMI was calculated by the formula: Weight (kg)/Height2 (m2). Normal BMI was taken as 18-25 kg/m2. Patients with BMI values of 25-30 kg/m2 were classified as overweight; and those with BMI ≥30 kg/m2 were considered obese.

Waist circumference (cm) was measured parallel to the midpoint between the lower limit of the 12th costa and the ischial spine. The limits were accepted as >102 cm in men, and >88 cm in women (ATP: adult treatment panel III criteria).

4. Sample collection

Among the 1500 patients visiting the Department of Medicine, Faculty of Medicine, Benghazi University hospital for medical check up, 650 subjects were taken for the study. 200 subjects taken as controls(100 –males; 100-females) and 250 (100-males; 150-females) subjects formed the obese group and 200 formed the diabetes group(100 males and 100 females).Fasting blood samples were collected in vacutainer tubes with a gel separator and in heparinized tubes for HbA1C measurements and were centrifugated at 2000 rpm for 15 min at 4°C after an incubation period of 30 min. All biochemical variables were measured on the same day of the blood collection. Remaining serum specimens were stored at −20°C until analysis of adiponectin, leptin and resistin levels.

5. Biochemical methods

Serum glucose, total cholesterol (TC), HDL-cholesterol (HDL-C), triglyceride (TG) were measured by an enzymatic colorimetric method.Serum adiponectin levels were measured by enzyme linked immunosorbent assay (ELISA) with a sensitivity of 3 ng/ml. Serum leptin levels were measured by an active human leptin ELISA (DSL, Diagnostic System Laboratories, USA) with a sensitivity of 0.05 ng/ml. Serum resistin levels were measured by ELISA (Linco Research, USA) with a sensitivity of 0.16 ng/ml.

6. Calculations

Low-density lipoprotein-cholesterol (LDL-C) was calculated using the Friedewald formula. Standing height and body weight were measured with the subjects dressed in light indoor clothing without shoes. Body mass index (BMI) was calculated as weight divided by the square of the height (kg/m^2).

7. Statistical analyses

Statistical analysis was performed using SPSS for Windows (Statistical Package for the Social Sciences, version 20.0; SSPS Inc. Chicago, IL, USA). The normal distribution of the variables was evaluated using the Shapiro-Wilk test. The Mann-Whitney U test was used for the comparison of variables which were not normally distributed, and the independent Student's t-test for the comparison of variables which were normally distributed. The Pearson and Spearman tests were used for the evaluation of correlations among the variables according to the distribution of variables. $P<0.05$ was accepted as indicative of statistical significance. The results of variables with a normal distribution were expressed as mean ± SD and those with a non-Gaussian distribution were expressed as median (25th–75th percentile).

8. Ethical considerations

The study was carried out in accordance with the Declaration of Helsinki. Informed consent was obtained from all the patients for the initial study. The protocol was approved by the Medical Ethics Committee of the Faculty of Medicine, Benghazi University, Benghazi,Libya. Additional informed consent was obtained for the present study.

Results: Table.1. shows the differences in waist circumferences reported for various ethnic groups

Country or Ethnic group	Sex	Waist Circumference(cm)
*South Asian	Men	>94
	women	>80
*Chinese	Men	>90
	Women	>80
*Japanese	Men	>90
	Women	>80
*Europid	*Men	>94
	Women	>80
**Libyan	Men	>93
	Women	>90

Source *Adapted from Zimmet and Alberti [2006] [8]; ** present study

Table 1. Ethnic differences in Waist circumferences

Indicator	Cut off Points	Risk of Metabolic complications
Waist circumference	>94cm(M), >80cm(W)	Increased
Waist circumference	>102cm(M), >88cm(W)	Substantially increased
W/H ratio	>0.90(M), >0.85(w)	Substantially increased

M: men; W: women

Table 2. World Health Organization (WHO) cut off points and risk of Metabolic complications[9]

The mean BMI in Libyan adults is reported to be 27.7 kg/m2 (26.4 kg/m2 in men and 29 kg/m2 in women), and the mean waist circumference is 93.3 cm. [10] In the present study compared to other ethnic groups Libyan Men and women have higher BMI and Waist circumference carrying higher risk for metabolic complications as well as for chronic diseases. (BMI 25-30; (29.5) and 30 to 35 (34.5)respectively in normal as well as obese controls). Waist circumference 104cm; 114 cm for normal and obese subjects respectively; Waist circumference to Hip circumference; 0.97 for both men and women subjects.(W/H ratio). The normal control group had higher BMI as well as higher waist circumference indicating both subcutaneous fat and visceral fat are increased in the subjects studied.

	Chinese	*Malay*	*Asian Indian*	*Libyan*	*P Anova*
Males-Total Adiponectin(μg/ml)	*3.10±1.79*	*2.97±1.80*	*2.97±1.75*	*1.97±1.05*	*0.01*
Females(Total Adiponectin(μg/ml)	*4.60±2.50*	*4.28±2.52*	*3.83±1.95*	*2.45±1.10*	*0.001*

*Adapted from Chin Meng Khoo et al.[11] ** present study

*P value for comparison between the ethnic groups in men; †P value for comparison between the ethnic groups in women. The values for adiponectin for both Libyan men and women were comparatively lower than the values reported for other ethnic groups like Chinese, Malay, Asian Indian groups.

Table 3. Ethnic variation in Serum Adiponectin levels

	Control-normal	Obese controls	Diabetes	*P-value*	Adjusted P-value
Leptin, ng/mL	13.90 ± 3.16	*28.10 ± 5.00	**32.25±6.50	*0.000 **0.000	P<0.001
Adiponectin, µg/mL	2.01± 1.05	1.90± 0.75	*5.45±1.05	**0.009	P<0.01
Resistin, ng/mL	6.80 ± 3.70	*18.46 ± 8.80	**24.45±9.50	*0.0039 **0.000	P<0.01 P<0.001

Table 4. Serum Adiponectin, Leptin and Resistin levels in normal, obese and Diabetic Libyan patients

The serum levels of adiponectin did not show significant difference in their values between controls and obese subjects.The adiponectin level in diabetic subjects is significantly higher than the control subjects. The serum levels of leptin and resistin were significantly higher for obese and T2DM compared to normal controls.

	Control	Obese	Diabetes	p.value
Body mass index(kg/m^2)	29.5 (25.5-30.0)	*34.5 (30 – 35)	**36.5 (35-37.5)	*<0.001 **<0.001
Waist circumference(cm)	104	* 112	**120	*<0.001 **<0.001
FastingBlood glucose(mg/dL)	89.50±15.50	105.50±20.50	*155.50±24.50	*<0.001
Glycated hemoglobin(%)	5.50±1.05	6.45±1.25	*8.90±1.50	*<0.001
Total Cholesterol (mg/dL)	128.45±18.40	148.20±24.50	*175.50±25.50	*<0.001
HDL-cholesterol(mg/dL	37.45±4.50	35.50±5.50	*32.50±6.50	<0.05
LDL cholesterol (mg/dL)	95.45±12.50	105.5±14.00	*125.00±7.50	*<0.05
Non-HDL cholesterol(mg/dL)	91.00±7.50	*112.70±8.00	*143.00±12.50	<0.05
Triglycerides(mg/dL)	99.50±10.50	105.50±12.00	*145.00±25.50	<0.01

Table 5. Serum glucose, glycated hemoglobin (HbA1c) and Lipid Profile in the Libyan Subjects

There was no marked differences between the control group and obese group with respect to the serum levels of glucose, HbA1c, total cholesterol, HDL-cholesterol, LDL-cholesterol and triglycerides. There were marked increases in total cholesterol, LDL cholesterol, triglycerides with a marked fall in HDL cholesterol in diabetec subjects (dyslipidemia)

A marked increase was observed in non-HDL cholesterol in obese and diabetics compared to the control group.

The levels of serum total cholesterol and HDL cholesterol are comparatively lower for local Libyan subjects when compared to South Asians and Non South Asians.

	*Non-south Asians	*South Asians	**Libyan	P value
Total cholesterol (mg/dL)	207.60±30.45	199.88±28.45	*128.45±18.40	0.0028 <0.01
HDL cholesterol (mg/dL)	47.55±6.50	41.45±8.50	*37.5.±5.50	0.033 <0.05
Triglcyerides(mg/dL)	145.12±24.50	140.6±25.50	145.5±12.20	0.45

*France et al [12] ** present study

Table 6. Serum lipid profile in different ethnic groups

9. Discussion

Of the anthropometric measures Body mass index (BMI), waist circumference and waist-hip ratio, waist circumference were reported to be more closely related to abdominal obesity and T2DM. Majority of the studies supported the view that there is no optimal cut-off point that can be universally applied. It was suggested that country or region-specific cut off points may be used. [13-14]

Data available in the literature suggest that lower waist circumference and waist-hip ratio cut off point for Asians-85cm and 80 cm, W/H ratio 0.9 and 0.8 for men and women, respectively. [15-17] A study from Tunisia provided a cut-off point for waist circumference (for obesity, diabetes,and CVD) of 85 cm for both men and women, based on sensitivity being equal to specificity.[18]. The values for BMI and WC for Arab Nations are reported to be similar to European population.[19]

Obesity is a major public health concern for Libya. It is reported that about 30% of Libyan adults are obese. About 64% of Libyan adults are either overweight or obese. In the present study BMI values for control subjects were 29.5, 34.5 for obese subjects and 36.50 for T2DM subjects. WC values for control was 104cm,114 cm for obese subjects and 120 for T2DM subjects. These values clearly indicate that majority of the population are either over-weight or obese. This is supported by data that obesity related diseases like type 2 diabetes (T2DM), hypertension, poly cystic ovarian disease (PCOD) are on the rise in Libya. [7, 20-22]. There is a dire need for finding risk markers for obesity and obesity related disorders.

There is a shift in focus to find out whether ethnic diversity could be a factor in the distribution pattern of adiposity variation in different populations. Few studies have stated that adipocytokines particularly adiponectin values differ for different population indicating that adiponectin could be taken as a biomarker of ethnic heterogeneity. When compared to other population serum adiponectin values were comparatively lower for Libyan subjects. Serum leptin and resistin levels were higher for obese and T2DM subjects compared to control ones.Paradoxically the serum levels of adiponectin were higher for T2DM subjects contrary to reports that there is hypoadiponectinemia in T2DM. Hyperadiponectinemia reported quite contrary to the earlier observations is suggested to be due to the presence of severe insulin resistance possibly to genetically defective insulin receptors. [23]

This finding emphasizes that insulin receptor has a critical role regulating adiponectin synthesis as well as clearance. Patients who have anti-insulin receptor antibodies may be responsible for severe insulin resistance (Type B IR) who show a significant increase in serum adiponectin levels. Such a finding brings out considerable focus on the adiponectin –insulin sensitivity concept. Rather it opens up for more avenues of research to exactly elicit the adiponectin's role in insulin sensitivity and suggests that insulin effect on adiponectin metabolism is undermined.[23]

In the present study T2DM Libyan patients showed marked increase in serum adiponectin levels compared to the control subjects. These subjects had higher insulin levels and insulin resistance shown by HOMA index. The duration of diabetes in these patients is 10 years or more.The results are not shown here.

This finding appears unique to Libyan diabetic subjects. It is reported earlier that adiponectin levels in Libyan subjects are comparatively lower when compared to European or western population in general. Therefore serum adiponectin levels seem to be determined by ethnic heterogeneity reflected by the distribution of adipose tissue and its genetic regulation of adiponectin's synthesis, secretion and degradation. Possibly the reportedly higher BMI in the population with a higher basal insulin levels (accompanied by insulin resistance) might have an suppressive effect on adiponectin formation or clearance.

Insulin resistance(IR) is now generally accepted to be the primary metabolic defect of T2DM [24]. IR is defined as a state that requires more insulin to obtain the biological effects achieved by a lower amount of insulin in the normal state [25].

In contrast to other adipokines, circulating levels of adiponectin correlate inversely with body fat and IR in humans [26] and rodent models [25].). It circulates at high levels in human plasma accounting for approximately 0.01% (0.5-30 μg/mL) of all plasma protein in normal individuals [27], 1000-fold higher than other hormones such as leptin and insulin. Gender has an effect on concentrations of adiponectin, with females having higher levels than males [28]. It is also well known that adiponectin levels increase with age, however the cause for this increase is still unknown [29]

The molecule adiponectin is a 244-amino-acid long adipokine secreted from adipocytes. The gene product is a 30kD protein [30], however this is not found in circulation. Adiponectin automatically self-binds to form larger structures and there are different multimeric forms including low molecular weight (LMW) trimers, middle molecular weight (MMW) hexamers, high molecular weight (HMW) oligomeric structures and finally globular adiponectin (gC1q domain)[27]. It has been proposed that this globular fragment is generated by proteolytic cleavage of adiponectin multimers by leukocyte elastase secreted from activated monocytes and/or neutrophils [24]; however the pathophysiological importance of this cleavage remains to be determined. Structurally, the globular form of adiponectin lacks the collagenous domain necessary for multimerization. Adipocytes secrete both the low-molecular weight and high-molecular weight forms of adiponectin in vivo and in vitro. Thus, the low-molecular weight and high-molecular weight forms of adiponectin are the predominant forms in serum whilst smaller complexes such as the trimer are virtually undetectable. [31].

10. Monomeric structure

There are four distinct regions of adiponectin. The protein starts with a short signal sequence which acts to target the hormone for secretion outside the cell, then it leads into a short region that is variable between species, followed by an amino-acid region that shows similarity with collagenous protein, and finally ending with a globular domain. The three dimensional structure of its C-terminal globular domain is similar to that of tumor necrosis factor–alpha (TNF-α), even though there is no sequence homology at the primary structure level. [32].

11. Higher order structures

Initially, three adiponectin molecules associate through disulphide bonds within the collagenous domains of each monomer to form bouquet-like higher order structure, a homotrimer. The trimers continue to self-associate and form hexamers [33].

The levels of the higher order structures are sexually dimorphic [34], where females have increased proportions of the high-molecular weight forms. The varying forms have altered biological activity and therefore may also have separate functions. The gC1q domain and the trimeric forms of adiponectin activate AMP Kinase in skeletal muscle and lead to increased fatty acid oxidation and reduction in glucose concentrations, whereas the hexameric and full length HMW forms are thought to activate nuclear factor kappa B (NF-κB) pathways [35]. The proportion of HMW adiponectin within adipose tissue is higher than in blood plasma, suggesting regulation at the level of secretion and is a mechanism of adiponectin complex distribution. All isoforms of the molecule are stable in circulation having a relatively longer half life (half-life of ~15hrs) [24].

12. Receptors and signaling

Two receptors have been identified that bind adiponectin: Adipo R1 and Adipo R2. AdipoR1 was first identified when encoding cDNA was isolated from human skeletal cDNA library by screening for adiponectin binding [36]. The AdipoR2 was identified later due to its striking homology to AdipoR1. Both are surface membrane proteins [36] and have homology to G protein-coupled receptors.. These receptors contain seven transmembrane domains, but are structurally and functionally distinct from other known GPCRs (G-protein-coupled receptors[37]. The receptors have different affinities to the various molecular forms of adiponectin. AdipoR1 and AdipoR2 are found in liver, muscle and adipose tissue in humans; however AdipoR1 is predominantly expressed in skeletal muscle whereas AdipoR2 is more predominant in the liver [36]. AdipoR1 is a high-affinity receptor for globular adiponectin as well as having a lower affinity for full length adiponectin. In contrast the AdipoR2 receptor has an equal intermediate affinity for globular and full length HMW adiponectin [36]. The receptors affect a very important cellular metabolic rate control point, by targeting AMP-activated protein Kinase (AMPK), downstream. AMPK is a stress induced kinase that is activated in response to depleting Adenosine triphosphate (ATP) or increasing Adenosine monophosphate (AMP) levels. AMPK activates ATP and generates catabolic processes such as fatty acid breakdown and glycolysis and shuts down ATP-consuming processes such as lipogenesis [37]. Expression of these receptors is correlated with insulin levels [24]. A review of studies involving the adiponectin receptors suggests that they may have an important role in adiponectin physiology. Key findings suggest that changes in expression of AdipoR isoforms in skeletal muscle (rather than total circulating adiponectin concentrations) may be of physiological importance [38]. More recently, by means of expression cloning, T-cadherin has been recognized as an adiponectin receptor on vascular endothelial cells and smooth muscle [36]. The expression of this cadherin molecule is known to be correlated with atherosclerosis [33].By genomic sequence analysis, Saito et al. determined that the ADIPOQ gene spans 16 kb,contains 3 exons and 2 introns and the promoter lacks a TATA box(a sequence involved in the process of transcription). The exon-intron organization of this gene was very similar to that of obese gene,encoding leptin. Saito et al. reported that the ADIPOQ gene was located on human chromosome band 3q27using chromosome mapping of this gene by fluorescence in situ hybridization (FISH) taking genomic DNA fragment as a probe [39]. It is reported that a mutation in this gene is associated with low serum adiponectin levels and T2DM[41].

It has been reported that blood concentrations of adiponectin fall from 20-50% in humans and mice respectively with the administration of insulin, thus implying that the effect of insulin to lower adiponectin levels may involve inhibition of adipocyte secretion. Plasma adiponectin levels have also been shown to be decreased in an obese rhesus monkey model that frequently develops Type 2 Diabetes [42] Many prospective studies [43-45] have shown that lower adiponectin levels are associated with a higher incidence of diabetes in humans and more importantly the decrease in plasma adiponectin levels was in parallel with the decrease in insulin sensitivity [25]. This finding is further supported by a recent analysis of 13 prospective studies, which found that higher adiponectin levels were associated with a lower risk of Type 2 Diabetes across diverse populations [45-46].

The levels of serum total cholesterol and triglycerides are comparatively lower for local Libyan subjects when compared to South Asians and Non South Asians.[47] The serum level of total HDL cholesterol is also low in Libyan subjects probably due to the lowered levels of total cholesterol and triglycerides.[47].

A marked increase was observed in non-HDL cholesterol in obese individuals compared to the control group.[48] and there was a marked fall in HDL cholesterol indicating that dyslipidemia is prevalent in local Libyan subjects

This preliminary study indicates that the distribution of fat in Libyan population varies from other populations. There is a marked increase in total as well as abdominal adiposity indicated by anthropometric measurements. The serum level of adiponectin is low in this population along with comparatively HDL cholesterol with a marked increase in non-HDL cholesterol. Therefore further studies are being carried out to bring out the nature unique ethnic diversity in the population as well as to recommend that an overall reduction of body weight in the population need to be considered to lower risk of metabolic disorders.

Apart from these observations the serum levels of adiponectin were found to be lower for the Libyan subjects and its level was increased in T2DM subjects.

This observation seems to suggest whether serum adiponectin level in Libyan subjects can be taken as a biomarker of ethinic heterogeneity.

Acknowledgements

This research was supported by a grant from the National Agency for Scientific Research, Tripoli.Libya.

Author details

Fatum Elshaari[1], F.A. Elshaari[1], D.S. Sheriff[1*], A.A. Alshaari[2] and S. Omer Sheriff[3]

*Address all correspondence to: dhastagir@yahoo.ca

1 Department of Biochemistry,Faculty of Medicine, Benghazi University, Benghazi, Libya

2 Department of Medicine, Faculty of Medicine, Benghazi University, Benghazi, Libya

3 Faculty of Dentistry, IMU,Kuala Lumpur, Malaysia

The authors declare that there is no conflict of interest that could be perceived as prejudicing the impartiality of the research reported.

References

[1] Scott M. Grundy,1 Ian J. Neeland,2 Aslan T. Turer,2 and Gloria Lena Vega1. Clinical Study Waist Circumference as Measure of Abdominal Fat Compartments. Journal of Obesity2013, 454285, 9 pages.http://dx.doi.org/10.1155/2013/454285.

[2] Mente A, Razak F, Blankenberg S, Vuksan V, Davis AD, Miller R et al., "Ethnic variation in adiponectin and leptin levels and their association with adiposity and insulin resistance," Diabetes Care2010;33:1629–1634, 2010.

[3] Carey, D. G., Jenkins, A. B., Campbell, L. V., Freund, J. & Chrisholm, D. J."Abdominal Fat and Insulin Resistance in Normal and Over-Weight Women: Direct Measurements Reveal a Strong Relationship in Subjects at Both Low and High Risk of NIDDM,"Diabetes1996;45: 633-8.

[4] Preis S.R., Massaro J.M, Robins R.J. Hoffmann U, Ramachandran S. V, Thomas Irlbeck V.et al. "Abdominal Subcutaneous and Visceral Adipose Tissue and Insulin Resistance in the Framington Heart Study," Obesity 2010; 18 : 2191-2198.

[5] Kadowaki T, Sekikawa A, Okamura T, Takamiya T, Kashiwagi A, Zaky WR, et al "Higher levels of adiponectin in American than in Japanese men despite obesity," Metabolism 2006;55:1561–1563.

[6] Lazar MA: Resistin-and Obesity-associated metabolic diseases. Horm Metab Res 2007, 39:710-716

[7] Rafik R. Elmehdawi* and Abdulwahab M. Albarsha. Obesity in Libya: a review. Libyan J Med 2012, 7: 19086

[8] Alberti KGMM, Zimmet PZ. Definition, diagnosis and classification of diabetes mellitus and its complications. Part 1: diagnosis and classification of diabetes mellitus. Provisional report of a WHO consultation. *Diabetic Med.*1988; 15: 539-553.

[9] Ministry of Health-Libya. National Survey of Non-Communicable Disease Risk Factors. 2009. Tripoli: Ministry of Health-Libya.(Reference for BMI for Libya)

[10] WHO. Physical status: the use and interpretation of anthropometry. Report of a WHO expert consultation. Geneva, World Health Organization (WHO), 1995.

[11] Chin Meng K, Sarina S, Siska T, Daphne G, Yi Wu, Jeannette L, Rob M. van Dam, and Shyong T,et al. Ethnicity Modifies the Relationships of Insulin Resistance, Inflammation, and Adiponectin With Obesity in a Multiethnic Asian Population. Diabetes Care. May 2011; 34(5): 1120–1126.

[12] France M.W., Kwok,S, McElduff.P., Seneviratne, C.J. Ethnic trends in lipid tests in general practice. Q.J.Med 2003;96:919-923.

[13] Qiao Q, Nyamdorj R. The optimal cutoff values and their performance of waist circumference and waist-to-hip ratio for diagnosing type II diabetes. European Journal of Clinical Nutrition, 2010b, 64(1):23-29.

[14] WHO. Obesity: Preventing and managing the global epidemic. Report of a WHO Consultation (TRS 894). Geneva, World Health Organization (WHO), 2000

[15] Wang J, Thornton JC, Russell M, et al. Asians have lower body mass index (BMI) but higher percent body fat than do whites: comparisons of anthropometric measurements. American Journal of Clinical Nutrition 1994;60(1):23-28.

[16] Misra, A.; Chowbey, P.K.; Makkar, B.M.; Vikram, N.K.; Wasir, J.S.; Chadha, D.et al Consensus statement for diagnosis of obesity, abdominal obesity and the metabolic

syndrome for Asian Indians and recommendations for physical activity, medical and surgical management. J. Assoc. Physicians India 2009, 57, 163–170.

[17] S Kalra1,2, M Mercuri2,3 and S S Anand2,3,4 Measures of body fat in South Asian adults Nutrition & Diabetes 2013; 3, e69; doi:10.1038/nutd.2013.10

[18] Benghazi diabetes and endocrine center. Statistics. 2009. Benghazi: Ministry of Health-Libya.

[19] Dakhil FO, Zew M, Ahmad M, Aboudabus F, El Jaroushi A, El Badri A, et al. Pattern of hypertension in Ibn Sina hypertension clinic, benghazi-libya. Garyounis Med J. 1998–2000; 19: 56–60.

[20] Najem FI, Elmehdawi RR, Swalem AM. Clinical and biochemical characteristics of polycystic ovary syndrome in Benghazi-Libya: a retrospective study. Libyan J Med. AOP: 071018.

[21] Bouguerra R, Alberti H, Smida H et al. Waist circumference cut-off points for identification of abdominal obesity among the Tunisian adult population. *Diabetes, Obesity and Metabolism,*2007, 9(6):859-868.

[22] Al-Lawati JA, Jousilahti P. Body mass index, waist circumference and waist-to-hip ratio cut-off points for categorisation of obesity among Omani Arabs. *Public Health Nutrition,* 2008, 11(1):102-108.

[23] Semple RK, Halberg NH, Burling K, Soos MA, Schraw T, Jian'an Luan, et al. Paradoxical Elevation of High–Molecular Weight Adiponectin in Acquired Extreme Insulin Resistance Due to Insulin Receptor Antibodies Diabetes 2007;56:1712–171723.

[24] Smith SA Central role of the adipocyte in the insulin-sensitizing and cardiovascular risk modifying actions of the thiazolidinediones. Biochimie 2003;85:1219-1230

[25] Kadowaki T, Yamauchi T, Kubota N, Hara K, Ueki K and Tobe K : Adiponectin and adiponectin receptors in insulin resistance, diabetes, and the metabolic syndrome. J Clin Invest 2006;116:1784-1792

[26] Whitehead JP, Richards AA, Hickman IJ, Macdonald GA and Prins JB :Adiponectin--a key adipokine in the metabolic syndrome. Diabetes Obes Metab. 2006;8:264-280

[27] Yatagai T, Nagasaka S, Taniguchi A, Fukushima M, Nakamura T, Kuroe A, et al: Hypoadiponectinemia is associated with visceral fat accumulation and insulin resistance in Japanese men with type 2 diabetes mellitus. Metabolism.2003;52:1274-1278.

[28] Magkos F and Sidossis LS: Recent advances in the measurement of adiponectin isoform distribution. Curr Opin Clin Nutr Metab Care 2007;10:571-575.

[29] Xu A, Chan KW, Hoo RL, Wang Y, Tan KC, Zhang J, et al : Testosterone selectively reduces the high molecular weight form of adiponectin by inhibiting its secretion from adipocytes. J Biol Chem. 2005;280:18073-18080.

[30] Sattar N, Wannamethee SG and Forouhi NG: Novel biochemical risk factors for type 2 diabetes: pathogenic insights or prediction possibilities? Diabetologia. 2008;51:926-940

[31] Scherer PE, Williams S, Fogliano M, Baldini G and Lodish HF (1995): A novel serum protein similar to C1q, produced exclusively in adipocytes. J Biol Chem 1995; 270 : 26746–26749

[32] Pajvani UB, Hawkins M, Combs TP, Rajala MW, Doebber T, Berger JP, et al : Complex distribution, not absolute amount of adiponectin, correlates with thiazolidinedione-mediated improvement in insulin sensitivity. J Biol Chem 2004;279:12152-12162.

[33] Arita Y, Kihara S and Ouchi N : Paradoxical decrease of an adipose-specific protein, adiponectin, in obesity. Biochem Biophys Res Commun 1999;257:79 – 83.

[34] Tilg H and Moschen AR: Adipocytokines: mediators linking adipose tissue, inflammation and immunity. Nat Rev Immunol. 2006;6:772-783

[35] Xu A, Chan KW, Hoo RL, Wang Y, Tan KC, Zhang J, et al : Testosterone selectively reduces the high molecular weight form of adiponectin by inhibiting its secretion from adipocytes. J Biol Chem. 2005;280:18073-18080.

[36] Hug C, Wang J, Ahmad NS, Bogan JS, Tsao TS and Lodish HF: T-cadherin is a receptor for hexameric and high molecular-weight forms of Acrp30/adiponectin. Proc Natl Acad Sci U S A 2004;101:10308-10313.

[37] Takeuchi T, Adachi Y, Ohtsuki Y and Furihata M: Adiponectin receptors, with special focus on the role of the third receptor, T-cadherin, in vascular disease. Med Mol Morphol. 2007;40:115-20

[38] Yamauchi, T., Kamon, J., Ito, Y. et al. : Cloning of adiponectin receptors that mediate antidiabetic metabolic effects. Nature (London) 2003;423: 762–769

[39] Shetty S, Kusminski CM and Scherer PE. Adiponectin in health and disease: evaluation of adiponectin-targeted drug development strategies. Trends Pharmacol Sci. 2009;30:234-9

[40] Saito, K., Tobe, T., Minoshima, S., Asakawa, S., Sumiya, J., Yoda, M.,etal.: Organization of the gene for gelatin-binding protein (GBP28). Gene; 1999; 229: 67-73

[41] Kondo, H., Shimomura, I., Matsukawa, Y., Kumada, M., Takahashi, M., Matsuda, M. et al. Association of adiponectin mutation with type 2 diabetes: a candidate gene for the insulin resistance syndrome. Diabetes 2002; 51: 2325-2328

[42] Klssebah, A. H., Sonnenberg, G. E., Myklebust, J., Goldstein, M., Broman, K., James, R. G.,et al Quantitative trait loci on chromosomes 3 and 17 influence phenotypes of the metabolic syndrome. Proc Natl Acad Sei USA2006; 97: 14478-14483

[43] Jalovaara K, Santaniemi M, Timonen M, Jokelainen J, Kesaniemi YA,Ukkola O, et al : Low serum adiponectin level as a predictor of impaired glucose regulation and type

2 diabetes mellitus in a middle-aged Finnish population. Metabolism. 2008;57:1130-1134.

[44] Spranger J, Kroke A, Mohlig M, Bergmann MM, Ristow M, Boeing H, et al: Adiponectin and protection against type 2 diabetes mellitus. Lancet 2003;361:226-228.

[45] Li S, Shin HJ, Ding EL and van Dam RM: Adiponectin levels and risk of type 2 diabetes: a systematic review and meta-analysis. JAMA. 2009;302:179-188.

[46] Yu JG, Javorschi S, Hevener AL, Kruszynska YT, Norman RA, Sinha M, et al. The effect of thiazolidinediones on plasma adiponectin levels in normal, obese, and type 2 diabetic subjects. Diabetes. 2002;51:2968-74

[47] France M.W., Kwok,S, McElduff.P., Seneviratne, C.J. Ethnic trends in lipid tests in general practice. Q.J.Med 2003;96:919-923.

[48] Varbo A., Benn M., Tybjærg-Hansen A., Jørgensen A.B., Frikke-Schmidt R., Nordestgaard B.G.; Remnant cholesterol as a causal risk factor for ischemic heart disease. J Am Coll Cardiol. 2013;61:427-436.

Chapter 5

Clinical Trials on Diabetes Mellitus

Blas Gil Extremera, Pilar Jiménez López, Alberto Jesús Guarnido Ramírez, Elizabet García Peñalver, Maria Luz Abarca Martínez and Isabel Mérida Fernández

Additional information is available at the end of the chapter

http://dx.doi.org/10.5772/59130

1. Introduction

Today in the clinical practice Diabetes Mellitus (DM) has supplanted syphilis and tuberculosis as the big masquerade. Now, from the professional view, many physicians are involved in hard challenges, controversies concerning diabetic patients: insulin resistance, management of the disease, diabetic pregnant women, carbohydrate disorders, diabetic foot, diabetes and surgery, pharmacological aspects, psychological and sociological problems, new modalities of treatment and many others and important clinical questions. Diabetes mellitus, the most common endocrine disorder, is characterized by several metabolic abnormalities and numerous long-term complications affecting mostly the kidneys, peripheral nerves, blood vessels, organ vision, and central nervous system; also, we must not forget that it is the main cause of morbidity and mortality in the Western and developed countries.

Since the discovery of insulin in 1921 by Banting and Best, and McLeod, it has been employed in the treatment of DM [1]. By the time, the manufacturing process of insulin has improved becoming free of impurities or associated to hormonal products (glucagon, polypeptide pancreatic, proinsulin) until obtaining purified insulin.

Insulin was obtained from a bovine source; and particularly porcine insulin differs only from the human insulin in one aminoacid. Later in the clinical practice, biosynthetic and semi-synthetic human insulin were introduced, having a structure identical to the native human insulin, and, for that circumstance without antigenic power. The semi-synthetic insulin comes from laboratory transpeptidation of porcine insulin (exchange of alanine by threonine of aminoacid B_{30}), while biosynthetic insulin is obtained by means of genetic recombination process from bacterias (*Escherichia coli*) or yeasts. Today, biosynthetic insulin is the most frequently used in some countries.

On the other hand, insulin is a polypeptide hormone synthesized in the beta cells of the islets of Langerhans of the endocrine pancreas, and it is necessary for normal metabolization of glucose by most cells of the body. In diabetic persons the capacity of body cells to use glucose is inhibited, thereby increasing blood sugar levels (hyperglycemia). When high levels of glucose are present in the blood, the excess must be excreted in the urine (glycosuria). The symptoms derived from the disease are increased urinary volume, thirst, itching, hunger, weight loss, and weakness; in medical expression the classical findings are well known: polyuria, polydipsia, polyphagia, slimming, and asthenia [2, 3].

Diabetes affects an estimate of 366 million people worldwide, with type 2 diabetes mellitus (T2DM) accounting for more than 90% of the cases. Renal insufficiency is a common comorbidity condition in T2DM patients with chronic kidney disease (CKD,) defined as kidney damage or an estimated glomerular filtration rate (eGFR) < 60 mL/min/1.73m^2 for > 3 months. The kidney is both the origin and victim of elevated blood pressure. Hypertension is a pathogenic factor that contributes to the deterioration of kidney function. Therefore, management of hypertension (salt reduction intake adequate diet, exercise and antihypertensive drugs) has become the most important intervention control all modalities of chronic kidney disease (CKD). The role of hypertension in renal disease is crucial. The aged world population is increasing. The ageing is the most common risk factor for the development of hypertension and diabetes, as well as CKD [4].

2. Historical evocation

Diabetes was known some millenniums before the Christian era, and it was in India where the disease was more deeply studied during the ancient age. The first data come from the *Ayurveda,* texts concerning medicine writings (sankrit texts). The word *Ayurveda* means knowledge or "science life"; it has profound roots on the philosophy and Hinduistic spirituality; it was developed between years 3000 and 500 b.C. on the valley rivers of the Indian civilization. Its knowledge was transmitted orally from generation to generation through the verses known as *vedas*. At that time some documents showed detailed information about unquenchable thirst –polydipsia-in the diabetic patients, increased urine –polyuria-, and sugar in urine –glycosuria-. Instead of sweetened and viscous consistency of the urine, they described other symptoms such as halitosis, digestive and respiratory disorders, somnolence, tuberculosis, and forunculosis. The autochthonous black ants indirectly helped to detect this pathology. The physicians observed how ants and flies congregated around the urine being attracted by its taste. Based on that circumstance, it was called honey urine. Also, they pointed out that diabetes were more frequent in obese people, usually taking rice and sweeten food.

The majority of historians accept the papyrus form of 1862 close to the ruins of Luxor, the ancient sacred city of Thebes. The well-known document, a roll of papyrus by two meters long and thirty centimeters large, is a vast compendium with the totality of knowledge at the pharaohs era like at current texts of medicine. The physician-priest recommended, as treatment, fatty of calf, beer, leaf of mint, hippopotamus's blood and offering sacrifice to gods. The

http://dx.doi.org/10.5772/59130

antiquity of this document is about 3500 years; it was acquired and analyzed by the German Egyptologist George M. Ebers (1837-1898). It is currently kept in good conditions at the library of the University of Leipzig. The first description of diabetes appeared in this papyrus where polyuria was described. Celsus in the 1st century of our era established from his personal experience the "painless polyuria with dangerous emaciation". Areteus of Capadocia (century II), a Greek physician named the disease *diabetes;* in greek, *diabainein* means "to pass through", or "running throw" which is in relation to severe diuresis favourable to final outcome; and from Latin, *mellitus* (sweetened with honey). Claudius *Galenus* (3rdcentury) considered diabetes as a kidney disease. Thomas Willis (1621-1675) in 1675 found in the patients the sweetness of the urine, and William Cullen (1710-1790) proposed the term *mellitus*. The hereditary character of the disease was postulated by R. Morton in his text *Phthisiologia* (1689). Another historical event was made by P. Langerhans (1847-1888) when he described the pancreatic islets. Allen (1914) with an uniqueness criteria considered diabetes as a hereditary disorder of carbohydrate metabolism resulting in insufficient production of insulin. Since the discovery of insulin by Frederick Grant Banting, Charles Herbert Best and John Richard MacLeod, Nobel Prizes of Medicine in 1923, the prognosis of the disease is improving, although the *prevalence* still rises progressively from 5 % at age 20 to older people > 75 years.

The Canadian physiologist Frederick Grant Banting (1891-1941) and the medical student Charles Herbert Best (1899-1978) isolated insulin in Toronto in 1922. At that point, the new era on the treatment of diabetes was started. The results of the work by the German internist Oskar Minkowski (1858-1931) and Joseph von Mering (1894-1908) of removing the pancreas, led to the conclusion that the cause of diabetes resides in the lack of internal secretion of the Langerhans's islets placed in the pancreas.

Many researchers have dedicated their efforts to obtain the hormone against diabetes. In 1909, the Belgian Jean de Meyer named *insulin* the substance produced by the islets of Langerhans. Particularly, the internist Georg Ludwig Zülzer (1870-1949) was able to isolate after 1903 an effective compound. Nevertheless, two circumstances led him to abandon his work: a) uncontrollable toxic allergic reactions; and, b) overdose impossible to recognize for the absence of method of blood glucose determination. On July, 1921, the director of the Physiology Institute of Toronto, John James Richard MacLeod (1876-1935) provided to the young physician Frederick Grant Banting with a laboratory and ten dogs, and 21-year-old *student* Charles Herbert Best as his assistant. Banting and Best had been working to obtain insulin from a saline solution of triturated islets of pancreas. The extract was administered to diabetic dogs, by intravenous injection; simultaneously Best carried out continuous determinations of sugar in blood. This work made possible the new measuring methods that need only 0.2 ml of blood instead of 25 ml. After this finding Banting and Best studied better and easier procedures to obtain the hormone from cow fetus of four months. They discovered that the active substance was better extracted with acetone instead of acidulous alcohol. The decisive experiments were carried out between the 7 and 14th August of 1921.

After the first and successful achievements, MacLeod decided to interrupt any other investigation and focus on the insulin project: purification, control and manufacturing. The chemist James Bertram Collip (1892-1965) was able to obtain huge amounts of insulin and to success to its standardization. The latter is of capital importance because overdose can produce muscle spasm due to hypoglycemia.

Since the end of the 19thcentury, researchers have found the relationship between the pancreas and the metabolic disease –diabetes-. Some of them pointed out that the clinical problems are produced by the lack of a hormonal substance secreted by the endocrine pancreas or Langerhan's islets, although the German Oskar Minkowski (1858-1931) and others investigators failed to isolate this hormone. Edward Albert Sharpey-Schafer (1850-1935) coined the word "insulin"; he considered that insulin controls the hydrocarbonate metabolism and that the absence of insulin will be followed by hyperglycemia and an increase of glucose in urine. After that conclusion, pancreatic extract was given to diabetic patients; but unfortunately, this attempt was unsuccessful because the hormone was destroyed by the proteolytic enzymes. Also, the technical procedures for blood and urine glucose determinations available were rudimentary and with little accuracy. After numerous attempts, researchers obtained more purified insulin to be used in the clinical practice. Insulin was used for the first time in 1922 in a 14-year-old diabetic boy, who presented good results; it was the first publication concerning the efficacy of insulin in humans and was published in the prestigious journal *Canadian Medical Association Journal*.

One year later, in 1923, the Medicine Nobel Prize was awarded to Banting and MacLeod for his crucial medical milestone. In 1926, Jakob Abel found the synthesis of insulin; this finding was published in the *Proceedings of the National Academy of Sciences*, Washington, with the article entitled *Crystalline insulin*. After that, the era of insulin was started.

As it is well known, there are two modalities of the disease: insulin dependent diabetes mellitus or IDDM (type I) found in young people requiring daily insulin injection; although most cases of IDDM appear before age 20, the disease can develop late in life. In these patients, the necessary insulin is not secreted by the pancreas and hence must be managed by parenteral way. On the other hand, Type II, non-insulin dependent diabetes mellitus (NIDDM), adult onset diabetes, can be controlled by strict dietary restriction of carbohydrates, oral hypoglycemic agents (blood-sugar-lowering) and also insulin in some particular patients. The situation coming from sluggish pancreatic insulin secretion and concomitant tissue resistance to secreted insulin worsens insulin secretion by the beta cells. Anyway, despite the previous classification as juvenile or adult diabetes, either type can be observed at any age; however, NIDDM is the most common clinical presentation found in up to 90 percent of all forms of diabetes. The risk factors predisponing to type 2 diabetes are pointed out in table 1.

From the clinical point of view, to get a suitable control of the disease (blood glucose, glycated hemoglobin, lipids profile, body weight, and quality of life) it is crucial to ensure successful outcomes [table 2]. We must realize that subjects with asymptomatic, undiagnosed diabetes not unusually develop serious complications. Despite the absence of fasting hyperglycemia large-scale screening with glucose tolerance test should be established in many cases. Nowadays, the goals of therapy with insulin or oral agents for varied circumstances is frequently hazardous [5]. This particular point explains the urgent necessity to find better drugs (more effective and well tolerated). The way to reach this goal is, undoubtedly, the *clinical investigation;* in others words, *clinical trials* [6].

http://dx.doi.org/10.5772/59130

Family antecedents of diabetes (parents)
Obesity (Body Mass Index BMI >25 kg/m^2
Sedentarism
Race/ethnicity
Previously identified impaired fasting glucose (IFG), or impaired glucose tolerance (IGT)
Gravid diabetes mellitus (GDM)
HDL cholesterol < 35 mg/dl and/or triglyceride level > 250 mg/dl
Previous vascular disease
Acanthosis nigricans or polycistic ovary syndrome

Table 1. Risk factors predisposing to type 2 diabetes mellitus.

1. Symptoms of diabetes –polyuria, polyphagia, polydipsia, slimming or asthenia- plus random blood glucose level 200 mg/dl. Or
2. Fasting plasma glucose > 126 mg/ dl. Or
3. Two-hour plasma glucose (200 mg/dl) during an oral glucose tolerance test.
1) Random is considered at any time since the last meal
2) Fasting is defined as no food intake for previous 12 hours
3) Two-hours plasma glucose > 200 mg/dl during glucose tolerance test

Table 2. Clinical and laboratory criteria for diagnosis of diabetes mellitus

In 1912, two Boston researchers, F. G Benedict and Elliot P. Joslin, founder of the Joslin Diabetes Center –Boston-iniciated extensive metabolic balance studies in diabetic patients whose circulating blood glucose levels were high; they intended to control the disease by an strict dietary restriction of carbohydrates. And now, more than a century after the creation of the former institution, it continues the tradition of excellence recognized everywhere as a diabetes research, treatment, and teaching center. It is focused to improve the lives of persons with diabetes today and in the future. We now know that the excreted sugar coming from exogenous and endogenous proteins is converted in our body by the liver into glucose. But, in spite of the hard investigations, nowadays diabetes remains a difficult clinical problem mostly in the Western and developed countries.

3. Personal overview

Based on this controversial clinical status and related to our conventional duty since March 1990, our group in Granada (Spain) has created a *Hypertension and Lipid Unit*, and during the large *interim* period (twenty four years) until now, we have carried out a huge work by participating in several international clinical studies –more than one hundred fifty-focused mostly on hypertension and diabetes, but also on lipid disorders and ischemic heart disease; many of them are well recognized everywhere by prestigious publications using acronyms titles for an easier identification of them: SYST-EUR, HYVET, CONVINCE, VALUE, ONTARGET, TRANSCEND, TECOS, STABILITY, SAVOR, ODISSEY, OMNEON, LIXILAN, as well as other works in process and others scheduled to start in the near future.

Our participation in clinical trials about diabetes represents a big and continual effort in the most relevant clinical research of this important and crucial area. We believe and hope that the abstract's information (clinical and pedagogical) contained in this article will be suitable to many physicians (practitioners, internists, cardiologists, endocrinologists), chemists, nurses and others health professionals. Unfortunately, nowadays the knowledge concerning clinical trials and it relevance for research and health is very poor not only for physicians but also for the general population. We would like that the present book and particularly this chapter will offer some attractive and available information for a better knowledge of diabetes mellitus and current medical challenges.

From this particular contribution we present to the reader a conventional design of clinical trials commonly used everywhere. *Sensu lato*, the primary objective is to provide better benefits to diabetic patients by the new non commercialized drugs (phases II, III of clinical trials) matched to ordinary ones or placebo. To reach the aim of this research it is mandatory to have a huge financial support coming from pharmaceutical companies, with the indispensable contribution of investigators, patients, data managers, physicians, auxiliary staff, technical support, computer experts, nurses, etc. In summary, the following twenty items represents a schematic example common in many clinical trials in which we participated.

4. Conventional clinical trial design

A clinical trial is intended to produce credible results answering the questions raised about a drug or treatment without exposing patients to unnecessary risks.

It thus requires rigorous scientific methodology:

- In choosing the options in the methodology (study design, protocol, development, calculation of sample size, statistical analysis) which are the subject of another work in this collection.
- In conducting the trial: this is the objective of the rules of Good Clinical Practice (in research): use of procedures that leave little room for improvisation, validated techniques, suitable working methods, qualified staff, a paper trail documenting all steps, data that can be verified post hoc, which are the subject of this book.

A clinical trial is a project which involves different tasks and the final quality of its conclusions depends on the wakest link in the chain of events. Therefore, it is important to make a major effort in ensuring the quality of each area of interest involved, i.e. quality of documents,

http://dx.doi.org/10.5772/59130

medical products, monitoring, follow-up of adverse events, and the computerized data processing. In addition, the quality of trial should be "auditable" at all times, and hence the need for quality in archieving all documents [table3].

	Screening	**Run-in**	**Randomization**	**Randomized**	**Post-trial**
	V1	**V2**	**V3**	**Treatment**	
	W-3	**W-2**	**Day 1**	**Phase**	
				V4....	
				Day 6	
Screening period					
Single-blind placebo run-in		X	X		
Double-blind Treatment period			X	X	
TRIAL PROCEDURES					
Obtain informed consent. Inclusion/exclusion criteria	X				
Medical history	X				
Weight	X	X	X	X	
Physical examination					
12-lead electrocardiogram (ECG)			X	X	
Adverse event monitoring		X	X	X	
Vital signs (pulse, rate and blood pressure (measured duplicate)	X	X	X	X	
INSTRUCTIONS/ COUNSELING					
Diet and exercise					
Dispense glucose meter					
Introduction on dose recording					
OTHER MONITORING TEST					
CENTRAL LABORATORY TESTS					
Hematology	X	X	X	X	

	Screening	Run-in	Randomization	Randomized	Post-trial
	V1	V2	V3	Treatment	
	W-3	W-2	Day 1	Phase	
				V4....	
				Day 6	
Chemistry panel	X	X	X		
Lipid Panel Fasting plasma Glucose (FPG)	X	X	X	X	
Hemoglobin A1c (A1c)	X	X	X		
Urinalysis	X				
STUDY MEDICATION					
Dispense single-blind		X	X		
Placebo medication	X				
Medication compliance	X	X	X		

V1: visit 1; V2: visit 2, W-3: week 3; W-2: week 2; FPG: fasting plasma glucose.

Table 3. Conventional Model of Trial Flowchart

1.	**PRINCIPLES**	
	1.1.	Declaration of principle
	1.2.	Organization charts
	1.3.	Definitions of function
	1.4.	Writing, management and revising procedures
	1.5.	Principles of planning studies
2.	**DOCUMENTS**	
	2.1.	Investigator's brochure
	2.2.	Protocol* (standard plan, approved cycle, amendments)
	2.3.	Case report forms* (standard pages, approval channel)
	2.4.	Operations manual
	2.5.	Study report
3.	**PROTECTION OF PERSONS***	
	3.1.	Submission of project to a committee
	3.2.	Writing the documents to obtain consent

http://dx.doi.org/10.5772/59130

4.	**MONITORING***	
	4.1.	Initial visit(s)
	4.2.	Meeting to set up project
	4.3.	Intermediate visits
	4.4.	Final visit
	4.5.	Phone contacts
5.	**SERIOUS ADVERSE EVENTS**	
	5.1.	Definition of serious adverse events*
	5.2.	Collection, documentation of cases and follow-up
	5.3.	Reporting*
	5.4.	Causal relationship
	5.5.	Corrective measures
	5.6.	Crisis management
6.	**THE STUDY DRUG**	
	6.1.	Obtaining a standard drug (reference therapy)
	6.2.	Double-blind methodology
	6.3.	Jury of resemblance
	6.4.	Packaging*
	6.5.	Randomization list*
	6.6.	Labelling*
	6.7.	Release of finished product (pharmaceutical and for use)*
	6.8.	Dispatch – Reception*
	6.9.	Expiry date*
	6.10.	Drug accountability
	6.11.	Dispensing
	6.12.	Destruction
7.	**DATA**	
	7.1.	Progression cycle of CRFs
	7.2.	Deferred correction of data*
	7.3.	Coding
	7.4.	Computer entry of data
	7.5.	Test to validate data
	7.6.	Comprising a data base
	7.7.	Safeguards and protection

	7.8.	Computer systems (validation, documentation, use, security)
	7.9.	Statistical analysis
8.	**AUDIT AND INSPECTION**	
	8.1.	Audit of a study site
	8.2.	Audit of a study file
	8.3.	Systems audit
	8.4.	Preparation for inspection
9.	**LABORATORY VALUES**	
	9.1.	List of compulsory test
	9.2.	Quality control of assays
	9.3.	Centralized laboratory
10.	**DEVELOMENT**	
	10.1.	Designing a development plan
	10.2.	Monitoring a development plan
	10.3.	Coordination of a multicenter trial
	10.4.	Termination of a study center's participation
	10.5.	Termination of a trial
	10.6.	Termination of a product development
11.	**REGULATORY AFFAIRS**	
	11.1.	Declaration or request for authorization of a trial*
	11.2.	Relations with the competent authorities
	11.3.	Submission for registration
	11.4.	Insurance*
	11.5.	Import / export of drugs for clinical trials
	11.6.	Periodic reports
12.	**MISCELLANEOUS**	
	12.1.	Monitoring training programs
	12.2.	Trial with no direct individual benefit
	12.3.	Relations with sub-contractors
	12.4.	Corrective measures in case a document is lost
	12.5.	Publication
	12.6.	Abbreviations
	12.7.	Definitions
	12.8.	Archieving*

http://dx.doi.org/10.5772/59130

The procedures for the most part can be written by referring to the following plan.

1.	**Introduction**
–	Title of procedure and name of company
–	Objetive (summary in a few lines)
–	Other procedures simultaneously involved
–	Personnel involved
–	Date and number of ongoing version with the wording: "replaces previous version of..."
–	Date of application
–	Name of person responsible who approved this version.
2.	**Responsibilities: "Who?"**
–	Status of persons(s) responsible for carrying out each task stipulated in the procedure (by job title and not by name)
–	Status of person responsible for seeing that a procedure was carried out.
3.	**Operations**
–	What?
	Definition of the task
	Where does the operation begin and end?
–	Where?
	In-house or on-site; parent company or subsidiary?
–	When?
	Start: "as soon as..." (receipt of a document...)
	End: minimum, maximum duration
	Chronological flow-chart of events
–	How?
	Systematic description of steps and methods to be used (equipment, personnel, documents)
	Options, or variations planned (specify circumstances)
	Unplanned: How and whom to refer to?
4.	**Verification of tasks performed**
–	One or more checklist (dated and signed)
–	Model and circulation of report or written note
–	Distribution list
–	Measures to be taken when a check reveals non-compliance
5.	**History**
–	Dates of validity of different versions and a very succinct presentation of the reasons for the revision (one or two lines per version)

CORE PROTOCOL	
1.	Objectives and hypotheses
–	Primary
–	Secondary

2.	Study Endpoints: Primary, Key secondary endpoints.
3.	Evidence of a personally signed and dated informed consent document indicating that the patient has been well informed about all aspects of the study.
4.	Subject/patients:
	4.1. Inclusion Criteria. Subject eligibility should be reviewed and documented by an appropriate qualified scientific study team before inclusion in the trial.
	4.2. Exclusion Criteria.
5.	Trial Design and Duration
6.	Pre-randomization visit.
	6.1. Randomization visit. Following completion of the run-in period, subjects will be randomized for active drug and in some cases for placebo. The goal for blood glucose, glycated 6.2. hemoglobin or other biological parameters has been established by any protocol submitted for investigation. For example, group 1 (drugs), group 2 (drugs or placebo).
7.	Trial Visits. General information. Informed Consent
8.	Follow-up of subjects.
9.	Drug supplies.
	These items include formulation and packaging, preparation and dispensing, administration, doses adjustments, drug storage, and accountability.
10.	Study Procedures.
	The specific procedures, including laboratory test to be performed at all study visits. Blood draw must be taken in the morning before 12.00 p.m.; ECG, and others parameters, and, in some cases, X-Ray, or other diagnostic imaging procedures. It must be taken in the same day in order to offer more facilities to patients.
11.	Data Collection.
	The case report forms to be used are designed to collect an appropriate amount of data necessary for the study.
12.	Administrative and Regulatory Details.
13.	Analysis of the End-point.
14.	Quality Control.
15.	Committees.
	The Coordinating Office and investigators will follow the principles of *Good Clinical Practice*. According with law, the trial information will be recorded in all electronic or papers forms and keep it during 10-15 years after the end of the study.
.	The Committee structure is very similar from one trial to another. The members of the committees will be detailed at the end of the publication, and also an appendix for acknowledgments will be provided
	On the other side, the members of the Data Monitoring Committee are not investigators of the trial. A National Coordinator for each country is desirable. The Steering Committee is responsible for agreeing the protocol, any change to the protocol and for the general running of the trial. The monitoring and statistical Committee (Data Monitoring Committee) will be responsible for quality control of the data, monitoring recruitment and other important aspects of the investigation.
16.	Data analysis / Statistical Methods. Steering Committee, Scientific Committee.
17.	Ethical aspects.
	Ethical conduct of the study.

http://dx.doi.org/10.5772/59130

	Subject information and consent.
	Subject recruitment.
18.	Definition of the end of trial.
19.	Periodical audit.
	During the study frequent external audit to the data and investigators will be done.

5. Diabetes mellitus a medical challenge

Type 2 Diabetes Mellitus (DM) accounts for more than 90% of all diabetes. This disorder is a worldwide epidemic affecting an estimate of 366 million adults aged 20-79 years, according to data from 2011. The prevalence of this metabolic disorder in adult population is expected to go from 8.3% to an estimate of 9.9% by 2030, resulting in an increase in the number of people with diabetes worldwide up to 552 million.

Unfortunately, many people are unaware that they have diabetes. The figures reveal that over six million Americans are undiagnosed. The proportion is very similar in other Western countries. The disease is commonly discovered when the typical symptoms, previously mentioned, are developed and high blood sugar levels are found, defined as a daytime level greater than 200 milligrams per deciliter or a fasting level greater than 120 milligrams per deciliter. In some cases oral glucose tolerance test is required for undiagnosed people.

The relationship between glycemia and the risk of microvascular disease has been well-established. The results of the *Diabetes Control and Complications Trial* (DCCT), the *United Kingdom Prospective Diabetes Study* (UKPDS) [7], and the *Action in Diabetes and Vascular Disease: Preterax and Diamicron Modified-Release Controlled Evaluation* (ADVANCE) *Trial* [8], demonstrated that patients with DM treated to lower glycemic targets have reduced rates of microvascular complications (e.g., retinopathy and nephropathy). However, results of more recent trials including ADVANCE, the *Action to Control Cardiovascular Risk in Diabetes* (ACCORD), and *Veterans Affairs Diabetes Trial* (VADT) [9] aimed for an A1c <6.0, and ADVANCE aimed for an A1c<6.5%. These and other data have more recently led to a movement away from blanket prescriptive targets for A1C (e.g. <6.5% or <7%) and to the growing consensus among diabetes experts that glycemic targets and glucose-lowering therapies should be individualized. Age, weight, and comorbidities such as established cardiovascular disease, and kidney or liver disease are among the patient's factors that should be considered by physicians, nurses, family, and others. Diet, exercise, and education remain the main stay of treatment for diabetic patients in order to avoid serious complications [10]. In addition, there are several classes of oral antihyperglycemic agents (AHA) available for use as monotherapy or as combination therapy, including the dipeptidylpeptidase (DPP-4) inhibitor class, which is administered either once or twice daily [11, 12, 13].

In general, medication adherence in chronic diseases, such as diabetes may be low, ranging from 36% to 93%. Side effects associated with oral antihyperglycemic agents therapies, including hypoglycemia, (sulfonylureas, meglitinides, insulin), weight gain, (sulfonylureas, meglitinides, insulin, hypersensitivity reactions, thiazolidinediones) and gastrointestinal intolerance, nausea, vomiting (metformin, alpha-glucosidase inhibitors) are common patient-reported reasons for poor medication adherence. Many studies have demonstrated that adherence to antihyperglycemic agents therapy is related to the number of pills prescribed: several studies have reported that, when patients were prescribed multiple drugs to treat diabetes, adherence significantly decreased, with reductions ranging from 15% to 54%. A prospective study showed a mean adherence of 79% for a triple-daily regimen, 65% for a twice-daily regimen, and 38% for a thrice-daily regimen. Some data from osteoporosis therapies indicate that, compared to a once-daily regimen, a once-weekly treatment can increase medication adherence and compliance. Therefore, a once-weekly oral AHA therapy might improve treatment adherence in many patients with these metabolic disorders.

6. Epidemiology and social relevance of diabetes

It's well established that diabetes mellitus is a serious health problem in the worldwide population and the most frequent metabolic disease, but, it is hard to know the real incidence in the general population. There are several causes to hold up the adequate epidemiological knowledge: a) the number of studies is limited and difficult to compare among them; b) in many patients diagnosis of DM is not established mostly in older people with very poor symptoms because of the absence of the conventional common disorders: polyuria, polydipsia, polyphagia, weight loss, and asthenia; c) unfortunately, in several cases the diagnosis of diabetes is not reported in the death certificate.

The prevalence in the European countries varies between 2% and 19.5% per 100.000 inhabitants/year; but the incidence of diabetes increases with age and other factors such as more expectancy life, obesity, increase of glucose intake, and a better and early detection of the disease. Another important feature of the disease is it chronic and progressive character that need treatment for life, acute and chronic complications, and high morbidity and mortality rate. Unfortunately, the current trend towards the increasing incidence worldwide is a reality; with this preface diabetes will be a leading cause of clinical problems for the foreseeable future.

We must not forget that DM includes a group of common metabolic disorders characterized by the presence of hyperglycemia usually followed by glycosuria. There is a number of types of diabetes related to a complex interaction between genetic factors, environmental influence, and lifestyle of patients. The consequences of the metabolic dysregulation secondary to this disorder lead to changes in different organ systems and affect the health and future of many patients. For example, this disease is the leading cause of end-stage renal disease, lower extremity amputations, adult blindness, and chronic heart failure. The therapeutic procedures are aimed at controlling diabetes; in other words, glycemic < 100 mg/dl, negative glycosuria and glycated hemoglobin < 6%.

All patients must be put on an appropriate diet personally designed to help them to reach and maintain normal body weight and to restrict their intake of carbohydrates and fats. They must be encouraged to exercise daily (at least 30 minutes walking), which improves the movement of glucose into muscle cells and blunts the rise in blood glucose that follows carbohydrate

http://dx.doi.org/10.5772/59130

ingestion. In all cases, the objective of diabetes treatment is to keep the level of blood sugar within normal values (90-100 mg/dl) as well as to reduce metabolic complications, such as diabetic ketoacidosis, hypoglycemia, hyperosmolar coma, or lactic acidosis, and late complications such as circulatory abnormalities, nephropathy, neuropathy, foot ulcers, frequent infections, and retinopathy (retinal changes leading to blindness).

Recent researches into the area of treatment include pancreas transplantation and implantable mechanical insulin infusion system, new medication, as oral hypoglycemic agents, different modalities of insulin, and recent monoclonal antibodies given by intradermal injection way.

From another point of view, it's well known that some clinical trials have demonstrated how angiotensin – converting enzyme (ACE) inhibitors decrease mortality for stroke, myocardial infarction, and other heart problems in patients with cardiovascular disease or high risk diabetes. Nevertheless, up to 20% of patients –mostly women-are unable to tolerate captopril, enalapril, ramipril or others ACE drugs mainly due to persistent and improductive cough, or even other side effects such as hypotension, renal dysfunction or angioneurotic edema, according to our personal experience [14, 15]. *The Action in Diabetes and Vascular Disease: preterAx and DiamicroN Controlled Evaluation* (ADVANCE) Trial, using perindopril combined with gliclazide was designed to assess outcome of macrovascular and microvascular disease on diabetic patients [15]. Ramipril did not affect heart failure events in low-risk patients according to the findings reported in the DREAM Study [16]. It's possible to believe that when the absolute risk of heart failure is low, angiotensin-converting enzyme inhibitors and angiotensin-receptor blockers are not able to reduce the incidence of heart failure. Myocardial infarction rate was lower in TRASCEND study compared to HOPE trial. It is possibly due to that patients included in the TRASCEND study were at lower risk compared with those admitted in HOPE (Heart Outcomes Prevention Evaluation) Study Ongoing Trial [17]; the population of women was about 40% in the TRASCEND study while only 2% was reported in ONTARGET trial, and other previous studies of ACE inhibitors.

It is also important to realize, according to numerous clinical experiences and data from TRASCEND study, that telmisartan (angiotensin-receptor blockers) could be regarded as a potential treatment for patients with vascular disease or high-risk diabetes when the patients are unable to tolerate antihypertensive drugs as ACE inhibitors.

Concerning hypertension and based on data from many large-scale clinical trials, international guidelines recommend two drugs with subsequent complementary mechanisms of action to control BP in most patients, with initial combination therapy when Systolic Blood Pressure (SBP) is 150 mmHg or Diastolic Blood Pressure (DBP) is > 100 mmHg above target [18, 19]. These guidelines also favour the use of a fixed dose combination for the clinical practice [20].

From the clinical point of view, it is significant to understand the strong pathophysiological relationship between diabetes and hypertension. The latter is predicted to rise dramatically with a number of cases expected to reach 1560 million worldwide by 2025 [21]. Unfortunately, this is coupled with low rates of BP control (target <130/80 mmHg), despite the increased use of antihypertensive treatment. It must be emphasized an early and sustained BP control in order to reduce the long-term burden associated with this condition. To address challenges for now and the future, some international guidelines recommend early treatment with agents that have complementary mechanism of action. These combinations have benefits related to compliance, efficacy and safety for the patients.

The difficulty in getting good metabolic and clinical control of BP in many patients, may result in the development of acute clinical disorders or chronic complications. Physicians must keep in mind when the patient develops acute confusional states or coma; these events could be due to DM *per se*, or other pathologies developed in those patients, such as hepatic failure, renal disease, stroke, respiratory distress, poisoning or drug overdose; the distinction between coma secondary to inadequate level of insulin, and non diabetic disease is crucial for the prognosis of the patients.

7. Acute metabolic complications

Patients with diabetes are susceptible to four acute metabolic complications: hypoglycemia, ketoacidosis, hyperosmolar and lactic acidosis. All of them can result in coma. The two first are complications of IDDM, while the other two are usually developed in the setting of NIDDM. These clinical situations must be considered completely different from severe disorders that occur not related to DM *per se* such as stroke, acute heart failure, hepatic dysfunction, in others words: *coma* in *diabetic patients* is completely different for *diabetic coma*.

Unfortunately, a lot of patients developed coma situations despite the treatments available, generally caused by incorrect dose, or medication missed dose. This is the relevant point to consider other possibilities, and the way is clinical trial.

Diabetic ketoacidosis. It is often caused by cessation of insulin administration but it may result from physical (infection, surgery, traumatism) or emotional stress despite continued insulin therapy. Several complications can be present in diabetic ketoacidosis: erosive gastritis or acute gastric dilatation manifested by pain, vomiting of blood, or weight lost, cerebral edema with or without neurological signs or coma, increased potassium serum (cardiac arrest); myocardial infarction, respiratory distress syndrome, or thrombosis events.

Hyperosmolar coma. This modality of acute diabetes complication is usually due to NIDDM. It is characterized by a profound dehydration resulting from a sustained hyperglycemic diuresis by situations in which the patient is unable to drink enough water to keep up normal urinary excretion of detritus. This situation commonly occurs in elderly patients often living alone or in a nursing home. They develop stroke or bacterial infection that worsens adequate water intake. Hyperosmolar coma can also be caused by peritoneal dialysis or hemodialysis, the use of osmotic agents such as manitol and urea. Clinically, patients show extreme hyperglycemia, hyperosmolality and central nervous system disorders (seizure activity, transient stroke, hemiplegia or clouded sensorium and coma). Pneumonia, gram-negative sepsis or others infections are also very common. Bleeding probably caused by disseminated intravascular coagulation, acute pancreatitis and widespread thrombosis is usually found at necropsy.

http://dx.doi.org/10.5772/59130

Lactic acidosis. It is a serious clinical finding that can occur because of an increase in endogenous lactic acid, the final step of the carbohydrate metabolism. That causes profound effects on the respiratory, cardiac and nervous systems. The blood pH drop suddenly and is accompanied by an increase in respiratory ventilation (Adolph Kussmaul, 1822-1902), depression of cardiac contractility, pulmonary edema and altered central nervous system function manifested with headache, lethargy, stupor, or in such patients even coma. The prognosis is very bad and most of the patients die soon.

8. Late complications

Diabetic patients are susceptible to developing several complications responsible for morbidity and early mortality; some of them do not present problems, whereas in others, complications appear early, usually after the appearance of the hyperglycemic symptoms developed between 15 and 20 years after the onset of the disease [table 4]. The clinical findings showed the following circulatory abnormalities: atherosclerosis, coronary artery disease, stroke, heart failure, peripheral vascular disease and left ventricular failure.

Microvascular Complications
Ocular disease
Retinopathy
Proliferative
Nonproliferative
Neuropathy
Mono-and polyneuropathy
Nephropathy
Macrovascular complications
Coronary artery disease
Peripheral vascular disease
Stroke
Others
Infections
Dermatology problems
Genitourinary (sexual dysfunction)
Cataracts
Psychological disorders
Glaucoma

Table 4. Late complications developed in diabetic patients

8.1. Diabetic retinopathy

Is a relevant cause of blindness; however a high number of diabetic patients never lose the vision. When the occlusion of retinal capillaries occurs, it results in a subsequent formation of saccular and fusiform aneurysm and arteriovenous shunt. Hemorrhages into the inner retinal surface are dot-shaped; conversely, bleeding into the superficial larger nerve fiber produces flame-shaped, blot-shaped or linear lesions. Cotton-wool spots can be observed by angiography, and sudden increase of the number of these lesions has an ominous prognostic sign and is the beginning of rapid progress of retinopathy. Hard exudates are common findings and are probably related to leakage of protein and lipids from damaged capillaries. The lesions must be summarized into two categories: *simple* (microaneurysms, dilated veins, hard exudates, arteriovenous shunts, hemorrhage, cotton-wool spots, increased capillary permeability and capillary closure, and dilation) and *proliferative*: new vessels, vitreous hemorrhage, retinitis proliferans (scar) and retinal detachment.

8.2. Renal disease

Despite the worldwide importance of diabetic nephropathy as a cause of mortality and morbidity, many questions still remain about treatment aimed at delaying its harmful effects [22, 23]. So far, there is little scientific evidence to support strict glycemic control at this stage, although common sense dictates that wild swings of control should be avoided. Protein restriction may have a role but the studies to support this have not been forthcoming.

9. Circulatory changes

We recognize hypertension and DM as common disorders, but there is much evidence to suggest that the two occur together more frequently than by chance. Development of hypertension greatly worsens the prognosis of diabetic patients. Raised BP accelerates the progress of diabetic nephropathy, and possibly retinopathy, while the harmful cardiovascular effects of the two disorders are at least additional. There are a number of reasons why hypertension and diabetes may be associated, and these are discussed in this contribution.

Life expectancy is reduced in diabetic patients, both insulin-dependent (IDDM) and non-insulin dependent (NIDDM), and the leading causes of death are cardiovascular complications. The excess mortality cannot be explained by the diabetic state *per se*. Based on the Whitehall study of more than 17.000 civil servants followed for 15 years, Jarrett and Shipley suggested that diabetes and cardiovascular disease may not be causally linked at all but might rather share a common, possibly genetic antecedent. Among the known risk factors for cardiovascular disease in diabetes, hypertension has attracted much interest. The prevalence of hypertension is increased in diabetic patients, IDDM and NIDDM, and hypertension is known to be a powerful risk factor for cardiovascular disease in diabetes, insulin treated or not.

It's well known that hypertension has also a consistent relation to coronary heart disease and other risk factors which are not only found by the presence of proteinuria. Furthermore, the

http://dx.doi.org/10.5772/59130

clinical significance of hypertension as an important risk factor was recently strongly supported by two independent studies on IDDM patients, demonstrating an improved survival rate in the decade following the introduction of efficient antihypertensive drugs.

Hypertension is a community problem everywhere with hazardous solution. It is the major risk factor for development and progression of the disease in non-diabetic and diabetic chronic kidney disease. About one billion people worldwide have high BP (defined as > 140/90 mmHg), but the number is higher considering the present criteria of >130/80 mmHg, and it is expected to increase up to 1.56 billion patients by 2025. The predicted prevalence of hypertension will increase by 24 per cent in developed countries.

Hypertension control rate, defined as BP level < 130/80 mmHg, is substantially lower in patients with CKD, particularly in those with diabetes and chronic renal failure. This is illustrated by the National Kidney Foundation's (USA) Kidney Early Evaluation Program (KEEP), a US-based health screening program for individuals at a high risk for kidney disease.

Hypertension is the most prevalent cardiovascular disease in the world and a major public health issue. Cardiovascular disease is the leading cause of mortality worldwide and is expected to increase with the general ageing of the world's population. The goal of antihypertensive therapy is to reduce the incidence of blood pressure-related morbid events and cardiovascular mortality.

It is well established that heart is an important target organ in hypertension. Continuous high BP level is associated with myocardial problems, such as left ventricular hypertrophy and increases the burden of coronary artery disease (CAD). These forms of damage may result in congestive heart failure, CAD manifestations, arrhythmias and sudden cardiac death. The event rates of cardiovascular disease in Japan, for example, differ from those in Europe and the United States. Mortality from CAD in the Japanese country is one-third that of the United States, and mortality from cerebrovascular disease is 1.5 times higher in Japan than that reported in the United States. Hypertension is the most common cause of disease and is even more prevalent in the Japanese population than in the Western countries. The percentage of cerebral bleeding is two or three times greater than in Caucasian people from Europe and the United States, and cerebral infarction is mostly caused by lacunar type ischemic stroke owing to hypertensive small vessel disease. The incidence of athero-thrombotic infarction or cardio-embolic infarction is currently increasing in Japan, and the dominant pathogenetic factor for stroke is changing from small arterial disease to large arterial disease in Japanese hypertensive patients. These differences may be partly explained by differences in the lifestyle of Japanese and Western populations, which are reflected in body mass index (mean BMI: 23.25 and 28-30 kg/m^2, respectively). However, most of mortality-morbidity trials have been carried out in the Western countries, in which none or only a minority of East Asian patients were included. Owing to the scarcity of large-scale trials in East Asian people, it remains to be determined whether the results from similar clinical trials in Western societies are internationally applicable to East Asian races or the Japanese population, or whether genetic background can cause different pharmacokinetic and pharmacodynamic responses to the same drug.

There is a clear and substantial evidence in juvenile onset IDDM that strict BP control by reducing and maintaining levels under 130/80 mmHg or a mean arterial pressure of 105 mmHg remains the only effective treatment for the physician to try to slow the development of end stage renal failure and the need for renal support. In practical terms, the use of a combination of drugs including diuretics will be often required. The newer classes of drugs such as ACE inhibitor or calcium channel blockers have a clear advantage in their side-effect profile over betablockers in diabetics, because they are safer and better tolerated. The primary goal remains effective in BP control and often beta-blockers may need to be added to the regime to achieve this.

In patients with IDDM aged older than sixty and in diabetics with nephropathy who are non-insulin dependent, there is no definitive scientific evidence that prognosis is improved and that the progression to end stage disease is slowed after antihypertensive treatment. It is reasonable for the physician to assume that aggressive treatment of BP in this group is justified from data of several studies in younger patients. A crucial question remains about the degree of BP reduction required and in particular whether it is necessary or indeed harmful to aggressively reduce systolic BP in this group. Accurate long-term clinical trials with measurement of cardiovascular end points as well as the slowing of GFR decline and reduction of proteinuria need to be carried out. Indeed, it is important to reach normal BP levels especially on the stage of incipient nephropathy in order to obtain better therapeutic results in patients.

Large scale, long-term multicenter studies in both IDDM and NIDDM patients with proteinuria will be required to give a clear answer to the question of whether there is a selective benefit of the ACE inhibitor group over a suitable hypotensive agent such as a calcium channel blockers. So far, there is some evidence that ACE inhibitors used in the evolution of nephropathy or when employed later in combination with diuretics are effective in reducing protein excretion which may be separate from their BP lowering capacities. These data, make them a reasonable choice in the antihypertensive regime of diabetics with nephropathy. This property to reduce proteinuria without reducing BP has not been shown with any other antihypertensive agents and until and unless such evidence is forthcoming, the careful use of ACE inhibitors in combination with diuretics can be recommended in diabetic nephropathy. As many of these patients will have occult or manifest cardiovascular dysfunction, this approach may be beneficial also in improving cardiac performance. Future studies, especially in non insulin-dependent patients should evaluate the potential benefit of reducing morbidity and mortality from cardiovascular disease with the newer antihypertensive drugs, such as ARA II.

Coexisting hypertension and diabetes act as additive risk factors to accelerate vascular complications. The incidence of coronary and cerebral vascular diseases is much higher in hypertensive than in normotensive diabetic patients. Mortality rates in diabetic patients with systolic BP exceeding 160 mmHg is four times higher than that of other diabetic individuals. Whereas antihypertensive therapy has been clearly shown to retard deterioration of renal function and urinary albumin excretion, evidence that pharmacological control of BP reduces overall mortality in the diabetic population without overt nephropathy is strikingly lacking. Thus, current recommendations for drug intervention in diabetics with hypertension rely on data derived from the general hypertensive population. Specific adjustments in drug selection

http://dx.doi.org/10.5772/59130

and dosage need to be made for drug effects which might be of particular significance in the diabetic patient. Nevertheless, a recent alarming retrospective study from the Joslin Clinic demonstrated that antihypertensive treatment is associated with a marked increase in cardiovascular mortality in diabetic hypertensive patients. The most obvious implication of this finding is the need for large scale prospective studies in diabetic hypertensive individuals to assess the risks and benefits in treating hypertension in this population. Some of the newest strategies for BP control must be examined and compared with these retrospective findings. Until further information becomes available, much attention should be given to careful drug selection, therapy monitoring, and judicious and continuous assessment of coexisting risk factors in the course of treatment of high BP in diabetes.

10. Etiology of chronic diabetes complications

The cause of diabetic complications is still unknown and probably multifactorial. Chronic complications of DM affect many organ systems and are responsible for the majority of morbidity and mortality. Special attention must be given to the metabolic conversion of glucose to sorbitol. This one is implicated in the pathogenesis of neuropathy, retinopathy, aortic disease, nephropathy and lens damage (cataracts). Another mechanism of possible pathogenetic relevance is glycation of proteins. The effect of glycation on hemoglobin is well known; in addition, other proteins are altered by the same mechanism such as plasma albumin, fibrin, collagen, lipoproteins, and low protein. Retinopathy, nephropathy and neuropathy are considered common disorders of microvascular complications; and stroke, gangrene, and myocardial infarction for macrovascular complications [table 4].

11. Can diabetic complications be prevented?

This is an important and fascinating question strongly related with the patient prognosis. Hyperglycemia or other aspects of the abnormal metabolism of diabetes are responsible for the development of complications; additional factors, which maybe genetic, have also a pathogenic influence. The clinical practice shows the mistery; how diabetic patients suffering for decades from poor control are free of late complications; however typical complications can be found at the time of diabetes diagnosis, even in the absence of fasting hyperglycemia. Intensive therapy for all diabetic patients with strict dietary control is essential. The role of the family doctor, specialist and other professionals –nurses, nutritionists, auxiliary persons, etc-, are very important for these particular patients.

12. Miscellaneous findings on diabetes

Because diabetes affects almost every body systems, the patients can develop several symptoms and complications. The chapter of I*nfections* is large. In some cases this finding may not occur more frequently than in non diabetic population, but it seem to be more severe probably because in diabetic patients leukocyte function is impaired and subsequently accompanied by poor control. Also this population is particularly prone to four unusual infections with strong relationship with diabetes –focus on skin, urinary tract, lungs, and bloodstream. *Malignant external otitis*, usually due to *Pseudomonas aeruginosa* tends to appear in older population and is characterized by severe pain in the ear, fever, and leukocytosis. The facial nerve becomes paralyzed in 50% of the cases, but other crucial nerves can be involved. *Emphysematous cholecystitis* tends to affect diabetic men and diagnosis is established when gas is seen in the gallbladder wall or during non invasive imaging examination.

Hypertriglyceridemia is common in diabetics and is related to overproduction of VLDL (*Very Low Density Lipoprotein*) in the liver and to a defect of metabolization on the peripheral tissues. The latter is due to a deficiency of lipoprotein lipase, an insulin-dependent-enzyme. It is important to know that some patients have high level of lipids profile even when diabetic disease is controlled; probably these cases have a primary familial hyperlipoproteinemia, a circumstance independent of DM. Of course, these patients must be treated for lipids disorder –hypertriglyceridemia and lipids hypercholesterolemia with HMG-CoA reductase inhibitors such as lovastatin, pravastatin, simvastatin, fluvastatin, atorvastatin, rosuvastatin, as mode of action that reduces cholesterol synthesis and increases LDL receptors; ezetimibe reduces the absorption of lipids from diet at the intestinal level; and fibric acid derivatives –↓ LPD and tryglyceride, hydrolysis, VLDL synthesis, ↑ LDL catabolism. Patients can also suffer from a variety of skin lesions: necrobiosis lipoidica diabeticorum, candida albicans, vaginal moniliasis, in women, hypertrophy of fat, bullosis diabeticorum, diabetic dermopathy, atrophy of adipose tissue, Dupuytren's contractures, and schleroderma. Additional illnesses such as the prevalence of eating disorders can be seen particularly in young women.

13. Physical examinations of diabetic patients

Either complete physical examination or brief physical examination will be performed at the time points specified in the Time and Events Table.

The complete physical examination will include evaluation of the following organ or body systems:

- Skin (including injection site)
- Head, eyes, ears, nose, and throat
- Thyroid
- Respiratory system
- CV system, BP
- Abdomen (liver, spleen)
- Lymph nodes (neck, axilas, inguinal)

- Central nervous system
- Extremities

The brief physical examination will include evaluation of the following organ or body systems:

- Skin (including injection site)
- Respiratory system
- CV system
- Abdomen (liver, spleen)
- Central nervous system

14. Conclusions

The term of diabetes mellitus includes a group of some metabolic disorders characterized by hyperglycemia with secondary damage to multiple organ systems such as end–stage renal disease, lower extremities amputations, and adult blindness. The way to ameliorate this crucial situation is to obtain better drugs for an early treatment of the patients. The clinical trials, is so far, the best procedure to offer more efficient treatments to the increasing diabetic population, thanks to the procedures of clinical trials [24, 25].

Acknowledgements

We thank Mrs. Esperanza Velasco Rodríguez for help in the English translation. Financial sources: Department of Medicine. FIBAO ("Foundation of Basic Investigation Alejandro Otero"); and of course, to our patients for the altruistic and caring participation in the studies.

Author details

Blas Gil Extremera[1*], Pilar Jiménez López[2], Alberto Jesús Guarnido Ramírez[2], Elizabet García Peñalver[2], Maria Luz Abarca Martínez[2] and Isabel Mérida Fernández[2]

*Address all correspondence to: blasgil@ugr.es

1 University of Granada, Spain

2 University Hospital "San Cecilio", Granada, Spain

References

[1] Gil Extremera B. Los premios Nobel de Medicina. InScience Communications (Edit). Madrid, España., 2012.

[2] Pedro Pons A. Patología y Clínica Médicas. Enfermedades de la sangre y de las glándulas endocrinas. (Tomo V), Salvat S.A. (Edit.) Barcelona. España 1976

[3] Gil Extremera B. La medicina, pasado y presente. Alhulia (Edit), Granada. España (2008).

[4] Bakris GL, and Ritz E, on behalf of the World Kidney Day Steering Committee. The message for World Kidney Day 2009: Hypertension and Kidney disease –a marriage that should be prevent. J. Hum. Hypertens. 2009; 23: 222-225.

[5] American Diabetes Association. Clinical Practice Recommendations. Diabetes Care 2006; 29: 531-537.

[6] Inzucchi S E, Bergenstal RM, Buse JB, et al. Management of Hyperglycemia in Type 2 Diabetes: A patient-Centered Approach. Diabetes Care 2012; 35: 2012

[7] UK Prospective Diabetes Study (UKPDS) Group. Intensive blood-glucose control with sulfonylureas or insulin compared with conventional treatment and risk of complications in patients with type 2 diabetes (UKPDS 33). Lancet 1998; 352: 837-853

[8] Patel A. MacMahon S. Chalmers J, et al. Intensive blood glucose control and vascular outcomes in patients with type 2 diabetes. ADVANCE Collaborative Group. N Engl J Med 2008; 358: 2560-2577

[9] Gerstein HC, Miller ME, Byington RP, et al. Effect of intensive glucose lowering in type 2 diabetes. Action to Control Cardiovascular Risk in Diabetes Study Group. N Engl J Med 2008; 358: 2545-2559

[10] Shamoon H, Duffy H, Fleischer N, et al. The Diabetes Control and Complications Trial Research Group. The Effect of intensive treatment of diabetes on the development and progression of long-term complications in insulin-dependent diabetes mellitus. N Engl J Med 1993; 329: 977-986

[11] Reaven PD, Moritz TE, Schwenke DC, et al. Intensive glucose-lowering therapy reduces cardiovascular disease events in veterans affairs diabetes trial participants with lower calcified coronary atherosclerosis. Veterans Affairs Diabetes Trial. Diabetes 2009; 58: 2642-2648

[12] Drucker DJ, Sherman SI, Gorelick FS, et al. Incretin-based therapies for the treatment of type 2 diabetes: evaluation of the risks and benefits. Diabetes Care 2010;33:428-433

[13] Xu L, Man CD, Charbonnel B, et al. Effect of sitagliptin, a dipeptidyl peptidase-4 inhibitor, on beta-cell function in patients with type 2 diabetes: a model-based approach-Diabetes Obes Metab 2008; 10: 1212-1220

[14] The Heart Outcomes Prevention Evaluation (HOPE) Study investigators. Effects of ramipril on cardiovascular and microvascular outcomes in people with diabetes mellitus: results of the HOPE study and MICRO-HOPE substudy. Lancet 2000; 355: 253-259

[15] Patel A, Mahon S, Chalmers J, et al. ADVANCE Collaborative Group. Effects of a fixed combination of perindopril and indapamide on macrovascular and microvascular outcomes in patients with type 2 diabetes, insulin (the ADVANCE trial): a randomized controlled trial. Lancet 2007; 370: 829-840

[16] DREAM Trials investigators. Effect of ramipril on the incidence of diabetes. N Engl J Med 2006; 355: 1551-1562

[17] Yusuf S. Gerstein HS, Hoogwerf B, et al, for the HOPE study Investigators. Ramipril and the development of diabetes. JAMA 2001; 286:1882-1285

[18] Bulpitt Ch, Beckett NS, Cooke J, Dumitrascu DL, Gil Extremera B, Nachev C, Nunes M, Peters R, Staessen JA and Thijs L, on behalf of the Hypertension in the Very Elderly Trial (HYVET) Working Group. Results of the pilot study for the Hypertension in the Very Elderly Trial. J Hypertens 2003; 21: 2401-2409

[19] Gil Extremera B, Ma PT, Yulde J, et al. The adjunctive effect of telmisartan in patients with hypertension uncontrolled on current antihypertensive therapy. Inter J Clin Pract 2003; 57: 861-866

[20] Mancia G, de Backer G, Dominiczak et al. 2007 Guidelines for the Management of Arterial Hypertension: The Task Force for the Management of the European Society of hypertension (ESH) and of the European Society of Cardiology (ESC). J Hypertens 2007; 25: 1105-1187

[21] Kearney PM, Whelton M, Reynolds K, et al. Global burden of hypertension: analysis of worldwide data. Lancet 2005; 365: 217-223.

[22] Whiting DR, Guariguata L, Weil C, Shaw J. IDF diabetes atlas: global estimates of the prevalence of diabetes for 2011 and 2030. Diabetes Res Clin Pract 2011; 94: 311-321

[23] Gerstein HC, Miller ME, Byington RP, et al. Effects of intensive glucose lowering in type 2 diabetes. Action to Control Cardiovascular Risk in Diabetes Study Group. N Engl J Med 2008; 358: 2545-2549

[24] Spriet A, Dupin-Spriet T. Good practice of clinical drug trials. 3rd edit. S-Kurger, Basel. 2005

[25] Miralles García MªC, and Gil Extremera B. Diabetes Mellitus: (I):1989; 75: 361-376. Cuadro clínico y diagnóstico (II): 1989; 75: 461-474. Tratamiento (III): 1989; 75: 537-557. Complicaciones agudas y crónicas (IV). Actualidad Med 1990; 76: 47-54

Section 2

Treatment of Diabetes

Chapter 6

Pharmacological Treatments for Type 2 Diabetes

Roberto Pontarolo, Andréia Cristina Conegero Sanches, Astrid Wiens, Cássio Marques Perlin, Fernanda Stumpf Tonin, Helena Hiemisch Lobo Borba, Luana Lenzi and Suelem Tavares da Silva Penteado

Additional information is available at the end of the chapter

http://dx.doi.org/10.5772/59204

1. Introduction

Type 2 diabetes mellitus (T2DM) is the most common type of diabetes, which is defined as a chronic metabolic disorder characterized by hyperglycemia. In this disease, the body is able to produce insulin; however, its secretion is irregular and/or the body's cells fail to use and respond appropriately to this hormone (insulin resistance), leading to an accumulation of blood glucose [1, 2].

Although the reasons for the development of T2DM are still unknown, it is a multifactorial disease that involves a genetic predisposition as well as other factors, including a poor diet, sedentary lifestyle, age (45 or older), previous gestational diabetes, and overweight or obese physical conditions, which represent the most common risk factors for the development of insulin resistance [3, 4].

Epidemiologically, the number of individuals with T2DM (representing 85-95% of all cases of diabetes mellitus) in recent decades has increased rapidly worldwide. This disease usually affects adults, especially males, but an increase in the number of cases in children and adolescents has also been observed [5, 6]

The high incidence of T2DM is associated with economic development, aging populations, increasing urbanization, dietary changes, reduced physical activity and changes in lifestyle and other cultural patterns. It is estimated that more than 382 million people suffer from this disease worldwide (8.3% prevalence). In 2013, 5.1 million deaths were reportedly caused by diabetes. If these trends continue, it is estimated that by the year 2035, approximately 592 million people (1 in 10 adults) will be carriers of the disease [7-9].

Therefore, the increasing number of new cases of diabetes per year combined with high prevalence and mortality rates impose high costs socially and economically to the populations of all countries. In 2013, approximately 548 billion dollars were spent worldwide on diabetic patients. Thus, understanding this disease and all the variables involved, including prevention, diagnosis and treatment must be a priority [8].

The diagnosis of T2DM is based on summarized plasma glucose quantification criteria (either fasting or after a glucose tolerance test). Furthermore, the assessment of the amount of glycated hemoglobin (Hb_{A1c}) is included as a diagnostic option for diabetes. However, many individuals with T2DM are asymptomatic in the early stages of this disorder and only discover the disease after the onset of more severe symptoms and other complications. The first symptoms of T2DM may include polyuria, polydipsia, constant hunger, appearance of wounds with delayed healing, visual changes and frequent infections [10, 11].

When undiagnosed or poorly controlled, this disease is a risk factor for the onset of various complications at both the microvascular (nephropathy, retinopathy and neuropathy) and macrovascular (cardiovascular disease) level. Diabetes is one of the major factors that leads to blindness, kidney failure, lower limb amputation and development of cardiovascular disease, the latter being the primary cause of death worldwide [3, 11].

Therefore, simple lifestyle changes, including increased physical activity, diet modification and weight loss are recommended for the management of pre-diabetes and early diabetes. These changes have been shown to be effective in preventing or delaying the progression of T2DM or damage to target organs [4, 12].

The treatment of diabetes mainly targets glycemic control, thus aiming to relieve symptoms, improve the quality of life of patients, prevent further complications and reduce mortality. However, the use of other therapeutic treatments is needed as a strategy for reducing multi-factorial risks [3, 13].

The basic strategies for the treatment and control of diabetes mostly consist of a specific balanced diet, physical activity and proper use of medications (oral and/or insulin agents). Patient education coupled with self-care and support from family and physicians are essential procedures for the prevention of acute complications and reduction of long-term complications. Additionally, frequent tests (including blood pressure measurement and lipid profile), foot care (avoiding the appearance of lesions), stress control and reduction in the consumption of alcoholic beverages and tobacco are important actions related to disease control [1, 14, 15].

Compared with type 1 diabetes mellitus patients, the majority of type 2 patients typically do not require daily insulin doses. The disease can be treated with oral medications and changes in lifestyle until resistance becomes difficult to control, after which an insulin regimen is usually required [8].

Thus, drug treatment of T2DM is based on the knowledge of patient characteristics together with the severity of the hyperglycemia and availability of therapeutic options. Many oral drugs are used to control diabetes, such as metformin (biguanide), sulfonylureas and thiazolidinediones, which have been used for decades with satisfactory results. These antidiabetic drugs compose the most studied cast of oral pharmacologicals worldwide and play an important role in glycemic control; in addition, they are often recommended as the first option for the treatment of the disease by the American Diabetes Association (ADA) and European Association for the Study of Diabetes (EASD) [10, 15, 16]. Technological advances and new avenues of drug research have enabled the development of new drug therapies for the treatment of T2DM, and approximately 180 new drugs are currently under study [17, 18].

Typically, various drug classes can be used to control type 2 diabetes, including human insulin analogs, drugs that reduce insulin resistance (biguanides and thiazolidinediones or glitazones), secretagogues and their analogues (sulfonylureas, meglitinides, inhibitors of dipeptidyl peptidase IV (DPP-4) or agonists and analogues of glucagon-like peptide-1 (GLP-1)), and drugs that reduce the rate of carbohydrate degradation (alpha-glucosidase inhibitors). Dapagliflozin is one of the newer medications for glycemic control and was recently approved by the FDA (January 2014). Its mechanism of action inhibits the sodium-glucose cotransporter 2 (SGLT2), a protein responsible for glucose reabsorption in the kidney, which leads to the elimination of excess glucose in the urine [17, 18].

Multiple therapies, or a combination of oral hypoglycemic drugs and/or other drugs, are also an option for the control of diabetes mellitus [11, 19]. However, the therapeutic use of drugs is limited by factors such as their efficacy, adverse events, costs, side-effects, dose management problems, inflexible dosages, weight gain, etc.; therefore, such effects should be critically evaluated for each patient [19].

For example, weight loss is a priority in obese diabetics. If glycemic control is not achieved after 4-6 weeks of treatment with drugs that increase sensitivity to insulin action (such as biguanides and thiazolidinediones) medications may be given to control obesity, which include drugs that affect the appetite and induce satiety, such as orlistat. If necessary, drugs may also be used that retard the degradation of sugars in the diet (such as acarbose or miglitol) or drugs such as sulfonylureas or meglitinides that increase insulin secretion in the pancreas [20-23].

In terms of therapeutic classes, the action of biguanides, whose main representative is metformin, is related to decreased peripheral insulin sensitivity, reduced hepatic glucose output, and modified lipid metabolism. All of these effects contribute to the control of T2DM. The advantages of these drugs include the absence of hypoglycemia and its anorectic effect, which also aids in patient weight loss. The adverse effects of this class are few but include diarrhea, nausea, metallic taste and intestinal colic, which gradually decreases with continued use [16, 19, 23].

The class of sulfonylureas that act by directly stimulating insulin secretion (secretagogues) includes chlorpropamide, glibenclamide, gliclazide and glimepiride. These drugs have several adverse effects, including nausea and vomiting (gastrointestinal), hypoglycemia (glucose), leukopenia, agranulocytosis, thrombocytopenia and hemolytic anemia (hematological) and weight gain. Accordingly, the use of newer insulin secretagogues (glinides class, including mitiglinide, repaglinide and nateglinide) is suggested as an alternative for patients treated with sulfonylureas who have irregular meal times or late postprandial hypoglycemia. Because of their rapid absorption, the action of these drugs is initiated 30 minutes after administration [16, 22].

The thiazolidinedione drugs (pioglitazone and rosiglitazone) are oral hypoglycemic agents capable of increasing the sensitivity of liver, muscle and fat cells to insulin, which results in reduced peripheral resistance. This class is contraindicated in patients with hepatic dysfunction and heart conditions and adverse effects include upper respiratory tract infections, headaches, weight gain, anemia and edema [12, 16, 23].

With respect to alpha-glucosidase, competitive inhibitors such as acarbose, miglitol and voglibose act as antagonists of amylase and sucrose, thereby decreasing the intestinal absorption of glucose. These drugs are contraindicated in pregnant or lactating patients and in diabetic patients with renal or hepatic dysfunction [6, 18].

Another recent class of oral hypoglycemic drug is the DPP-4 inhibitors (sitagliptin, vildagliptin and saxagliptin), which act by increasing the levels of hormones that help to control glucose concentrations. These drugs have few adverse events, and incidences of hypoglycemia and weight gain are low [16, 23].

In addition to these oral medications, subcutaneous administration of exenatide (GLP-1 agonist) can stimulate insulin secretion (secretagogue). In addition to facilitating glycemic control, this medicine also helps in patient weight loss. Possible adverse events include nausea, vomiting and diarrhea [16, 23, 24]

For injectable drugs, the application of human insulin analogs (lispro, aspart and glargine) for the treatment of T2DM may be indicated for patients who no longer respond to diet combined with exercise and oral hypoglycemic agents or in more severe hyperglycemia cases. In addition to the different types of administration (including the innovation of inhalable insulin), this hormone may be used in combination with oral hypoglycemics [12, 25].

In short, with the emergence of new treatments for diabetes, various individualized treatment options are possible that consider ease of access, cost, mode of administration and patient characteristics.

Thus, the aim of this chapter is to evaluate the available treatments for T2DM as well as their mechanisms of action and adverse effects and describe the new drugs and therapeutic trends that are available. Such diabetes treatment updates for healthcare professionals and caregivers is essential for proper disease management and health promotion.

2. Biguanides

Metformin and phenformin are oral antidiabetic drugs of the biguanide class. Metformin is the drug of choice for the treatment of adults with type 2 diabetes because of its lower frequency of side effects. This drug is currently used by nearly one-third of the diabetic patients in Italy and is the most prescribed in the U.S. (> 40 million prescriptions in 2008). Phenformin is no longer marketed in many countries, although it is still available in Italy [26-28].

Both metformin and phenformin increase weight loss in obese non-diabetic patients without substantially reducing blood glucose levels. This weight loss is attributed to the drugs' anorectic effect and a slight reduction in the gastrointestinal absorption of carbohydrates [29]. Phenformin was withdrawn from clinical practice in the 1970s because of a greater tendency to develop severe and fatal adverse events, such as lactic acidosis.

2.1. Metformin

Metformin is sold in 500 and 850 mg tablets, and the maximum dosage is 2.5 g/day, although there are reports in the literature of dosages up to 3 g, which are always administered after meals to minimize gastrointestinal side effects [30]. It has been reported that this drug increases the number and improves the affinity of insulin receptors both in adipocytes and muscle. In muscle, glucose uptake increases from 15 to 40% and gluconeogenesis is stimulated. In adipocytes, metformin inhibits lipolysis and the availability of free fatty acids (FFA). Furthermore, metformin improves insulin action in the liver by reducing hepatic glucose production from 10 to 30%, and at the cellular level, it increases the tyrosine kinase activity of the insulin receptor in the muscles, which stimulates GLUT4 translocation and the activity of glycogen synthetase [31].

The use of metformin also improves the lipid profile by decreasing triglyceride levels by 20-25%, LDL-cholesterol by up to 10% and plasminogen activation inhibitor (PAI-1) by 20-30% and increasing HDL-cholesterol by 17%. Insulin secretion to stimuli may remain unchanged or decrease, and its anorectic effect helps in weight loss. In addition to being associated with weight reduction, its effectiveness in glycemic control is similar to that of sulfonylurea [32]. Another advantage is the absence of hypoglycemia because insulin secretion is not stimulated [33].

The isolated use of metformin in type 2 diabetes lowers blood glucose levels by approximately 25%, or 60 to 70 mg/dl, and glycosylated hemoglobin by 1.5 to 2% [31]. Intensive glucose control using metformin significantly decreases the risk of cardiovascular disease and diabetes mellitus-related mortality and is associated with less weight gain and a lack of treatment-induced hypoglycemia associated with insulin or sulfonylureas [34].

Metformin is absorbed in the intestine, excreted by the kidneys and minimally metabolized by the liver. Metformin has a low affinity for mitochondrial membranes and does not interfere with oxidative phosphorylation, and it is indicated as a monotherapy in obese or even glucose intolerant diabetics. Approximately 5 to 10% of patients each year fail to have an appropriate response to this drug. In these cases, metformin can be used in combination with sulfonylurea, acarbose, thiazolidinediones, repaglinide and/or insulin to achieve satisfactory control [35-40].

The most common side effects of metformin are diarrhea (15%), metallic taste and nausea, which often decrease with continued use of the medication. The occurrence of lactic acidosis is rare (0.03 to 0.4/1000/year) and occurs most often in people who have a contraindication to metformin, such as chronic liver disease (elevated transaminases 2-3 times the normal values) and heart, respiratory, or renal conditions (clearance < 70 ml/min or serum creatinine ≥ 1.5 mg/dL). The use of metformin is not advisable in people over 80, pregnant women, infants or alcoholics. In patients with proteinuria who are subjected to radiological examination containing iodine, it is prudent to provide adequate hydration and discontinue the medication a few days prior to such examinations [33]. This drug shows a synergistic effect with cimetidine and may decrease the absorption of vitamin B12 [30].

3. Thiazolidinediones

The thiazolidinediones (TZDs) are popularly known as glitazones, and representatives include the drug troglitazone (withdrawn from the market because of liver toxicity), rosiglitazone and pioglitazone (second generation TZDs).

TZDs are widely used in the treatment of type 2 diabetes and increase and sensitize insulin action in the liver, muscles and adipocytes, thereby decreasing peripheral resistance. They activate intracellular nuclear receptors (PPAR-gamma-peroxisome proliferator-activated receptor) that regulate the expression of genes encoding glucose and lipid metabolism and are responsible for glucose uptake mediated by insulin in the peripheral tissues and differentiation of preadipocytes into adipocytes. Additionally, these drugs inhibit peripheral lipolysis in adipocytes and assist in reducing the levels of free fatty acids and visceral adipose tissue, resulting in improved glycemic and metabolic parameters. These drugs show good results in terms of long-term glycemic control compared with other consecrated therapeutic options, such as sulfonylureas and metformin [41-43].

TZDs decrease glucose levels by approximately 20% but do not increase insulin secretion. They inhibit the oxidation of long-chain fatty acids in the liver, decreasing gluconeogenesis and the availability of free fatty acids. Although these drugs reduce triglycerides by 15 to 20% and increase HDL-cholesterol by 5 to 10%, the total cholesterol and LDL-cholesterol levels may not change or may increase from 10 to 15% [33]. When compared to metformin, troglitazone has a greater potentiating effect of peripheral insulin action and little effect on the reduction of hepatic glucose production. The association of thiazolidinedione with metformin is interesting because it produces additive effects [39].

TZDs also increase the expression of glucose transporters (GLUT4) and lipoprotein lipase and reduce the expression of leptin and tumor necrosis factor (TNF-alpha). These results make it one of the most widely prescribed classes for the treatment of T2DM [33, 44].

Side effects occur in less than 5% of patients, and they consist of upper respiratory tract infections, headaches, elevated transaminase levels, edema, weight gain and anemia. Hypoglycemia can occur when its use is concomitant with secretagogues or insulin. The drugs are contraindicated for use in children and pregnant women and in individuals with liver disease and elevated transaminase levels (2-3 times the reference values) [33].

3.1. Troglitazone

In mice subjected to arterial injury, troglitazone inhibited the growth of vascular smooth muscle cells and intimal hyperplasia, suggesting that TZDs decrease the progression of atherosclerosis. Diabetic patients treated with troglitazone show decreases in platelet adhesion, activation of plasminogen activator inhibitor (PAI-1) and blood pressure levels. These multiple effects strengthen its indication for the treatment of the metabolic syndrome. However, caution is advised with troglitazone treatment because of possible liver complications, including fatal cases. In addition, caution is required when troglitazone is used with cardiac patients because of the possibility of edema [33, 45, 46].

3.2. Pioglitazone

Pioglitazone may be used as a monotherapy or in combination with metformin (increasing the anti-hyperglycemic effect), sulfonylurea, meglitinide, or even insulin, especially in diabetic patients with metabolic syndrome. The dose varies from 15 to 45 mg, which can be administered once a day. Pioglitazone displays a similar mechanism of action and side effects as rosiglitazone and less liver toxicity than troglitazone. However, it can interact with other drugs that are metabolized by P_{45} enzymes and alter their serum levels. An example is a decrease of approximately 30% of the contraceptive effect of ethinyl estradiol and norethindrone. Therefore, the contraceptive dose should be increased in diabetic women who do not wish to become pregnant. Its pharmacokinetics are not altered by mild to moderate renal impairment, so dose modification is required [47].

3.3. Rosiglitazone

Rosiglitazone is more powerful and has less liver toxicity than troglitazone. Additionally, it does not induce metabolism by cytochrome P_{450} (CYP) 3A4; thus, there is no interaction with oral contraceptives such as digoxin, ranitidine, nifedipine, etc. The rosiglitazone dose varies from 4 to 8 mg, which can be administered once a day. Similar to pioglitazone, rosiglitazone's pharmacokinetics are not altered by mild to moderate renal impairment, so dose modification is required [48].

Recently published safety data have raised concerns related to a possible association between the chronic use of rosiglitazone and increased risk of cardiovascular events, which is consistent with the use of TZDs in clinical practice. In addition, recently published studies have indicated that there is a loss of bone mass and increased possibility of fracture in patients using these medications [42, 44, 49].

4. Meglitinides

Insulin secretagogue agents act by stimulating endogenous insulin secretion via pancreatic β cells, and they include classes of sulfonylureas and meglitinides used in the treatment of T2DM. Meglitinide analogues consist of a relatively new class of oral hypoglycemic, and their clinical use in adult patients with T2DM was approved in 2000. These drugs were developed to promote the rapid increase in insulin secretion from β cells and therefore affect postprandial glucose levels. The mechanism of action of meglitinides is quite similar to that of sulfonylureas; however, meglitinide analogues have the advantage of a reduced risk of hypoglycemia because of their shorter half-life. Meglitinides are secretagogues of short-acting insulin, and they act primarily on postprandial hyperglycemia. Because of their characteristics, the meglitinides are preferable to insulin secretagogues such as sulfonylureas, especially in elderly patients [50-53]. Representatives of the meglitinide class include repaglinide, nateglinide and mitiglinide derived from benzoic acid and the amino acid D-phenylalanine, whose action is initiated approximately 30 minutes after administration because of rapid absorption. The advantages of these drugs are that they have no interactions with other drugs and are not contraindicated in pregnancy, during lactation or in the presence of other pathologies [52, 54].

4.1. Repaglinide

Repaglinide was the first meglitinide analogue approved for use in adults with T2DM; it is the S(+) enantiomer of 2-ethoxy-4-(2-((3-methyl-1-(2-(1-piperidinyl) phenyl)-butyl) amino)-2-oxoethyl) benzoic acid and has a molecular weight of 452.6 Da [50]. Repaglinide stimulates insulin release in a rapid action style, thereby promoting a decrease in blood glucose levels. Because of the rapid action, repaglinide is one of the most commonly used antidiabetic drugs in patients who have high postprandial glycemia [55-57].

The mechanism of action by which the meglitinide analogue stimulates insulin secretion comes from blocking the ATP-dependent potassium channels (KATP) of pancreatic β-cells, which results in membrane depolarization and calcium influx through voltage-dependent calcium channels. This mechanism culminates in an increased influx of calcium into the β cells, which stimulates exocytosis of insulin-containing granules [50, 58].

With regard to pharmacokinetics, repaglinide, whose absorption is independent of concurrent food intake, is rapidly absorbed following oral administration with 63% bioavailability. The maximum concentration is reached approximately 45 minutes after administration (Tmax ~ 45 min), and the half-life of plasma elimination is relatively short (approximately 1 hour); therefore, the drug is eliminated from the body within 6 hours. The drug is metabolized in the liver via cytochrome P_{450} (CYP3A4), with approximately 90% of the metabolites excreted in the bile and only 8% secreted in the urine. Altogether, 2% of the drug is eliminated in an unchanged form, and because the metabolites are not biologically active, there is no effect on the blood glucose. There is a rapid elimination of repaglinide through the biliary tract and no apparent accumulation in the plasma after multiple doses [50, 59-61].

Hepatic metabolism via cytochrome P_{450} means that concentrations of repaglinide may be increased by concomitant use of substances that inhibit the CYP3A4 enzyme, such as certain antibiotics and steroids; however, the concomitant intake of CYP3A4-inducing agents, such as barbiturates and carbamazepine, can lead to an increased metabolism of the meglitinide analogue, thus reducing its concentrations [50, 59-61].

4.2. Nateglinide

Another insulin secretagogue agent that also belongs to the class of meglitinides corresponds to nateglinide. Similar to repaglinide, nateglinide ((N-[(trans-4-isopropylcyclohexyl)-carbonyl]-D-phenylalanine A-4166) phenylalanine derivative) acts through the inhibition of KATP and causes the depolarization of the plasma membrane of β cells. This culminates in the influx of calcium ions into the cell and subsequent secretion of insulin [50, 62].

Despite the similar mechanism of action of these two meglitinide analogues, in vitro studies have demonstrated that nateglinide inhibits KATP channels faster and with a shorter duration of action than repaglinide. In addition, the half-life of repaglinide at the receptor of action is approximately 3 minutes, whereas the half-life of nateglinide is 2 seconds. Therefore, the time required for nateglinide to dissociate from the receptor is 90 times faster than that of repaglinide, so nateglinide has a very fast and ephemeral effect on insulin release. In vitro experiments have demonstrated that the action of nateglinide is enhanced in the presence of glucose compared to that glyburide and repaglinide, so that the response of the KATP channel with nateglinide is significantly less in periods of euglycemia than in periods of hyperglycemia. Thus, the minimum total insulin exposure generated by this meglitinide analogue protects the body against hypoglycemic attacks and allows the patient greater flexibility in relation to the intervals between meals. Pharmacodynamic studies have demonstrated that when nateglinide is administered before meals in type 2 diabetic patients, a secretion of early stage insulin occurs that causes a significant dose-dependent reduction in postprandial hyperglycemia [50, 59, 63].

Regarding its pharmacokinetic properties, nateglinide is absorbed rapidly, with peak plasma concentrations reached within 1 hour. This drug is rapidly eliminated from the plasma, with a half-life of 1.8 hour. Because of the short half-life, nateglinide is not accumulated at any administration dose. The drug is metabolized mainly via the cytochrome P_{450} (CYP2C9 and CYP3A4) and is eliminated via the kidneys, with 10% eliminated unchanged in the urine and 20% eliminated unchanged in the bile [50, 59, 64].

Both repaglinide and nateglinide may be used as a monotherapy or in combination with other agents, such as metformin and glitazones. The meglitinides have similar abilities in reducing fasting blood glucose, postprandial levels of plasma glucose and early insulin secretion, and they improve the insulin sensitivity and function of pancreatic β cells. However, repaglinide was more effective in reducing the glycosylated hemoglobin Hb_{A1c} and is also preferred to nateglinide in patients with chronic renal disease because nateglinide has active metabolites that are eliminated by the kidneys [52, 63].

4.3. Mitiglinide

Mitiglinide ((-)-2(S)-benzyl-4-(cis-perhydroisoindol-2-yl) butyric acid) is the third meglitinide analogue and corresponds to a benzylsuccinic acid derivative. It presents a similar mechanism of action to the other two meglitinide analogs, and its selective action on KATP channels of pancreatic β cells promotes insulin secretion with few adverse effects on the cardiovascular system [58, 59, 65]. Similar to nateglinide, mitiglinide is often used in early stage diabetes mellitus because it induces a rapid and short duration of postprandial insulin secretion, mimicking the normal insulin secretion and glucose metabolism of healthy individuals and thereby promoting a reduced risk of hypoglycemia [66, 67]. A randomized clinical trial demonstrated a similar efficacy between mitiglinide and nateglinide when used as a monotherapy in patients treated with diet and exercise in the three months leading up to trial [68].

Mitiglinide is rapidly absorbed and eliminated by the body [66] and metabolized in the kidneys and liver and generates metabolites with little of the secretory activity of insulin. The half-life of mitiglinide is 1.48 h [54], and it has been shown to prevent increases in oxidative stress and inflammation markers after meals in patients with diabetes mellitus because of the suppression of postprandial hyperglycemia promoted by this drug [69]. Because of its characteristics, mitiglinide is currently considered an ideal drug for the treatment of T2DM and is widely used in clinical practice [54].

5. Alpha-glucosidase inhibitors

The competitive inhibitors of alpha-glucosidase, such as acarbose, miglitol and voglibose, are administered orally and inhibit alpha-glucosidase, which is an enzyme that converts polysaccharides (e.g., amylase, maltase and sucrase) into monosaccharides, thus acting as an antagonist enzyme. Therefore, such inhibitors decrease the intestinal absorption of glucose, particularly postprandial absorption that modulates insulin secretion [70]. The slower rise in postprandial blood glucose concentrations is potentially beneficial in both type 1 and type 2 diabetes. In older patients with type 2 diabetes, acarbose may also increase insulin sensitivity [71]. These inhibitor lower the incidence of cardiovascular events, and they have no systemic absorption [72].

In addition, alpha-glucosidase is inhibited competitively, and its availability for oligosaccharides derived from the diet is reduced. Thus, there is a reduced formation of monosaccharides and less insulin is required for metabolism, which leads to a reduction of glucose (because it is not absorbed) as well as postprandial insulin-induced increases [73]. These effects reflect a significant decrease in glycated hemoglobin, which was observed in a meta-analysis of 41 trials of alpha-glucosidase inhibitor therapy (primarily acarbose trials) in which beneficial effects were observed (compared with placebo) on Hb_{A1c} (-0.77 percentage points), fasting, and postload glucose and postload insulin levels. These benefits are more evident in highly hyperglycemic patients. Hyperglycemia in patients with mild or moderate glycemic control is less common than in those using other oral antidiabetic agents. In such cases, competitive inhibitors of alpha-glucosidase can be used in combination with insulin or any other oral hypoglycemic agents [74-76].

The most frequent side effects of alpha-glucosidase inhibitors are observed at the intestinal level and include flatulence, diarrhea, abdominal pain and elevated transaminases [35, 77-79]

The occurrence of hypoglycemia and an increase in body weight are rare because the agent does not stimulate insulin release or hypersecretion. These effects are only observed when miglitol is combined with other therapies, and its use is contraindicated in cases of inflammatory bowel disease, pregnancy, lactation, and hepatic or renal impairment. In one prospective study of 893 patients treated with acarbose, only 16 to 20% were still taking the drug after one year, and half of the patients had stopped the drug during year two because of the side effects [80].

Recently, a mixed-treatment comparison (MTC) meta-analysis showed that there was no significant increase in hypoglycemia risk or body weight with alpha-glucosidase inhibitors [81].

5.1. Acarbose

Acarbose has a microbial origin and is structurally similar to natural oligosaccharides, with an affinity 104-105 times higher than drugs of the same class of alpha-glucosidases. With regard to its pharmacokinetic aspects, acarbose is poorly absorbed in the intestine (less than 2%). The products produced by bacterial enzymes cleave acarbose, yielding intermediate 4-methyl pyrogallol, which is conjugated and excreted as sulfates or glucuronidate [75].

Several trials have demonstrated the efficacy of acarbose in patients with type 2 diabetes [35, 82-85]. In one trial, 96 patients who were inadequately controlled by diet alone were randomly assigned to receive either glyburide or acarbose, and their Hb_{A1c} values and fasting blood glucose concentrations fell by a similar amount; the postprandial blood glucose concentrations, however, remained high in the glyburide group but fell in the acarbose group [83]. A second trial evaluated 354 patients treated with diet alone or diet plus a sulfonylurea, metformin or insulin. Compared with the placebo, the addition of acarbose in each of these groups reduced the mean postprandial blood glucose concentration and lowered the Hb_{A1c} values [35]. In general, acarbose has resulted in a greater improvement of Hb_{A1c} values than in fasting blood glucose concentrations, which is consistent with its predominant effect on postprandial hyperglycemia [85].

In a randomized, double-blind, placebo-controlled trial [82], satisfactory control of fasting and postprandial glucose occurred with acarbose in T2DM. In a multicenter, randomized, double-blind, placebo-controlled clinical trial [83] conducted for patients with T2DM who were subjected to a specific diet and use of insulin, the patients showed decreased levels of blood glucose and glycated hemoglobin as well as a reduced daily requirement for insulin.

In a systematic review of the literature, it was concluded that acarbose inhibits postprandial hyperglycemia by lowering insulin levels after a glucose overload. However, it presents no advantages with respect to corporal weight or lipid metabolism, and there are no statistically significant effects on mortality, morbidity and quality of life in patients with T2DM. Compared with the placebo, acarbose reduces Hb_{A1c}, fasting plasma glucose and postprandial glucose. Compared with sulfonylureas, it reduces glycemic control and has major adverse effects, particularly gastrointestinal effects [76]. Thus, treatment with acarbose might have a favorable effect on endothelial function in type 2 diabetes patients with ischemic heart disease [86-90]

5.2. Voglibose

Voglibose also has a microbial origin, and only 3-5% of the drug is absorbed at the intestinal level. It is a potent inhibitor of alpha-glucosidase, but it is weaker than acarbose in the inhibition of sucrase and has little effect on pancreatic alpha-amylase [75]. Furthermore, voglibose decreases the level of postprandial glucose with very low risk of hypoglycemia, but it is associated with frequent gastrointestinal side effects [91].

5.3. Miglitol

Miglitol has a synthetic origin and unique pharmacokinetic properties. It is absorbed rapidly through a transport mechanism in the jejunum that is close to the mechanism of glucose, and it is quantitatively excreted unchanged by the kidneys. Miglitol differs from acarbose because it does not inhibit alpha-amylase but rather inhibits intestinal isomaltase [75].

Based on studies in which miglitol was given alone or in combination with insulin or a sulfonylurea, the efficacy was similar to that of a placebo [92-95]. Miglitol is also effective when combined with metformin [96]. Thus, miglitol can be expected to suppress postprandial glucose more strongly than acarbose [97], so it should reduce the incidence of cardiovascular events [98].

6. Sulfonylureas

Another class of drugs used in the treatment of T2DM are the sulfonylureas chlorpropamide, acetohexamide, tolazamide and tolbutamide (first generation), glibenclamide, glipizide, gliclazide (second generation) and glimepiride (third generation). This class has long been established in the treatment of diabetes, and it was the first oral glucose-lowering medication to be introduced into clinical practice in the 1950s and has since been recognized as a first-line therapy as either a monotherapy or in combination [85, 99]. In the United Kingdom, sulfonylureas have been the second-line choice after metformin [100]. Furthermore, sulfonylureas are the drug of choice for type 2 diabetics who do not benefit exclusively from diet and exercise [101, 102].

Sulfonylureas usually lower blood glucose concentrations by approximately 20% and Hb_{A1c} by 1 to 2% [103, 104]. Recently, a systematic review of double-blind randomized control trials found that sulfonylurea monotherapy reduced Hb_{A1c} by an average of 1.5% (16 mmol/mol) compared with that of placebo groups [99, 105]. These drugs are most effective in patients whose weight is normal or slightly increased. In contrast, insulin should be used in patients (regardless of age) who are underweight, losing weight, or ketotic despite adequate caloric intake. Some of these latter patients may actually have type 1 diabetes, which can be confirmed by the presence of islet cell antibodies [106, 107].

Sulfonylureas act as insulin secretagogues and exert their main action on islet β cells, stimulating insulin secretion and thereby reducing the plasma glucose concentration. The mechanism of action involves binding of the drug to the subunit SUR1 of the ATP-sensitive potassium channels in the plasma membranes of β cells; these channels are then closed, which leads to a change in the membrane voltage, calcium influx and exocytosis of insulin granules [108-111]. The ATP-sensitive potassium channels are also present in other tissues but often contain different types of SUR subunits (e.g., SUR1 in β cells, SUR2A in heart cells, SUR2B in smooth muscle cells). The sensitivity of these different types of channels to sulfonylureas is variable [110].

The net effect of sulfonylureas is an increased responsiveness of β cells to both glucose and non-glucose secretagogues (such as amino acids), resulting in more insulin being released at all blood glucose concentrations. Thus, sulfonylureas are useful only in patients with some β cell function. Sulfonylureas may also have extrapancreatic effects, which includes an increased tissue sensitivity to insulin; however, the clinical importance of these effects is minimal [101, 103].

The basal secretion and insulin secretory response to various stimuli are intensified in the early days of treatment with sulfonylureas. With long-term treatment, circulating insulin levels decline to levels that occurred before treatment; however, despite this reduction, the decreased plasma glucose levels are maintained. The mechanism for this response is still unknown but may be associated with reduced plasma glucose, which allows the circulating insulin to have more pronounced effects on their target tissues, as well as the impairment of insulin secretion by chronic hyperglycemia.

Sulfonylureas are well absorbed after oral administration by the gastrointestinal tract. However, the presence of food and hyperglycemia may reduce their absorption. The peak plasma concentrations occur within 2-4 hours, and the duration of the effect varies. All of these drugs bind tightly to plasma albumin and are involved in interactions with other drugs (e.g., salicylates and sulfonamides) such that there is competition for binding sites. All sulfonylureas are metabolized by the liver, and their active metabolites are mostly excreted in the urine; thus, their action is increased in elderly patients or those with renal or hepatic disease.

The choice of sulfonylurea is primarily dependent upon cost and availability because their efficacy is similar. However, because of the relatively high incidence of hypoglycemia in patients taking glyburide or chlorpropamide, shorter acting drugs should be used, especially in elderly patients [112]. In a patient who is not a candidate for metformin or cannot tolerate metformin as initial monotherapy, a shorter-duration sulfonylurea such as glipizide is suggested.

6.1. First-generation sulfonylureas

The first-generation sulfonylureas vary considerably in their half-lives and the extent of their metabolism. The acetohexamide half-life is short, but the drug is reduced to an active compound whose half-life is similar to that of tolazamide and tolbutamide (4 to 7 hours). If required, these drugs can be divided into daily doses. Chlorpropamide has a long half-life (24 to 48 hours) [113]

The action of chlorpropamide, acetohexamide, tolazamide and tolbutamide is long lasting, and there is substantial excretion in the urine. Therefore, these drugs can cause severe hypoglycemia in elderly patients who have experienced a progressive decline in glomerular filtration. These drugs cause flushing after alcohol consumption and exert similar effects to that of the diuretic hormone on the distal nephron, producing hyponatremia and water intoxication [113].

6.2. Second-generation sulfonylureas

The second-generation sulfonylureas (glibenclamide, glipizide and gliclazide) are more potent, but their hypoglycemic effects are not much improved, and they fail to control blood glucose, which is commonly observed with tolbutamide. All of these drugs contain the sulfonylurea molecule, but different substitutions result in differences in pharmacokinetics and duration of action. Glibenclamide should be avoided in the elderly and patients with mild renal impairment because of the risk of hypoglycemia because several of its metabolites are excreted in the urine and are moderately active [113].

The sulfonylureas cross the placenta and stimulate insulin release by fetal β cells, causing severe hypoglycemia at birth. Consequently, their use is contraindicated during pregnancy, and gestational diabetes is treated by diets supplemented with insulin when required [113].

In general, sulfonylureas are well tolerated. The observed side effects are hematological, including hypoglycemia, leukopenia, agranulocytosis, thrombocytopenia, and hemolytic anemia, gastrointestinal, including nausea, vomiting, and cholestatic jaundice (rare), and allergic reactions. Sulfonylureas may also cause weight gain, and their binding to plasma proteins can be potentiated by other drugs used concomitantly, which may cause hypoglycemia. This condition is the most problematic adverse event and may be prolonged, which can have severe consequences in elderly patients, patients treated with multiple drugs and those with impaired renal function. Moreover, sulfonylureas stimulate appetite and can occasionally cause allergic rashes and bone marrow injury [113].

Sulfonylureas have structural characteristics that allow them to be given in much lower doses than the first-generation sulfonylureas. Nevertheless, the different sulfonylureas are equally effective in lowering blood glucose concentrations. There are, however, differences in absorption, metabolism and effective dose [114], which is partly caused by the formation of active metabolites [115]. These drugs also cause greater suppression of overnight hepatic glucose output, thereby lowering fasting blood glucose concentrations. These benefits may be counterbalanced by an increased risk of hypoglycemia [112].

6.3. Glimepiride

The US Food and Drug Administration (FDA) approved glimepiride in 1995 for the treatment of T2DM alone and in combination with metformin or insulin. It has prolonged action and lasts over 24 hours. Glimepiride has advantages with respect to its clinical and pharmacological profile, and it has also been shown to cause a low incidence of severe hypoglycemia compared to other representatives of its class [116, 117].

Regarding hypoglycemia, the findings observed in certain studies differ. In a systematic review and meta-analysis [118], glimepiride was found to cause increased hypoglycemia compared to other sulfonylureas and even more than other secretagogues. In other studies, the long-acting sulfonylureas, such as chlorpropamide and glibenclamide, were shown to have an increased likelihood of causing hypoglycemia [112, 119]. In a UK survey, the rate of diagnosis of hypoglycemia was higher for glibenclamide compared to other representatives of the same class [120].

With regard to weight gain, in the UK Prospective Diabetes Study [34], the mean weight change after 10 years of follow up ranged from a minimum of 1.7 kg as a result of glibenclamide use to a maximum 2.6 kg with chlorpropamide use. Glimepiride was found to be neutral with respect to body weight, whereas other authors observed weight reduction [121, 122].

Sulfonylureas have different cross reactivities with cardiovascular ATP-dependent potassium channels. The closing of these channels by ischemic preconditioning can lead to cardiovascular mortality [123].

Several compounds increase the hypoglycemic effect of sulfonylureas, and several of these interactions are potentially important from a clinical standpoint. Non-steroidal anti-inflammatory agents (including azapropazone, phenylbutazone and salicylates), coumarin, certain uricosuric agents (e.g., sulfinpyrazone), alcohol, monoamine oxidase inhibitors, certain antibacterials (including sulfonamides, chloramphenicol, and trimethoprim) and certain antifungal agents (including miconazole and possibly fluconazole) produce severe hypoglycemia when administered with sulfonylureas. The probable basis for these interactions is the competition for metabolizing enzymes, but interference in plasma protein binding or excretion may also exert some effect. The agents that reduce the action of sulfonylureas include diuretics (thiazides and loop diuretics) and corticosteroids [113].

7. Anti-obesity medications

Obesity (body mass index (BMI) above 30 kg/m^2) is common in many diabetic patients, and it is important to highlight the rising prevalence of these two health conditions in the modern world [124]. Being obese or overweight produces important risk factors for type 2 diabetes and is associated with many serious health conditions, such as heart disorders and cancer, which lead to increased mortality, especially in individuals over 65. In patients previously diagnosed with type 2 diabetes, the presence of obesity can lead to a worsening of the metabolic disorders associated with diabetes, such as hyperglycemia, hypertension and hyperlipidemia [125, 126]. Thus, weight loss is required to improve glycemic control in the patient as well as to reduce the cardiovascular risk factors, which will likely reduce the risk of mortality in those individuals [127-129].

A systematic review published in 2011 [126] reported data from two clinical trials that showed a reduction of 30% to 50% in the incidence of diabetes in overweight and obese patients (with elevated plasma glucose levels) after behavioral interventions that lead to weight loss. However, the results arising from actions aimed at the prevention of obesity and changes in the obesogenic environment are often insufficient and produce insignificant weight loss that is usually regained over time. For these individuals, more invasive treatments are required to produce a sufficient weight reduction. Bariatric surgery has been a widely used intervention in obese patients because it promotes rapid and significant weight loss. However, the risks of surgery mean that this intervention is reserved for patients with morbid obesity. Thus, the FDA advises pharmacological intervention for patients with BMI ≥ 30 kg/m^2 (obese) or ≥ 27 kg/m2 (overweight) when in the presence of co-morbidities related to obesity [125, 130-132].

Numerous medications have been used for weight loss in recent decades; however, the occurrence of adverse side effects has restricted their current use [125]. In the 1990s, the drugs fenfluramine and dexfenfluramine (sympathomimetic amines that promote appetite suppression) were withdrawn from the market because of the risk of heart damage. The European Medicines Agency (EMA) suggested the withdrawal of various anti-obesity drugs, such as diethylpropion (amfepramone), mazindol and phentermine (also sympathomimetic amines inhibiting appetite), in the 2000s because of the high risk of adverse events. In 2006, rimonabant (first selective blocker of endocannabinoid receptor subtype 1-CB1) became available in 56 countries; however, because of its adverse psychiatric events, this drug was never approved by the FDA and was withdrawn from the European market in 2009. Additionally, after clinical trials assessing the safety and tolerability of sibutramine (an appetite suppressant that acts as a selective inhibitor of the reuptake of norepinephrine and serotonin), the FDA considered the option to restrict access to this substance or withdraw it from the market, causing the suspension of marketing authorization in 2010 [130, 133].

From the drugs approved before 2012, several sympathomimetic amines are available. These include phentermine, diethylpropion, benzphetamine and phendimetrazine, which are approved for short-term weight management (≤ 12 weeks), and orlistat (a potent reversible inhibitor of gastric and pancreatic lipase capable of preventing the absorption of up to 30% of dietary fat), which is the only anti-obesity drug for long-term use [130, 134, 135]. In 2012, the FDA approved two new drugs for obesity control: lorcaserin (agonist of the serotonin receptor 5-HT2C) and extended release phentermine-topiramate (association between a sympathomimetic amine appetite suppressant and an anticonvulsant). The mechanism responsible for weight loss when using extended release phentermine-topiramate is believed to be the subsequent increase in activity of the neurotransmitter gamma-aminobutyric acid (GABA), although the exact association mechanism remains unclear. Both drugs were approved for long-term use [131, 136, 137].

Depression is a common side effect observed in patients with type 2 diabetes, which may be associated with a lack of glycemic control, increased risk of complications, lack of adherence to treatment and even the presence of obesity or overweightness [137, 138]. A meta-analysis in 2001 by Anderson et al. showed that the prevalence of depression was twice as high in individuals with T2DM than in those without this health condition. Thus, reducing the incidence of depression and improving the quality of life of diabetic patients, especially those who are also obese, are highly relevant clinical objectives [139-141]. The treatment of depression in diabetics is usually accomplished by the use of serotonin reuptake inhibitors, such as fluoxetine and sertraline. These drugs not only act on depression but also promote weight loss, which is highly desired in obese or overweight diabetics [68, 142].

8. SGLT2 inhibitors

8.1. Dapagliflozin

Dapagliflozin was the first hypoglycemic agent of the new class of selective reversible inhibitors of sodium-glucose cotransporter 2 (SGLT2) approved in the US (April 2012) and demonstrates a new mechanism of action independent of insulin. This drug is recommended in adults aged 18 years or older with type 2 diabetes, both as a monotherapy and as a combination therapy with other hypoglycemic drugs, including insulin when diet and exercise does not provide adequate glycemic control [143-145].

The hypoglycemic effect occurs by reducing the reabsorption of glucose from the renal proximal tubule, which leads to increased urinary excretion of glucose with an associated loss of calories [143, 144]. On average, a daily dose of 10 mg dapagliflozin increases the amount of glucose excreted in the urine of a patient with type 2 diabetes to 50-80 g/day. This effect is observed with the first dose, and with chronic treatment, this increased excretion of glucose can be maintained for at least two years [146, 147].

In patients with type 2 diabetes, urinary loss of glucose works through a mechanism independent of insulin secretion and action [148-153] and has the potential to improve glycemic control, including control of Hb_{A1c}, fasting plasma glucose and postprandial glucose.

The selectivity of dapagliflozin for SGLT2 is 1000-3000 times greater than for SGLT1 [154].

Dapagliflozin is rapidly and extensively absorbed following oral administration. The oral bioavailability of a 10 mg dose is ≥ 75% and may be administered with or without food. It is extensively metabolized to inactive conjugates, predominantly dapagliflozin 3-*O*-glucuronide, which is then eliminated via the kidneys [146, 154].

Dapagliflozin's effectiveness is dependent on renal function and therefore should not be used by patients with moderate to severe renal impairment; dose adjustment is necessary for patients with mild renal failure or moderate hepatic impairment. Moreover, dapagliflozin should not be used in patients with severe hepatic impairment because exposure to dapagliflozin can be increased.

Interactions between dapagliflozin and other agents routinely used in the control of diabetes mellitus, including sulfonylureas, statins, warfarin and digoxin, were observed [154].

Dapagliflozin was generally well tolerated in clinical trials lasting 1 or 2 years and in studies lasting approximately 2 years [146]. Polyuria, nocturia and thirst may be experienced by some patients, and the increased excretion of glucose causes osmotic diuresis, which is similar to what is observed in patients with uncontrolled diabetes. The additional fluid loss of 300-400 ml/day is well tolerated by most patients [149, 155].

Genital infections are common in patients receiving dapagliflozin because glycosuria provides a favorable environment for the growth of microorganisms [146, 149, 155].

Dapagliflozin is recommended for patients with T2DM in the following situations [154]:

1. Monotherapy as an adjunct to diet and exercise when metformin is not tolerated;
2. Combined therapy
3. with metformin, diet and exercise, to improve glycemic control in patients when these measures alone do not achieve adequate glycemic control and there is little prospect of therapeutic response to metformin (e.g., high Hb_{A1c} levels);

4. with a sulfonylurea when sulfonylureas alone with diet and exercise do not provide adequate glycemic control; and

5. with insulin (alone, with metformin or a sulfonylurea or both) when existing therapy along with diet and exercise do not provide adequate glycemic control;

A number of other SGLT2 inhibitors are under investigation, including empagliflozin, canagliflozin and ipragliflozin. In addition, a non-selective SGLT inhibitor (LX4211) is under development. It is likely that these and other agents that share similar pharmacodynamic properties may become available in the coming years [146].

9. Insulins

In 1921, insulin was introduced as a therapeutic drug, which improved the quality and life expectancy of diabetics. The first available commercial insulin preparations corrected acute diabetic decompensation but were inefficient for chronic use because their duration was too short. Thus, diabetics were required to take four to five injections daily to achieve good metabolic control. Such short-acting insulin was the only commercially available type in 1935. Prolonging the action of insulin to over 24 hours could achieve the aim of decreasing the amount of daily injections, and it was achieved by incorporating certain substances, such as oily solutions, heavy metals (zinc) and protein (protamine). In 1950, by changing the concentration of protamine and decreasing the amount of zinc, the intermediate insulin called isophane or NPH ("Neutral Protamine Hagedorn" in honor of the scientist) became available. There were still more changes in the formula that affected the time of action, and in 1954, the family of insulins slow, semi-slow, or ultra-slow containing zinc instead of protamine was produced [156, 157].

The use of insulin is essential in the treatment of type 1 diabetes mellitus. In T2DM, it is reserved for patients with severe hyperglycemia with ketonemia or ketonuria, newly diagnosed diabetics or those who do not respond to treatment with diet, exercise, oral hypoglycemic agents and the anti-hyperglycemic action of insulin sensitizers [158].

A milestone in diabetes therapy occurred with the Diabetes Control and Complication Trial (DCCT), which showed that blood glucose levels close to normal drastically reduced or even prevented the complications of diabetes when the carrier of the disease was subjected to intensive insulin treatment and follow-up with a team of diabetes educators. According to the DCCT, to achieve this control, one proposal is to replace conventional insulin treatments (one or two daily applications of insulin) with an intensive treatment of up to four applications per day [159].

Currently, attempts to achieve good metabolic control in patients with diabetes include treatment with exogenous insulin, which is an effective therapy option in cases of partial and/or total deficiency of insulin secretion by the pancreas. It is estimated that 20-25% of all patients with diabetes are treated with insulin, and 5-10% of these patients are type 1 (who need this hormone to survive) and 15% are type 2 (who show severe insulin deficiency) [157].

Commercial insulin is a protein hormone with two linked chains of amino acids that cannot be administered orally because it is degraded by digestive and intestinal enzymes. Most commercial insulin is manufactured from bovine and porcine pancreases, which are similar to the human pancreas. Bovine and human insulin differ in three amino acids, whereas porcine insulin differs in one amino acid (amino acid thirty). Chemically synthesized insulin is also produced by recombinant DNA techniques that use bacterial cells or other tissues that are free from impurities and have a minor antigenic action [160, 161].

The pharmacokinetics of insulin varies according to its type and kind, injection technique, presence of insulin antibodies, site of injection and the individual [162].

Commercial preparations of insulin are classified according to duration as either short, intermediate or long acting, and the species of origin is also a classifier, with insulin derived from human, porcine, bovine and or porcine bovine mixtures. Because of differences in the amino acid sequences, the bovine and porcine insulins have different physicochemical properties to human insulin. Human insulin has become widely available following the advent and development of recombinant DNA techniques [163]. These techniques have led to different formulations of insulin that differ according to recombinant DNA production techniques, amino acid sequences, concentrations, solubility and time of onset and duration of biological action. However, insulin produced through recombinant DNA technology are more soluble in aqueous solutions. Currently, the commercially available forms are supplied at neutral pH, resulting in improved stability, which is essential for storage over several days at room temperature [164].

The long-acting analogues such as glargine and detemir appeared on the market in 2000 and 2004, respectively [165], and they show a relatively stable profile of action over time [166]. In January 2013, the European Commission authorized the introduction of a new generation of ultra-long insulin analogues. Degludec insulin is an ultra-long acting basal insulin analogue [167].

9.1. Short or ultra-rapid acting insulin

This group of insulins includes regular, lispro, aspart and glulisine analogues.

Regular insulin is usually administered subcutaneously and often in combination with intermediate-acting or long-lasting insulin. Special buffers are used so that a pump is not required to prevent crystallization because of its slow infusion. Monomers of this insulin present as hexamers that reduce the absorption rate. Normally, regular insulin is recommended for the treatment of diabetic ketoacidosis, and it is associated with human intermediate-acting insulin or basal analogs taken before meals [168]. This insulin should be administered 30-45 minutes before meals to reduce peak postprandial glycemia, and its action lasts between 2 and 4 hours, which contributes to postprandial hyperglycemia and hypoglycemia in the period between meals because regular insulin will peak after food has been metabolized [169].

Insulin lispro is a human insulin analog developed through genetic engineering by reversing the amino acids proline and lysine at positions 28 and 29 of the β chain, which results in the insulin sequence Lys (B28) Pro (B29). This insulin in its pharmaceutical preparation with phenol and zinc form stable hexamers [168], has a reduced tendency to self-aggregate at the site of subcutaneous injection, is absorbed more rapidly than regular human insulin, and mimics the physiological profile of insulin in response to a meal. In addition, its onset of action is between 5 and 15 minutes and duration of action is 1-2 hours [170]. The use of these analogues requires an additional dose in the afternoon to compensate for the hyperglycemia that results from an afternoon snack. There is evidence that insulin lispro reduces postprandial hyperglycemic peaks and the risk of hypoglycemia compared to regular insulin, especially at night [168, 171].

In aspart insulin, one proline amino acid is replaced by aspartic acid, which is negatively charged, at position 28 of the β chain, producing electrical repulsion between the insulin molecules and reducing their self-association tendency; in vials or cartridges, it occurs as hexamers, but in subcutaneous tissue, there is rapid dissociation to dimers and monomers, which ensures its rapid absorption and onset of action between 5 and 15 minutes and duration of action of 1 to 2 hours[168].

Insulin glulisine is another ultra-rapid insulin analogue obtained by the exchange of asparagine for lysine at position 3 of the β chain and lysine for glutamic acid at position 29 of the same chain. Thus far, there have been few studies with glulisine insulin, which appears to be similar to lispro and aspart in efficacy and hypoglycemic events. Because of its faster absorption, its administration should be performed only 5-10 minutes before meals to provide greater flexibility for the patient and thereby improve their quality of life. Its shorter half-life reduces the need to eat food 2-3 hours after its administration, which is necessary with regular insulin, whose longer half-life causes postprandial hypoglycemia [172].

A recent direct and indirect meta-analysis published by Sanches et al. (2013) for glycated hemoglobin reduction outcomes compared rapid action insulin (aspart, glulisine and lispro) with human insulin (regular), and the direct meta-analysis only showed a statistically significant difference for aspart, favoring the insulin analog. However, the results of indirect meta-analyses of Hb_{A1c} reduction outcomes showed that the result of rapid-acting insulin are consistent and the difference between them is not clinically significant. The ranking suggests that the probability of selecting the short-acting insulin brings the following provision: the first choice should be regular followed by glulisine, lispro and finally aspart. No significant differences were found in the comparison of tolerability outcomes in the rapid-acting insulin (aspart and lispro) and human insulin (regular) [173].

Recent studies have attempted to alter the pharmacokinetics of fast acting insulin analogues that are associated with recombinant human hyaluronidase, and they revealed that absorption was accelerated two-fold during the first half hour of exposure, which resulted in an onset of action between 13 and 25 minutes faster and a shorter duration of effect (40 to 49 minutes).

http://dx.doi.org/10.5772/59204

The ultra-rapid action arising from this association may be beneficial in furthering the control of postprandial blood glucose, and administering insulin lispro and hyaluronidase immediately before meals in patients with type 1 or 2 diabetes may be beneficial. Studies are being conducted for the commercial production of HUMALOG ® (Eli Lilly Nederland B.V) as part of an intensive basal-bolus insulin treatment for these patients [174].

9.2. Intermediate insulins

NPH insulin was released in 1946, and it is an insulin suspension in a zinc complex and protamine phosphate buffer. Its dosage is usually once a day before breakfast or twice a day. It has an absorption peak approximately 4-6 hours after subcutaneous administration, which is followed by a steady decline in plasma insulin concentrations [175].

The major disadvantages of NPH are the wide daily variations in the timing and duration of peaks among and between individuals, which, when compared to the timing and duration of long-acting analogs, may result in non-optimal metabolic control and an increased risk for nocturnal hypoglycemia. [172].

With respect to better glycemic control and safety when comparing the use of NPH with long-term insulin analogues, a meta-analysis published in 2013 showed that in type 2 diabetic patients, glycemic control does not seem to differ among different classes, although there is evidence for a possible reduced risk of nocturnal hypoglycemia.

Other information found in the study was that only detemir (and not glargine) may be associated with less of a weight gain than is associated with NPH [176]. In an indirect meta-analysis of long-term insulin, the results of reducing Hb_{A1c} are consistent with data from direct comparison meta-analyses and allowed a ranking of probability choice of insulins to improve the reduction of Hb_{A1c} as follows: NPH, glargine and detemir [173, 177].

9.3. Basal insulins

Glargine and detemir insulin analogs represent groups referred to as long-term or basal [168]. Detemir is produced by means of recombinant DNA technology with expression in *Saccharomyces cerevisiae* followed by chemical modification [178]. A fatty acid (myristic acid) is attached to the lysine at position 29, and it binds to circulating albumin, forming a complex that dissociates slowly, thereby prolonging its action time. Detemir is soluble at neutral pH but cannot be mixed with the rapid analogs. Detemir has shown potential benefits in body weight control, with weight loss or decreased weight gain in adults and in children and adolescents [179].

Glargine is synthesized from changes in the amino acid chain of human insulin through a substitution of asparagine by glycine at position A21 and the addition of two arginines at position B30. These modifications result in a unique pattern of release from the injection site, meaning that this analog precipitates in the subcutaneous tissue, allowing a gradual absorption into the bloodstream [180].

Basal insulin has been developed to promote basal levels of insulin over 24 hours and can be administered once a day or at bedtime. When comparing conventional long-acting insulin with glargine insulin, the insulin analog is observed to have a constant concentration profile without prominent peaks [181]. In addition, the onset is between 1 and 2 hours, plateau of biological action is between 4 and 6 hours and termination of effect is between 20 and 24 hours. Because of its slightly acidic pH, glargine cannot be mixed with other insulins in the same syringe; therefore, children may sometimes complain of a burning sensation at the application site [168]. The timing of administration of glargine appears to have no impact on its efficacy for glycemic control, but the administration should occur at approximately the same time each day so that its effectiveness as an insulin is maintained without peak action. If a dose is missed, 50% of the daily insulin will be missing that day [172].

In a direct meta-analysis comparing the insulin analogues (glargine and detemir) to NPH insulin in reducing glycated hemoglobin, the results were statistically significant and favored the twice-daily administration of detemir alone. The safety and tolerability results also showed minor differences between the insulin analogues and NPH insulin [173].

The insulin degludec belongs to a new class of insulin analogues and has a unique absorption mechanism that allows for an ultra-slow and stable pharmacokinetic profile. Its structure differs from human insulin at the β chain termination with removal of threonine at position B30 and a 16-carbon fatty acid attached to lysine at B29 by glutamic acid. This change allows for the formation of a deposit of soluble multi-hexamers, which accumulate in the subcutaneous tissue and have a slow release because of the dissociation of zinc ions; therefore, degludec insulin monomers are circulated in a slow and sustained fashion. In clinical trials, it was observed that the pharmacokinetic variations are four times smaller than in the other long-acting insulin analogues. Studies show that this insulin is related to a lower risk of nocturnal hypoglycemia, and because of these characteristics, administration can occur at intervals of up to 40 hours [182, 183].

New insulins, such as U300 and LY2605541 insulins, are still under investigation. Insulin glargine U300 is a new formulation containing glargine in a 300 U/mL concentration (the usual concentration is 100 U/mL). This change alters the pharmacokinetic and pharmacodynamic properties of glargine. For subcutaneous injections, a compact deposit of U300 is administered with a smaller deposit surface, and this produces a more gradual and prolonged release than conventional glargine; therefore, its pharmacokinetic profile is more regular and shows plasma concentrations even beyond 24 hours [184].

Another new insulin, LY2605541, is a long-acting insulin that is a modification of lispro insulin with a 20 kDa polyethylene glycol and half of lysine B28 through covalent urethane, which increases the hydrodynamic size of the insulin complex. This surface provides a greater delay in absorption and reduces the clearance, resulting in a prolongation of its action. This modified insulin has a low affinity for binding to the growth factor receptors linked to insulin, which reduces its mitogenic potential compared to human insulin. Its average life is 24-45 hours, and the duration of action may exceed 36 hours. Animal studies suggest selective action on hepatic metabolism [184].

9.4. Inhalable insulin

The benefit of injectable insulin is often limited because of the difficulty of convincing the patient to adhere to proper treatment, which is related to the need for multiple injections to ensure adequate glycemic control [185].

To alleviate this discomfort, the first inhalable insulin (Exubera®, Pfizer/Nektar) was approved in the U.S. in January 2006. Exubera® consists of a dry powder formulation containing 1 to 3 g of human insulin administered via a single inhaler lung [186]. The technology used in this product was the development of an inhaler for polyethylene glycol in a dry powder that releases the equivalent to 3 UI and 8 UI of short-acting insulin subcutaneously [187]. Exubera® has demonstrated efficacy and a low risk of hypoglycemia; however, there was a poor acceptance by the prescriber and patient. In April 2008, clinical trials showed the first case of cancer, and there were six subsequent cases of lung cancer and a case of primary malignant lung tumor in a patient who had a history of smoking. Other important aspects are coughing, decline of lung function, and increase of anti-insulin antibodies [188]. These facts led the manufacturer to withdraw Exubera® from the market.

The insulin AERx was developed by the Aradigm Corporation and Novo Nordisk. This system generates aerosol droplets from liquid insulin, and the devices guide the user to inhale the insulin. Moreover, it offers the ability to download data on the use of insulin, such as the frequency of inhalation, which can allow for the monitoring of treatment, which is important because of the experience with Exubera® [189].

AFREZZA™ (insulin Technosphere®) overcomes some of the barriers that contributed to the withdrawal of Exubera® from the market. Studies have shown that Technosphere® is a unique formulation of ultra-rapid insulin with a relatively short duration that effectively improves glycemic control without contributing to an increase in weight gain or hypoglycemia compared to other prandial insulins. Additionally, Technosphere® insulin has shown a favorable safety and tolerability profile in clinical studies to date [190]. Technosphere® insulin (TI) combines the post-dried recombinant human insulin (Mannkind Corp.) with the MedTone® Inhaler (Pharmaceutical Discovery Corp.) [191, 192.]. Recently the FDA approved this insulin; however, a continuation of the studies is required in the post-marketing period.

10. Conclusion

Despite the variety of drugs currently available for the treatment of type 2 diabetes, there was no observed decrease in the number of patients who have inadequate glycemic control keeps the last 10 years. This occurs for a variety of reasons, such as non-adherence to treatment, inappropriate prescribing of medication, lack of efficacy of medicine, among other reasons.

The search of glycemic control in patients with T2DM is still a challenge for patients and health professionals. Importantly, the success of drug treatment also depends on the association with non-pharmacological measures such as healthy diet and exercise.

Author details

Roberto Pontarolo[1], Andréia Cristina Conegero Sanches[2], Astrid Wiens[1], Cássio Marques Perlin[1], Fernanda Stumpf Tonin[1], Helena Hiemisch Lobo Borba[1], Luana Lenzi[1] and Suelem Tavares da Silva Penteado[1]

*Address all correspondence to: pontarolo@ufpr.br

1 Department of Pharmacy, Federal University of Paraná, Curitiba, Paraná, Brazil

2 Department of Medical and Pharmaceutical Sciences, State University of West of Paraná, Cascavel, Paraná, Brazil

References

[1] Alibasic E, Ramic E, Alic A. Prevention of diabetes in family medicine. Materia sociomedica 2013;25:80-2.

[2] Kahn SE, Cooper ME, Del Prato S. Pathophysiology and treatment of type 2 diabetes: perspectives on the past, present, and future. Lancet 2014;383:1068-83.

[3] Association AD. Standards of medical care in diabetes-2014. Diabetes care 2014;37 Suppl 1:S14-80.

[4] Shamseddeen H, Getty JZ, Hamdallah IN, Ali MR. Epidemiology and economic impact of obesity and type 2 diabetes. The Surgical clinics of North America 2011;91:1163-72, vii.

[5] Botero D, Wolfsdorf JI. Diabetes mellitus in children and adolescents. Archives of medical research 2005;36:281-90.

[6] Tahrani Aa, Bailey CJ, Del Prato S, Barnett AH. Management of type 2 diabetes: new and future developments in treatment. Lancet 2011;378:182-97.

[7] Chen L, Magliano DJ, Zimmet PZ. The worldwide epidemiology of type 2 diabetes mellitus: present and future perspectives. Nature reviews Endocrinology 2012;8:228-36.

[8] International Diabetes Federation. IDF Diabetes Atlas. 6 ed ed2013. 1-159 p.

[9] Hex N, Bartlett C, Wright D, Taylor M, Varley D. Estimating the current and future costs of Type 1 and Type 2 diabetes in the UK, including direct health costs and indirect societal and productivity costs. Diabetic medicine : a journal of the British Diabetic Association 2012;29:855-62.

[10] Adebayo O, Willis GC. The changing face of diabetes in America. Emergency medicine clinics of North America 2014;32:319-27.

[11] Boada CA, Martínez-Moreno JM. Current medical treatment of diabetes type 2 and long term morbidity: how to balance efficacy and safety? Nutrición hospitalaria 2013;28 Suppl 2:3-13.

[12] McLellan KCP, Wyne K, Villagomez ET, Hsueh Wa. Therapeutic interventions to reduce the risk of progression from prediabetes to type 2 diabetes mellitus. Therapeutics and clinical risk management 2014;10:173-88.

[13] Tuomi T, Santoro N, Caprio S, Cai M, Weng J, Groop L. The many faces of diabetes: a disease with increasing heterogeneity. Lancet 2014;383:1084-94.

[14] Nolan CJ, Damm P, Prentki M. Type 2 diabetes across generations: from pathophysiology to prevention and management. Lancet 2011;378:169-81.

[15] World Health Organization. Diabetes fact sheet: WHO Media Center; 2013. http://www.who.int/mediacentre/factsheets/fs312/en.(acessed 15 July 2014).

[16] Stein SA, Lamos EM, Davis SN. A review of the efficacy and safety of oral antidiabetic drugs. National Institute of Health 2014;12:153-75.

[17] PHARMA. Medicines in Development 2014. Biopharmaceutical Research Companies Are Developing 180 Medicines to Treat Diabetes and Related Conditions.

[18] Jayawardene D, Ward GM, O'Neal DN, Theverkalam G, MacIsaac AI, MacIsaac RJ. New Treatments for Type 2 Diabetes: Cardiovascular Protection Beyond Glucose Lowering? Heart, lung & circulation 2014:1-12.

[19] Rochester CD, Akiyode O. Novel and emerging diabetes mellitus drug therapies for the type 2 diabetes patient. World journal of diabetes 2014;5:305-15.

[20] Espeland Ma, Rejeski WJ, West DS, Bray Ga, Clark JM, Peters AL, et al. Intensive weight loss intervention in older individuals: results from the Action for Health in Diabetes Type 2 diabetes mellitus trial. Journal of the American Geriatrics Society 2013;61:912-22.

[21] Henry RR, Chilton R, Garvey WT. New options for the treatment of obesity and type 2 diabetes mellitus (narrative review). Journal of diabetes and its complications 2013;27:508-18.

[22] Ho J, Leung AKC, Rabi D. Hypoglycemic agents in the management of type 2 diabetes mellitus. Recent patents on endocrine, metabolic & immune drug discovery 2011;5:66-73.

[23] Irons BK, Minze MG. Drug treatment of type 2 diabetes mellitus in patients for whom metformin is contraindicated. Diabetes, metabolic syndrome and obesity : targets and therapy 2014;7:15-24.

[24] Dicker D. DPP-4 inhibitors: impact on glycemic control and cardiovascular risk factors. Diabetes care 2011;34 Suppl 2:S276-8.

[25] Wallia A, Molitch ME. Insulin therapy for type 2 diabetes mellitus. JAMA : the journal of the American Medical Association 2014;311:2315-25.

[26] L'uso dei Farmaci in Italia. Rapporto Nazionale anno 2007. http://www.agenziafarmaco.it/allegati/rapporto_osmed_2007.pdf. (acessed in 10 July 2014).

[27] American Diabetes Association. Standards of medical care in diabetes--2008. Diabetes care 2008 Jan;31 Suppl 1:S12-54.

[28] Top 200 generic drugs by total prescriptions. 2008. http://drugtopics.modernmedicine.com/drugtopics/data/articlestandard//drugtopics/222009/599844/article.pdf (acessed in 07 July 2014).

[29] Anderson J. Obesity. British medical journal 1972 Feb 26;1(5799):560-3.

[30] Cusi K, de Fronzo R. Metformin: a review of its metabolic effects. Diabetes Rev 1998;6:89-131.

[31] Santos RF, Nomizo R, Wajhenberg BL, Reaven GM, Azhar S. Changes in insulin receptor tyrosine kinase activity associated with metformin treatment of type 2 diabetes. Diabete & metabolisme 1995 Oct;21(4):274-80.

[32] Johansen K. Efficacy of metformin in the treatment of NIDDM. Meta-analysis. Diabetes care 1999 Jan;22(1):33-7.

[33] Araújo L, Britto MdS, Cruz T. Tratamento do Diabetes Mellitns do Tipo 2: Novas Opções. Arq Bras Endocrinol Metab 2000;44(6):509-18.

[34] Effect of intensive blood-glucose control with metformin on complications in overweight patients with type 2 diabetes (UKPDS 34). UK Prospective Diabetes Study (UKPDS) Group. Lancet 1998 Sep 12;352(9131):854-65.

[35] Chiasson JL, Josse RG, Hunt JA, Palmason C, Rodger NW, Ross SA, et al. The efficacy of acarbose in the treatment of patients with non-insulin-dependent diabetes mellitus. A multicenter controlled clinical trial. Annals of internal medicine 1994 Dec 15;121(12):928-35.

[36] DeFronzo RA, Goodman AM. Efficacy of metformin in patients with non-insulin-dependent diabetes mellitus. The Multicenter Metformin Study Group. The New England journal of medicine 1995 Aug 31;333(9):541-9.

[37] Hirsch IB. Metformin added to insulin therapy in poorly controlled type 2 diabetes. Diabetes care 1999 May;22(5):854.

[38] Hirsch, IB, Riddle, MC. Current therapies for diabetes. Endocr Clin North Am 1997;26:3.

[39] Inzucchi SE, Maggs DG, Spollett GR, Page SL, Rife FS, Walton V, et al. Efficacy and metabolic effects of metformin and troglitazone in type II diabetes mellitus. The New England journal of medicine 1998 Mar 26;338(13):867-72.

[40] Moses R, Slobodniuk R, Boyages S, Colagiuri S, Kidson W, Carter J, et al. Effect of repaglinide addition to metformin monotherapy on glycemic control in patients with type 2 diabetes. Diabetes care 1999 Jan;22(1):119-24.

[41] Flier JS. Diabetes. The missing link with obesity? Nature 2001 Jan 18;409(6818):292-3.

[42] Kahn SE, Haffner SM, Heise MA, Herman WH, Holman RR, Jones NP, et al. Glycemic durability of rosiglitazone, metformin, or glyburide monotherapy. The New England journal of medicine 2006 Dec 7;355(23):2427-43.

[43] Olokoba AB, Obateru OA, Olokoba LB. Type 2 diabetes mellitus: a review of current trends. Oman medical journal 2012 Jul;27(4):269-73.

[44] Silva AG, Lazaretti-Catro M. Diabetes melito, tiazolidinedionas e fraturas: uma história inacabada. Arq Bras Endocrinol Metab 2010;54(4):345-51.

[45] Horton ES, Whitehouse F, Ghazzi MN, Venable TC, Whitcomb RW. Troglitazone in combination with sulfonylurea restores glycemic control in patients with type 2 diabetes. The Troglitazone Study Group. Diabetes care 1998 Sep;21(9):1462-9.

[46] Iwamoto Y, Kosaka K, Kuzuya T, Akanuma Y, Shigeta Y, Kaneko T. Effect of combination therapy of troglitazone and sulphonylureas in patients with Type 2 diabetes who were poorly controlled by sulphonylurea therapy alone. Diabetic medicine : a journal of the British Diabetic Association 1996 Apr;13(4):365-70.

[47] Day C. Thiazolidinediones: a new class of antidiabetic drugs. Diabetic medicine : a journal of the British Diabetic Association 1999 Mar;16(3):179-92.

[48] Balfour JA, Plosker GL. Rosiglitazone. Drugs 1999 Jun;57(6):921-30; discussion 31-2.

[49] Grey A. Skeletal consequences of thiazolidinedione therapy. Osteoporosis international : a journal established as result of cooperation between the European Foundation for Osteoporosis and the National Osteoporosis Foundation of the USA 2008 Feb;19(2):129-37.

[50] Guardado-Mendoza R, Prioletta A, Jimenez-Ceja LM, Sosale A, Folli F. The role of nateglinide and repaglinide, derivatives of meglitinide, in the treatment of type 2 diabetes mellitus. Arch Med Sci 2013 Oct 31;9(5):936-43.

[51] Hemmingsen B, Schroll JB, Lund SS, Wetterslev J, Gluud C, Vaag A, et al. Sulphonylurea monotherapy for patients with type 2 diabetes mellitus. Cochrane Database Syst Rev 2013;4:CD009008.

[52] Iglesias P, Heras M, Diez JJ. Diabetes mellitus and kidney disease in the elderly. Nefrologia 2014 May 21;34(3):285-92.

[53] Kim CH, Park SH, Sim YB, Kim SS, Kim SJ, Lim SM, et al. Effects of nateglinide and repaglinide administered intracerebroventricularly on the CA3 hippocampal neuronal cell death and hyperglycemia induced by kainic acid in mice. Brain Res Bull 2014 May;104:36-41.

[54] Abe M, Okada K, Soma M. Antidiabetic agents in patients with chronic kidney disease and end-stage renal disease on dialysis: metabolism and clinical practice. Curr Drug Metab 2011 Jan;12(1):57-69.

[55] Ma J, Liu LY, Wu PH, Liao Y, Tao T, Liu W. Comparison of metformin and repaglinide monotherapy in the treatment of new onset type 2 diabetes mellitus in China. J Diabetes Res 2014;2014:294017.

[56] Papa G, Fedele V, Rizzo MR, Fioravanti M, Leotta C, Solerte SB, et al. Safety of type 2 diabetes treatment with repaglinide compared with glibenclamide in elderly people: A randomized, open-label, two-period, cross-over trial. Diabetes Care 2006 Aug; 29(8):1918-20.

[57] Stephens JW, Bodvarsdottir TB, Wareham K, Prior SL, Bracken RM, Lowe GD, et al. Effects of short-term therapy with glibenclamide and repaglinide on incretin hormones and oxidative damage associated with postprandial hyperglycaemia in people with type 2 diabetes mellitus. Diabetes Res Clin Pract 2011 Nov;94(2):199-206.

[58] Reimann F, Proks P, Ashcroft FM. Effects of mitiglinide (S 21403) on Kir6.2/SUR1, Kir6.2/SUR2A and Kir6.2/SUR2B types of ATP-sensitive potassium channel. Br J Pharmacol 2001 Apr;132(7):1542-8.

[59] Dornhorst A. Insulinotropic meglitinide analogues. Lancet 2001 Nov 17;358(9294): 1709-16.

[60] Hatorp V. Clinical pharmacokinetics and pharmacodynamics of repaglinide. Clin Pharmacokinet 2002;41(7):471-83.

[61] Hatorp V, Huang WC, Strange P. Repaglinide pharmacokinetics in healthy young adult and elderly subjects. Clin Ther 1999 Apr;21(4):702-10.

[62] Keilson L, Mather S, Walter YH, Subramanian S, McLeod JF. Synergistic effects of nateglinide and meal administration on insulin secretion in patients with type 2 diabetes mellitus. J Clin Endocrinol Metab 2000 Mar;85(3):1081-6.

[63] Tentolouris N, Voulgari C, Katsilambros N. A review of nateglinide in the management of patients with type 2 diabetes. Vasc Health Risk Manag 2007;3(6):797-807.

[64] Weaver ML, Orwig BA, Rodriguez LC, Graham ED, Chin JA, Shapiro MJ, et al. Pharmacokinetics and metabolism of nateglinide in humans. Drug Metab Dispos 2001 Apr;29(4 Pt 1):415-21.

[65] Zeng Y, Xie X, Duan J, Zhou T, Zhang Y, Yang M, et al. Perturbation of mitiglinide metabolism by chronic unpredicted mild stress in rats. Sci Rep 2014;4:3794.

[66] Konya H, Miuchi M, Konishi K, Nagai E, Ueyama T, Kusunoki Y, et al. Pleiotropic effects of mitiglinide in type 2 diabetes mellitus. J Int Med Res 2009 Nov-Dec;37(6): 1904-12.

[67] Shigeto M, Katsura M, Matsuda M, Ohkuma S, Kaku K. Nateglinide and mitiglinide, but not sulfonylureas, induce insulin secretion through a mechanism mediated by calcium release from endoplasmic reticulum. J Pharmacol Exp Ther 2007 Jul;322(1): 1-7.

[68] Li L, Yang M, Li Z, Yan X, Guo H, Pan H, et al. Efficacy and safety of mitiglinide versus nateglinide in newly diagnose patients with type 2 diabetes mellitus: a randomized double blind trial. Diabetes Obes Metab 2012 Feb;14(2):187-9.

[69] Assaloni R, Da Ros R, Quagliaro L, Piconi L, Maier A, Zuodar G, et al. Effects of S21403 (mitiglinide) on postprandial generation of oxidative stress and inflammation in type 2 diabetic patients. Diabetologia 2005 Sep;48(9):1919-24.

[70] van de Laar FA. Alpha-glucosidase inhibitors in the early treatment of type 2 diabetes. Vascular health and risk management 2008;4(6):1189-95.

[71] Meneilly GS, Ryan EA, Radziuk J, Lau DC, Yale JF, Morais J, et al. Effect of acarbose on insulin sensitivity in elderly patients with diabetes. Diabetes care 2000 Aug;23(8): 1162-7.

[72] Inzucchi SE, Bergenstal RM, Buse JB, Diamant M, Ferrannini E, Nauck M, et al. Management of hyperglycemia in type 2 diabetes: a patient-centered approach: position statement of the American Diabetes Association (ADA) and the European Association for the Study of Diabetes (EASD). Diabetes care 2012 Jun;35(6):1364-79.

[73] Rosak C, Mertes G. Critical evaluation of the role of acarbose in the treatment of diabetes: patient considerations. Diabetes, metabolic syndrome and obesity : targets and therapy 2012;5:357-67.

[74] Coniff R, Krol A. Acarbose: a review of US clinical experience. Clinical therapeutics 1997 Jan-Feb;19(1):16-26; discussion 2-3.

[75] Lebovitz HE. alpha-Glucosidase inhibitors. Endocrinology and metabolism clinics of North America 1997 Sep;26(3):539-51.

[76] van de Laar FA, Lucassen PL, Akkermans RP, van de Lisdonk EH, Rutten GE, van Weel C. Alpha-glucosidase inhibitors for patients with type 2 diabetes: results from a Cochrane systematic review and meta-analysis. Diabetes care 2005 Jan;28(1):154-63.

[77] Andrade R, Lucena M, Rodríguez-Mendizábal M. Hepatic injury caused by acarbose. Annals of internal medicine 1996;124:931.

[78] Carrascosa M, Pascual F, Aresti S. Acarbose-induced acute severe hepatotoxicity. Lancet 1997 Mar 8;349(9053):698-9.

[79] Fujimoto Y, Ohhira M, Miyokawa N, Kitamori S, Kohgo Y. Acarbose-induced hepatic injury. Lancet 1998 Jan 31;351(9099):340.

[80] Catalan VS, Couture JA, LeLorier J. Predictors of persistence of use of the novel antidiabetic agent acarbose. Archives of internal medicine 2001 Apr 23;161(8):1106-12.

[81] McIntosh B, Cameron C, Singh SR, Yu C, Ahuja T, Welton NJ, et al. Second-line therapy in patients with type 2 diabetes inadequately controlled with metformin monotherapy: a systematic review and mixed-treatment comparison meta-analysis. Open medicine : a peer-reviewed, independent, open-access journal 2011;5(1):e35-48.

[82] Braun D, Schönherr U, Mitzkat H. Efficacy of acarbose monotherapy in patients with type 2 diabetes: a double-blind study conducted in general practice. Endocrinol Metabol 1996;3:275-80.

[83] Coniff RF, Shapiro JA, Seaton TB, Hoogwerf BJ, Hunt JA. A double-blind placebo-controlled trial evaluating the safety and efficacy of acarbose for the treatment of patients with insulin-requiring type II diabetes. Diabetes care 1995 Jul;18(7):928-32.

[84] Hoffmann J, Spengler M. Efficacy of 24-week monotherapy with acarbose, glibenclamide, or placebo in NIDDM patients. The Essen Study. Diabetes care 1994 Jun;17(6): 561-6.

[85] Holman RR, Cull CA, Turner RC. A randomized double-blind trial of acarbose in type 2 diabetes shows improved glycemic control over 3 years (U.K. Prospective Diabetes Study 44). Diabetes care 1999 Jun;22(6):960-4.

[86] Chiasson JL, Josse RG, Gomis R, Hanefeld M, Karasik A, Laakso M, et al. Acarbose treatment and the risk of cardiovascular disease and hypertension in patients with impaired glucose tolerance: the STOP-NIDDM trial. JAMA : the journal of the American Medical Association 2003 Jul 23;290(4):486-94.

[87] Hanefeld M, Cagatay M, Petrowitsch T, Neuser D, Petzinna D, Rupp M. Acarbose reduces the risk for myocardial infarction in type 2 diabetic patients: meta-analysis of seven long-term studies. European heart journal 2004 Jan;25(1):10-6.

[88] Hirano M, Nakamura T, Obata JE, Fujioka D, Saito Y, Kawabata K, et al. Early improvement in carotid plaque echogenicity by acarbose in patients with acute coronary syndromes. Circulation journal : official journal of the Japanese Circulation Society 2012;76(6):1452-60.

[89] Shimabukuro M, Higa N, Chinen I, Yamakawa K, Takasu N. Effects of a single administration of acarbose on postprandial glucose excursion and endothelial dysfunction in type 2 diabetic patients: a randomized crossover study. The Journal of clinical endocrinology and metabolism 2006 Mar;91(3):837-42.

[90] Kitano D, Chiku M, Li Y, Okumura Y, Fukamachi D, Takayama T, et al. Miglitol improves postprandial endothelial dysfunction in patients with acute coronary syn-

drome and new-onset postprandial hyperglycemia. Cardiovascular diabetology 2013;12:92.

[91] Fujisawa T, Ikegami H, Inoue K, Kawabata Y, Ogihara T. Effect of two alpha-glucosidase inhibitors, voglibose and acarbose, on postprandial hyperglycemia correlates with subjective abdominal symptoms. Metabolism: clinical and experimental 2005 Mar;54(3):387-90.

[92] Johnston PS, Coniff RF, Hoogwerf BJ, Santiago JV, Pi-Sunyer FX, Krol A. Effects of the carbohydrase inhibitor miglitol in sulfonylurea-treated NIDDM patients. Diabetes care 1994 Jan;17(1):20-9.

[93] Johnston PS, Feig PU, Coniff RF, Krol A, Davidson JA, Haffner SM. Long-term titrated-dose alpha-glucosidase inhibition in non-insulin-requiring Hispanic NIDDM patients. Diabetes care 1998 Mar;21(3):409-15.

[94] Johnston PS, Lebovitz HE, Coniff RF, Simonson DC, Raskin P, Munera CL. Advantages of alpha-glucosidase inhibition as monotherapy in elderly type 2 diabetic patients. The Journal of clinical endocrinology and metabolism 1998 May;83(5):1515-22.

[95] Mitrakou A, Tountas N, Raptis AE, Bauer RJ, Schulz H, Raptis SA. Long-term effectiveness of a new alpha-glucosidase inhibitor (BAY m1099-miglitol) in insulin-treated type 2 diabetes mellitus. Diabetic medicine : a journal of the British Diabetic Association 1998 Aug;15(8):657-60.

[96] Chiasson JL, Naditch L, Miglitol Canadian University Investigator G. The synergistic effect of miglitol plus metformin combination therapy in the treatment of type 2 diabetes. Diabetes care 2001 Jun;24(6):989-94.

[97] Tsujino D, Nishimura R, Taki K, Morimoto A, Tajima N, Utsunomiya K. Comparing the efficacy of alpha-glucosidase inhibitors in suppressing postprandial hyperglycemia using continuous glucose monitoring: a pilot study-the MAJOR study. Diabetes technology & therapeutics 2011 Mar;13(3):303-8.

[98] Emoto T, Sawada T, Hashimoto M, Kageyama H, Terashita D, Mizoguchi T, et al. Effect of 3-month repeated administration of miglitol on vascular endothelial function in patients with diabetes mellitus and coronary artery disease. The American journal of cardiology 2012 Jan 1;109(1):42-6.

[99] Hirst JA, Farmer AJ, Dyar A, Lung TW, Stevens RJ. Estimating the effect of sulfonylurea on Hb_{A1c} in diabetes: a systematic review and meta-analysis. Diabetologia 2013 May;56(5):973-84.

[100] NICE. CG66 type 2 diabetes: full guideline. In: NICE clinical guideline 66. www.nice.org.uk/nicemedia/pdf/CG66NICEGuideline.pdf. 2008. (acessed in 03 July 2014).

[101] Langtry HD, Balfour JA. Glimepiride. A review of its use in the management of type 2 diabetes mellitus. Drugs 1998 Apr;55(4):563-84.

[102] Wannmacher L. Antidiabéticos orais: comparação entre diferentes intervenções. Uso Racional de medicamentos: temas relacionados Organização Pan-Americana da Saúde/Organização Mundial da Saúde 2005;2(11).

[103] Bressler R, Johnson DG. Pharmacological regulation of blood glucose levels in non-insulin-dependent diabetes mellitus. Archives of internal medicine 1997 Apr 28;157(8):836-48.

[104] Hermann LS, Schersten B, Bitzen PO, Kjellstrom T, Lindgarde F, Melander A. Therapeutic comparison of metformin and sulfonylurea, alone and in various combinations. A double-blind controlled study. Diabetes care 1994 Oct;17(10):1100-9.

[105] Nathan DM, Buse JB, Davidson MB, Ferrannini E, Holman RR, Sherwin R, et al. Medical management of hyperglycaemia in type 2 diabetes mellitus: a consensus algorithm for the initiation and adjustment of therapy: a consensus statement from the American Diabetes Association and the European Association for the Study of Diabetes. Diabetologia 2009 Jan;52(1):17-30.

[106] Irvine WJ, Sawers JS, Feek CM, Prescott RJ, Duncan LJ. The value of islet cell antibody in predicting secondary failure of oral hypoglycaemic agent therapy in Diabetes mellitus. Journal of clinical & laboratory immunology 1979 Apr;2(1):23-6.

[107] Kobayashi T, Itoh T, Kosaka K, Sato K, Tsuji K. Time course of islet cell antibodies and beta-cell function in non-insulin-dependent stage of type I diabetes. Diabetes 1987 Apr;36(4):510-7.

[108] Aguilar-Bryan L, Nichols CG, Wechsler SW, Clement JPt, Boyd AE, 3rd, Gonzalez G, et al. Cloning of the beta cell high-affinity sulfonylurea receptor: a regulator of insulin secretion. Science 1995 Apr 21;268(5209):423-6.

[109] Akalin S, Berntorp K, Ceriello A, Das AK, Kilpatrick ES, Koblik T, et al. Intensive glucose therapy and clinical implications of recent data: a consensus statement from the Global Task Force on Glycaemic Control. International journal of clinical practice 2009 Oct;63(10):1421-5.

[110] Ashcroft FM, Gribble FM. Tissue-specific effects of sulfonylureas: lessons from studies of cloned K(ATP) channels. Journal of diabetes and its complications 2000 Jul-Aug;14(4):192-6.

[111] Lee SJ, Eng C. Goals of glycemic control in frail older patients with diabetes. JAMA : the journal of the American Medical Association 2011 Apr 6;305(13):1350-1.

[112] Shorr RI, Ray WA, Daugherty JR, Griffin MR. Individual sulfonylureas and serious hypoglycemia in older people. Journal of the American Geriatrics Society 1996 Jul; 44(7):751-5.

[113] Rang H, Dale M, Ritter J. Farmacologia. Rio de Janeiro: Guanabara Koogan; 2012.

http://dx.doi.org/10.5772/59204

[114] Jonsson A, Rydberg T, Ekberg G, Hallengren B, Melander A. Slow elimination of glyburide in NIDDM subjects. Diabetes care 1994 Feb;17(2):142-5.

[115] Rydberg T, Jonsson A, Roder M, Melander A. Hypoglycemic activity of glyburide (glibenclamide) metabolites in humans. Diabetes care 1994 Sep;17(9):1026-30.

[116] Basit A, Riaz M, Fawwad A. Glimepiride: evidence-based facts, trends, and observations (GIFTS). [corrected]. Vascular health and risk management 2012;8:463-72.

[117] Holstein A, Plaschke A, Egberts E. Lower incidence of severe hypoglycaemia in patients with type 2 diabetes treated with glimepiride versus glibenclamide. Diabetes Metabolism research and review 2001;17:467-73.

[118] Gangji AS, Cukierman T, Gerstein HC, Goldsmith CH, Clase CM. A systematic review and meta-analysis of hypoglycemia and cardiovascular events: a comparison of glyburide with other secretagogues and with insulin. Diabetes care 2007 Feb;30(2): 389-94.

[119] Ferner RE, Neil HA. Sulphonylureas and hypoglycaemia. Br Med J (Clin Res Ed) 1988 Apr 2;296(6627):949-50.

[120] Ben-Ami H, Nagachandran P, Mendelson A, Edoute Y. Drug-induced hypoglycemic coma in 102 diabetic patients. Archives of internal medicine 1999 Feb 8;159(3):281-4.

[121] Bugos C, Austin M, Atherton T, Viereck C. Long-term treatment of type 2 diabetes mellitus with glimepiride is weight neutral: a meta-analysis. Diabetes Res Clin Pract 2000;50(1):S47.

[122] Martin S, Kolb H, Beuth J, van Leendert R, Schneider B, Scherbaum WA. Change in patients' body weight after 12 months of treatment with glimepiride or glibenclamide in Type 2 diabetes: a multicentre retrospective cohort study. Diabetologia 2003 Dec;46(12):1611-7.

[123] Lazdunski M. Ion channel effects of antidiabetic sulfonylureas. Hormone and metabolic research=Hormon-und Stoffwechselforschung=Hormones et metabolisme 1996 Sep;28(9):488-95.

[124] Norris SL, Zhang X, Avenell A, Gregg E, Schmid CH, Kim C, et al. Efficacy of pharmacotherapy for weight loss in adults with type 2 diabetes mellitus: a meta-analysis. Arch Intern Med 2004 Jul 12;164(13):1395-404.

[125] Eckel RH, Kahn SE, Ferrannini E, Goldfine AB, Nathan DM, Schwartz MW, et al. Obesity and type 2 diabetes: what can be unified and what needs to be individualized? Diabetes Care 2011 Jun;34(6):1424-30.

[126] Leblanc ES, O'Connor E, Whitlock EP, Patnode CD, Kapka T. Effectiveness of primary care-relevant treatments for obesity in adults: a systematic evidence review for the U.S. Preventive Services Task Force. Ann Intern Med 2011 Oct 4;155(7):434-47.

[127] Gibbs BB, Brancati FL, Chen H, Coday M, Jakicic JM, Lewis CE, et al. Effect of improved fitness beyond weight loss on cardiovascular risk factors in individuals with type 2 diabetes in the Look AHEAD study. Eur J Prev Cardiol 2014 May;21(5):608-17.

[128] Henry RR, Chilton R, Garvey WT. New options for the treatment of obesity and type 2 diabetes mellitus (narrative review). Journal of diabetes and its complications 2013 Sep-Oct;27(5):508-18.

[129] Stein SA, Lamos EM, Davis SN. A review of the efficacy and safety of oral antidiabetic drugs. Expert Opin Drug Saf 2013 Mar;12(2):153-75.

[130] Kang JG, Park CY. Anti-Obesity Drugs: A Review about Their Effects and Safety. Diabetes Metab J 2012 Feb;36(1):13-25.

[131] Kushner RF. Weight loss strategies for treatment of obesity. Prog Cardiovasc Dis 2014 Jan-Feb;56(4):465-72.

[132] Rodgers RJ, Tschop MH, Wilding JP. Anti-obesity drugs: past, present and future. Dis Model Mech 2012 Sep;5(5):621-6.

[133] Ioannides-Demos LL, Piccenna L, McNeil JJ. Pharmacotherapies for obesity: past, current, and future therapies. J Obes 2011;2011:179674.

[134] Walter CP, Bleske BE, Dorsch MP. Pharmacotherapy for weight loss: the cardiovascular effects of the old and new agents. J Clin Pharm Ther 2014 Jun 13.

[135] Yanovski SZ, Yanovski JA. Long-term drug treatment for obesity: a systematic and clinical review. JAMA 2014 Jan 1;311(1):74-86.

[136] Bray GA, Ryan DH. Update on obesity pharmacotherapy. Ann N Y Acad Sci 2014 Apr;1311:1-13.

[137] Mahgerefteh B, Vigue M, Freestone Z, Silver S, Nguyen Q. New drug therapies for the treatment of overweight and obese patients. Am Health Drug Benefits 2013 Sep; 6(7):423-30.

[138] Ye Z, Chen L, Yang Z, Li Q, Huang Y, He M, et al. Metabolic effects of fluoxetine in adults with type 2 diabetes mellitus: a meta-analysis of randomized placebo-controlled trials. PLoS One 2011;6(7):e21551.

[139] Anderson RJ, Freedland KE, Clouse RE, Lustman PJ. The prevalence of comorbid depression in adults with diabetes: a meta-analysis. Diabetes Care 2001 Jun;24(6): 1069-78.

[140] Knol MJ, Twisk JW, Beekman AT, Heine RJ, Snoek FJ, Pouwer F. Depression as a risk factor for the onset of type 2 diabetes mellitus. A meta-analysis. Diabetologia 2006 May;49(5):837-45.

[141] Impact of intensive lifestyle intervention on depression and health-related quality of life in type 2 diabetes: the Look AHEAD Trial. Diabetes Care 2014 Jun;37(6):1544-53.

[142] Mancini MC, Halpern A. Pharmacological treatment of obesity. Arq Bras Endocrinol Metabol 2006 Apr;50(2):377-89.

[143] Komoroski B, Vachharajani N, Boulton D, Kornhauser D, Geraldes M, Li L, et al. Dapagliflozin, a novel SGLT2 inhibitor, induces dose-dependent glucosuria in healthy subjects. Clinical pharmacology and therapeutics 2009 May;85(5):520-6.

[144] List JF, Whaley JM. Glucose dynamics and mechanistic implications of SGLT2 inhibitors in animals and humans. Kidney international Supplement 2011 Mar(120):S20-7.

[145] Orme M, Fenici P, Lomon ID, Wygant G, Townsend R, Roudaut M. A systematic review and mixed-treatment comparison of dapagliflozin with existing anti-diabetes treatments for those with type 2 diabetes mellitus inadequately controlled by sulfonylurea monotherapy. Diabetology & metabolic syndrome 2014;6:73.

[146] Kilov G, Leow S, Thomas M. SGLT2 inhibition with dapagliflozin--a novel approach for the management of type 2 diabetes. Australian family physician 2013 Oct;42(10):706-10.

[147] Plosker GL. Dapagliflozin: a review of its use in type 2 diabetes mellitus. Drugs 2012 Dec 3;72(17):2289-312.

[148] Bailey CJ, Gross JL, Pieters A, Bastien A, List JF. Effect of dapagliflozin in patients with type 2 diabetes who have inadequate glycaemic control with metformin: a randomised, double-blind, placebo-controlled trial. Lancet 2010 Jun 26;375(9733):2223-33.

[149] Ferrannini E, Ramos SJ, Salsali A, Tang W, List JF. Dapagliflozin monotherapy in type 2 diabetic patients with inadequate glycemic control by diet and exercise: a randomized, double-blind, placebo-controlled, phase 3 trial. Diabetes care 2010;33:2217-24.

[150] Wilding J, Woo V, Pahor A, Sugg J, Langkilde A, Parikh S. Effect of dapagliflozin, a novel insulin-independent treatment, over 48 weeks in patients with type 2 diabetes poorly controlled with insulin. Diabetologia 2010;53((Suppl 1)):Abstract s348.

[151] List JF, Woo V, Morales E, Tang W, Fiedorek FT. Sodium-glucose cotransport inhibition with dapagliflozin in type 2 diabetes. Diabetes care 2009 Apr;32(4):650-7.

[152] Strojek K, Yoon KH, Hruba V, Elze M, Langkilde AM, Parikh S. Effect of dapagliflozin in patients with type 2 diabetes who have inadequate glycaemic control with glimepiride: a randomized, 24-week, double-blind, placebo-controlled trial. Diabetes, obesity & metabolism 2011 Oct;13(10):928-38.

[153] Wilding JP, Norwood P, T'Joen C, Bastien A, List JF, Fiedorek FT. A study of dapagliflozin in patients with type 2 diabetes receiving high doses of insulin plus insulin sensitizers: applicability of a novel insulin-independent treatment. Diabetes care 2009 Sep;32(9):1656-62.

[154] Squibb B-M. FORXIGA (dapagliflozin propanediol monohydrate) product information. Noble Park, VIC: Bristol-Myers Squibb Pty Ltd 2012.

[155] Gerich JE, Bastien A. Development of the sodium-glucose co-transporter 2 inhibitor dapagliflozin for the treatment of patients with type 2 diabetes mellitus. Expert review of clinical pharmacology 2011 Nov;4(6):669-83.

[156] Costa A, Almeida Neto J. Manual de diabetes: alimentação, medicamentos, exercícios. 3 ed São Paulo, Sarvier 1998.

[157] Pupo A. Insulina. Rev Assoc Med Bras 1986;32(11/12):205-7.

[158] Berger M, Jorgens V, Muhlhauser I. Rationale for the use of insulin therapy alone as the pharmacological treatment of type 2 diabetes. Diabetes care 1999 Apr;22 Suppl 3:C71-5.

[159] Wajchenberg B. Tratamento insulínico do diabetes insulinodependente ou do tipo I. Terapêutica em diabetes 1995;2(1).

[160] British Medical Association and Royal Pharmaceutical Society of Great Britain. British National Formulary. BNF 58. Septembre 2009.

[161] Souza C, Zanetti M. Administração de insulina: uma abordagem fundamental na educação em diabetes. Revista Escola de Enfermagem da USP 2000;34(3):264-70.

[162] American Diabetes Association. Medical management of type 1 diabetes. 3ed Alexandria, Clinical Education Series 1998.

[163] Davis S, Granner D. Insulina, Hipoglicemiantes Orais e a Farmacologia do Pâncreas Endócrino. In: Goodman, L S; Gilman, A (eds) In: As Bases Farmacológicas da Terapêutica Rio de Janeiro – RJ, McGraw-Hill, cap 61, p 1263-1290, 10º Ed 2005.

[164] Katzung B. Farmacologia. Hormônios pancreáticos e fármacos antidiabéticos. 9 Ed 2003:579-97.

[165] Jovanovic L, Pettitt DJ. Treatment with insulin and its analogs in pregnancies complicated by diabetes. Diabetes care 2007 Jul;30 Suppl 2:S220-4.

[166] Rolla A. Pharmacokinetic and pharmacodynamic advantages of insulin analogues and premixed insulin analogues over human insulins: impact on efficacy and safety. The American journal of medicine 2008 Jun;121(6 Suppl):S9-S19.

[167] European Medicines Agency. http://www.ema.europa.eu/ema/index.jsp?curl=pages/medicines/human/medicines/002498/human_med_001609.jsp&mid=WC0b01ac058001d124. (Acessed in 15 July 2014).

[168] Pires A, Chacra A. A evolução da insulinoterapia no diabetes melito tipo 1. Endocrinol Metab 2008;52 (2):268-78.

[169] Sociedade Brasileira de Diabetes. Diretrizes da Sociedade Brasileira de Diabetes. Tratamento e acompanhamento do diabetes melittos Rio de Janeiro, 2007. http://

www.anad.org.br/profissionais/images/Diretrizes_SBD_2007.pdf. (acessed in 10 July 2014).

[170] Wajchenberg AR, Forti, AC, Ferreira, SRG, Oliveira, O, Lopes, CF, Lerário, AC, Sena, RC, Kayath, MJ. Menor incidência de hipoglicemia noturna com o uso de insulina lispro comparada à insulina humana regular no tratamento de pacientes com diabetes do tipo 1.. Arq bras endocrinol metab 2000;44(2):133-8.

[171] Recasens E, Morínigo R, Casamitjana R, Nicoletti C, Ramon, FGE, Conget I. Insulin lispro is as effective as regular insulin in optimising metabolic control and preserving β-cell function at onset of type 1 diabetes mellitus. Diabetes Research and Clinical Practice 2003; 60(3):153-9.

[172] Schmid H. New options in insulin therapy. Jornal de Pediatria 2007;83(5):S146-54.

[173] Sanches A, Correr C, Venson R, Gonçalves P, Garcia M, Piantavini M, et al. Insulin analogues versus human insulin in type 1 diabetes: direct and indirect meta-analyses of efficacy and safety. Braz J of Pharm Scie 2013;49(3):501-9.

[174] Morrow L, Muchmore DB, Hompesch M, Ludington EA, Vaughn DE. Comparative pharmacokinetics and insulin action for three rapid-acting insulin analogs injected subcutaneously with and without hyaluronidase. Diabetes care 2013 Feb;36(2):273-5.

[175] Home PD, Rosskamp R, Forjanic-Klapproth J, Dressler A, Bartusch-Marrain P, Egger T, et al. A randomized multicentre trial of insulin glargine compared with NPH insulin in people with type 1 diabetes. Diabetes/Metabolism Research and Reviews 2005;21(6):545-53.

[176] Monami M, Marchionni N, Mannucci E. Long-acting insulin analogues versus NPH human insulin in type 2 diabetes: a meta-analysis. Diabetes Res Clin Pract 2008 Aug; 81(2):184-9.

[177] Sanches AC, Correr CJ, Venson R, Pontarolo R. Revisiting the efficacy of long-acting insulin analogues on adults with type 1 diabetes using mixed-treatment comparisons. Diabetes Res Clin Pract 2011 Dec;94(3):333-9.

[178] Kurtzhals P. Pharmacology of insulin detemir. Endocrinol Metab Clin North Am 2007;36 (suppl 1):14-20.

[179] Soran H, Younis NI. Insulin detemir: a new basal insulin analogue. Diabetes Obesity and Metabolism 2006;8:26-30.

[180] Rollin G, Punales N, Geremia C, Ce.; VG, Tschiedel B. Utilização da insulina glargina em crianças menores de oito anos de idade. Arquivos Brasileiros de Endocrinologia & Metabologia 2009;53(6):721-25.

[181] Vazquez-Carrera M, Silvestre JS. Insulin analogues in the management of diabetes. Methods & Findings in Experimental & Clinical Pharmacology 2004;26(6):445.

[182] Luis D, Romero E. Análogos De Insulina: Modificaciones En La Estrutura, Consecuencias Moleculares Y Metabolólicas. Semergen 2013;39(1):34-40.

[183] Simó R. Nueva insulina basal de acción ultralenta: insulina degludec. Av Diabetol 2013;29(1):4-11.

[184] Owens DR, Zinman B, Bolli GB. Insulins today and beyond. Lancet 2001 Sep 1;358(9283):739-46.

[185] Bailey CJ, Barnett, A. H. Inhaled insulin: new formulation, new trial. The Lanced 2010;375:2199-201.

[186] Siekmeier R, Scheuch G. Inhaled insulin--does it become reality? Journal of physiology and pharmacology : an official journal of the Polish Physiological Society 2008 Dec;59 Suppl 6:81-113.

[187] Mastrandrea LD. Inhaled insulin: overview of a novel route of insulin administration. Vascular health and risk management 2010;6:47-58.

[188] Arnolds S, Heise T. Inhaled insulin. Best practice & research Clinical endocrinology & metabolism 2007 Dec;21(4):555-71.

[189] Tibaldi JM. Evolution of insulin development: focus on key parameters. Advances in therapy 2012 Jul;29(7):590-619.

[190] Neumiller JJ, Campbell RK. Technosphere insulin: an inhaled prandial insulin product. BioDrugs : clinical immunotherapeutics, biopharmaceuticals and gene therapy 2010 Jun;24(3):165-72.

[191] Mastrandrea LD. Inhaled insulin: overview of a novel route of insulin administration. Vascular Health and Risk Management 2010;6:47-58.

[192] Tibaldi JM. Evolution of Insulin Development: Focus on Key Parameters. Adv Ther 2012;29(7):590–619.

Chapter 7

The Preventive and Therapeutic Effect of Caloric Restriction Therapy on Type 2 Diabetes Mellitus

Shuhang Xu, Guofang Chen, Li Chunrui and Chao Liu

Additional information is available at the end of the chapter

http://dx.doi.org/10.5772/59281

1. Introduction

1.1. The definition of caloric restriction therapy

Caloric restriction (CR) is to treat some diseases by restricting the intake of calorie or the content of a particular ingredient of the diet, while ensuring the basic nutritional need [1]. It was used to increase average and maximum lifespan in ancient times [2], however, in last 100 years CR effect on improvement of T2DM has been established by many researchers, because it can improve the metabolic parameters and pancreas islet function of type 2 diabetic patients [3]. The treatment efficacy and safety has been clear.

1.2. The main forms of caloric restriction therapy

Nowadays, CR is only used in basic and clinical researches, and its form is disunity. The earliest form of this method used in the study is called fasting, which means apastia, and the participators should never eat anything except drink water. This method was eliminated because of its uncertain adverse reactions [4]. According to the different restricted objects of CR, it can be divided into low-calorie restriction diet, low-carbohydrate restriction diet, low-fat restriction diet and so on; according to the different frequency of CR, we can divide it into continuous CR, intermittent CR (followed CR for 2 days per week and normal diet at the other times) or every other day CR (followed CR one day and a normal diet the next day); and it can also been divided into short-term CR (≤9 days) and long-term CR (>9 days) according to the length of restriction duration. Moreover, low-calorie restriction could be divided into low-caloric diet (LCD) and very-low-caloric diet (VLCD). All of them may improve the state of T2DM, control the blood glucose stably and reduce its morbidity, but the differences of the treatment efficacy among them are not clear until now.

2. The preventive effect of CR on T2DM

As a lifestyle intervention method, it is very important to make sure whether this therapy can prevent T2DM from occurrence in the high risk persons. Tuomilehto et al. [5] had assigned 552 middle-aged, overweight subjects with impaired glucose tolerance to either the intervention group or the control group. Each subject in the intervention group received individualized counseling aimed at reducing weight, total intake of fat, and intake of saturated fat and increasing intake of fiber and physical activity. After 3.2 years follow-up, they found that the cumulative incidence of diabetes was 11 percent (95% confidence interval, 6% to 15%) in the intervention group and 23% (95% confidence interval, 17% to 29%) in the control group, moreover, during the trial, the risk of diabetes was reduced by 58% ($P<0.001$) in the intervention group. The next year, another larger sample follow-up study focused on the lifestyle intervention on diabetes prevention, including CR, exercise, et al. Three years follow-up later, CR reduced the incidence by 58% (95% confidence interval, 48% to 66%), as compared with placebo [6]. These studies provided satisfactory evidences on the preventive effect of CR on T2DM.

3. The therapeutical effect of CR on T2DM

3.1. The short-term therapeutical effect of CR on T2DM

CR has shown to be helpful for the blood glucose control and the improvement of pancreatic islet function. It produces multiple beneficial effects on metabolic parameters in type 2 diabetic patients by virtue of both calorie restriction and weight loss. Animal experiments confirmed that CR regulates the process of glucose metabolism in a variety of tissues (adipose tissue, liver, pancreas, skeletal muscle, et al) [7]. In clinical trials, the blood glucose of the participators decreased to normal range within a few days, and to the lowest point after 1-2 weeks [8]. In another short-term study of 14 obese patients with T2DM using VLCDs, marked improvement was seen in glycosylated HbA1c [9]. It fell from 7.4±0.3% to 6.0±0.2% after 8 weeks VLCD [10]. As a consequence, CR was thought to improve glucose metabolism in type 2 diabetics. Besides, the fasting plasma insulin/C-peptide levels of patients with T2DM fell after CR, and thus improved the insulin sensibility [11]. Generally, Blood pressure, triglycerides, total cholesterol and LDL-C were reduced, while only HDL-C varied [12, 13].

3.2. The long-term therapeutical effect of CR on T2DM

Whether CR improves the state of T2DM for a long time has been the major concern for many researchers. Unick et al. [14] chose 5145 type 2 diabetic patients randomized to an intensive lifestyle intervention and diabetes support and education. The lifestyle intervention group received a behavioral weight loss program that included group and individual meetings, a ≥10% weight loss goal, calorie restriction, and increased physical activity. Diabetes support and education received a less intense educational intervention.After four years follow-up, body weight, blood glucose and lipid profile improved significantly in the intervention group, suggesting that CR may obtain an optimal long-term metabolic control in T2DM patients.

Because of the poor compliance of patients with long-term CR, there are few researches in this area, and more researchers begin to concentrate on the long-term effect of short-term CR on T2DM patients. In a clinical study, 40 obese patients with T2DM and symptomatic hyperglycaemia were selected despite combination oral anti-diabetic therapy+/-insulin, and given 8 weeks of VLCD therapy (750kcal/d), followed by standard diet and exercise advice at 2-3 month intervals up to 1 year [15]. After 8 weeks of VLCD, body weight and body mass index (BMI) fell significantly, with favourable reductions in blood pressure, fructosamine and HbA1c. Sustained improvements were evident after 1 year, with minimal weight regain. Unexpectedly, glycemic control tended to deteriorate. In another study, 18 insulin-treated T2DM patients were treated with 30 days VLCD (450kCal/day) with the cessation of all glucose-lowering medication, and then followed for 18 months [16]. Caloric intake was slowly increased to eucaloric and glucose-lowering medication can be restarted if necessary. After 18 months follow-up, the use of insulin was significantly reduced: 18 out of 18 patients on day 0, 5 out of 18 patients at 18 months. Moreover, although patients using insulin at 18 months had regained weight a little, but still had a better cardiovascular risk profile compared with this parameter before CR (Table 1). In spite of favourable outcomes, these shorter term CR studies still require more data to clarify the long-term therapeutical effect of CR on metabolic disorders.

3.3. The studies of special crowd for CR

Metabolic disorders including obesity and diabetes are more prevalent in children and adolescents. However, most of them cannot obtain a satisfactory blood glucose control since pharmacologic agents currently approved for use in children and adolescents with T2DM (metformin and insulin) are less optimal. Therefore, in hope of a better glucose control in children, lifestyle intervention attracted many interests. A chart review of 20 children (mean age 14.5±0.4 years) who consumed a ketogenic VLCD in the treatment of T2DM was conducted [17]. Eventually, VLCD allowed insulin and oral agents to be discontinued in all but one subject who was not compliant, and no other subjects required resumption of medications during the course of the diet on the condition that the metabolic parameters such as blood glucose and blood pressure were well controlled. More importantly, this study monitored the metabolic profiles to ensure that the patients were not at risk for developing electrolyte disturbances or ketoacidosis. Fortunately, none experienced nausea, vomiting, dehydration, or other side effects, such as orthostatic dizziness, muscle cramps, fatigue or halitosis previously reported in pediatric studies.

The efficacy and safety of CR in the elderly were also investigated. Recently, a total of 5145 individuals with T2DM (1053 aged 65 to 76 and 4092 aged 45 to 64) were chosen to compare the effects of 4 years of intensive lifestyle intervention in older and younger individuals [18]. Both groups were respectively divided into two subgroups and given either lifestyle intervention (include CR and exercise) or health education. After 4 years follow-up, lifestyle intervention was favourable to a better control of blood glucose, blood pressure. Surprisingly, the elderly group gained more benefits than the younger group. Therefore, CR may be considered to be a treatment to metabolic disorders.

4. The mechanism of CR of treating T2DM

In recent years, a number of studies have expounded the possible mechanisms from different sides of the CR studies.

4.1. Weight loss

It was thought that the effect of CR on blood glucose was similar to bariatric surgery, because both of them base on weight loss. Insulin sensitivity and blood glucose are improved after weight loss. However, it is still uncertain. An important issue is that blood glucose of patients fell before weight loss during 40 days VLCD [19]. Studies haven't been consistent with the effect of CR on obese patients with type 2 diabetes either. Bergman et al. [20] had compared the effect of CR on patients with normal BMI ($22.8\pm0.42kg/m^2$) and obesity ($36.1\pm1.548kg/m^2$), and found that both groups had a drop of hepatic glucose production volume after 12-48 hours CR, with a better improvement of the insulin sensitivity in normal BMI group. Recently, Unick et al. [14] divided the participators into overweight group, mildly obese group, moderately obese group and severely obese group according to their body weight, then they were treated with CR. The result showed that the overweight group lose less weight than other groups, but the change of other metabolic indicators was similar. This may show the change of body weight and metabolic indicators is not always parallel. So whether the effect of CR on the control of blood glucose was dependent on the weight loss is unclear now.

4.2. Glycometabolism

Firstly, CR inhibits gluconeogenesis, leading to the decrease of hepatic glucose output, thus reducing the glucose source; it increased fatty acid oxidation in the liver, and then produces ketones, which can improve the tolerance of hungry by inhibiting the appetite impulsion from hypothalamus; glucose metabolism and consumption in liver and muscles also increase after CR [21]. Secondly, CR increases the insulin sensitivity and reduces insulin resistance. When patients were recruited to evaluate the effect of VCLD, insulin resistance index significantly decreased eventually [22, 23]. However, it is still controversial. No contribution of CR on insulin sensitivity was found after 14 severely obese patients with T2DM were treated with VLCD for 7 days [10]. The short duration of VLCD and special population chosen may be responsible for this unsatisfactory result. Finally, CR improves pancreas islet function. The insulin secretion and the area under the insulin curve of OGTT increased after CR [24]. The first phase insulin secretion, which represents acute insulin response, increased after CR as well. Therefore, CR was thought to improve pancreas islet function.

Figure 1 shows the effects of CR on glycometabolism. CR leads to glycogen depletion in muscle and liver, and restriction of carbohydrate leads to lipolysis and the formation of ketone bodies by the liver. Together, hepatic glucose output is reduced via inhibition of gluconeogenesis and glycogenolysis. Meanwhile, high protein stimulates insulin secretion and increases satiety. Circulating ketone bodies probably contribute to tolerability of the diet by suppressing appetite in the hypothalamus. Weight loss and diminution of fat depots in the liver, muscle and peri-visceral space lead to reductions in insulin resistance. Improved insulin sensitivity, dynamic insulin secretion and reduced hepatic glucose output lead to reductions in blood glucose levels.

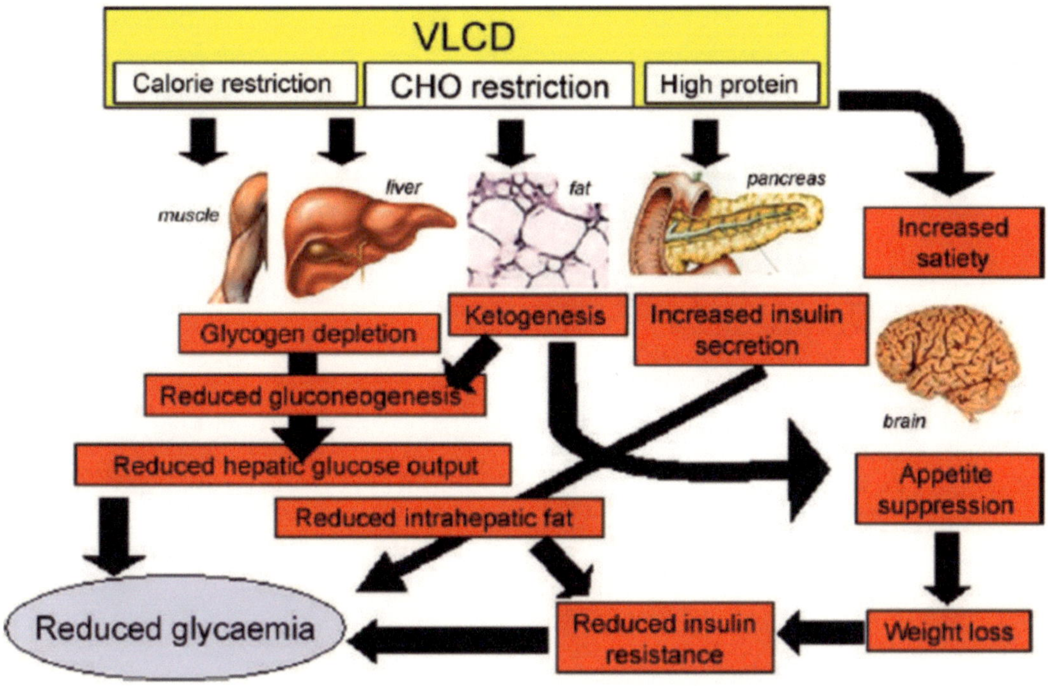

Figure 1. The effects of calorie restriction on glycometabolism. VLCD, very low calorie diet; CHO, carbohydrate.

4.3. Inflammatory response and oxidative stress

CR is "a new environment" to the human body. It causes lower blood glucose, insulin level, fat content and body weight. This helps human more tolerant to stress, thus some chronic diseases (T2DM, et al) could be prevented or treated [25]. Figure 2 has shown the effects of CR on oxidative stress. CR results in an increase in the level and activation of _adenine nucleotide translocase (ANT) and uncoupling protein (UCPs) to reduce the mitochondrial membrane potential, which induces a decrease in superoxide radical production at complex 1 of the electron transport chain. Less damage to the lipids in the mitochondrial membrane is further reduced by increases in the membrane lipid saturation. Increases in superoxide dismutase convert superoxide into hydrogen peroxide and increased levels of glutathione peroxidase (GPX) and catalase convert this to water reducing the product of the toxic hydroxyl radical (OH-) [26]. Lower levels of OH reduce the oxidative damage to proteins and DNA, which is further ameliorated by enhanced levels of degradation and base excision repair respectively. Animal experiments also confirmed that the oxygen free radicals in mice reduced and the β-hydroxybutyrate, which could act as an antioxidant, was increased after CR. In some clinical studies, some inflammatory factors (such as tumor necrosis factor-α, interleukin-6, interleukin-8) decreased significantly after CR.

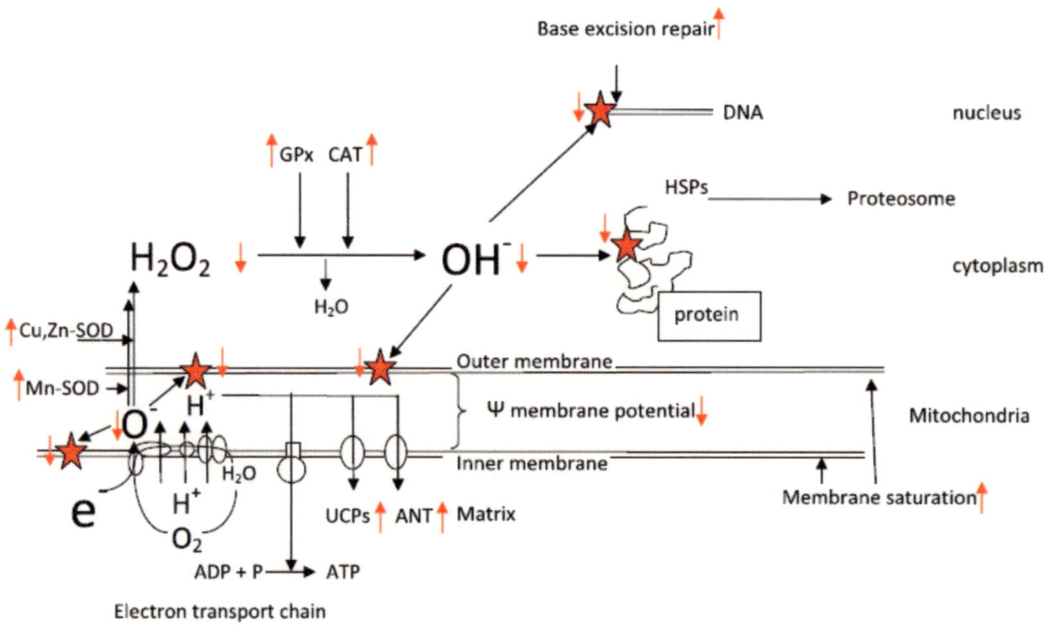

Figure 2. The effects of calorie restriction on oxidative stress.

4.4. Adiponectin

In 2011, Qiao et al. [27] found adiponectin gene expression increased in CR mice. Adiponectin in circulation could regulate various metabolic processes, including anti-inflammatory, insulin sensitivity and resistance, et al. It becomes another possible mechanism.

5. The differences among various forms of CR

Nowadays, the regime of CR in various studies is still not uniform. This causes imparity of CR effect. A systematic review published in 2004 showed that a very low calorie diet was associated with the most weight loss after 12 months in one small study with beneficial effects on asthma. There was no evidence that low carbohydrate diets were associated with greater long-term weight loss than low calorie diets. Nevertheless, they were associated with greater lowering of fasting plasma glucose and HbA1c than low calorie diets, with more adverse events, such as increasing risk of arhythmia, osteoporosis or kidney stones [28]. Until now, there are few evidences from large-scale follow-up studies to clarify the differences among various CR forms.

6. The adverse reactions of CR

Strict caloric restriction may increase risk of hypoglycemia. There are not enough evidences that CR causes arrhythmia or electrolyte disorders in the studies reported until now [29]. The risk of gallstones may be higher in the first few days because of inadequate intake of fat. Bone density decreases during CR without any data showing it increases fracture risk. The most remarkable adverse reaction is increase of uric acid during CR, but only few study found it induced gout. CR may induce the onset of ketosis, which may depend on the total intake of carbohydrate rather than calorie [30]. However, the level of ketone bodies in serum during CR is generally 0.33-0.71mmol/l, which is far below the level during ketoacidosis (>25mmol/l), even though it is abnormal.

Other possible adverse effects include mild dizziness, headache, fatigue, cold, dry skin, transient rash, changes of defecate habits, hair loss, cramps, menstrual disorders and short-term elevated transaminases [31]. Yet for all that, these adverse effects are all slight, and can be treated easily. Generally, CR is relatively safe in patients with type 2 diabetes, but more long-term adverse effects needed to be observed.

7. The prospect forecast of CR used in T2DM

As a type of lifestyle interventions, CR may play a pivotal role in the therapeutic strategy to maintain optimal glycemic control and prevent complications in the patients with type 2 diabetes. In the light of the unreasonable lifestyle nowadays, CR should be paid enough attention to because it provides more choices for the prevention and treatment of T2DM. Existing studies cannot ensure uniform regime of CR for different state of T2DM. Large-scale and forceful researches are required to clarify the differences among all the forms of CR and the long-term adverse effects.

Author details

Shuhang Xu[1,2], Guofang Chen[1,2], Li Chunrui[3] and Chao Liu[1,2*]

*Address all correspondence to: liuchao@nfmcn.com

1 Endocrine and Diabetes Center, Jiangsu Province Hospital on Integration of Chinese and Western Medicine, Nanjing, China

2 University of Traditional Chinese Medicine, Jiangsu Branch of China Academy of Chinese Medical Science, Nanjing, China

3 Department of Endocrinology, Weifang Municipal Official Hospital, Weifang, China

References

[1] Varady KA, Hellerstein MK. Alternate-day Fasting and Chronic Disease Prevention: A Review of Human and Animal Trials. American Journal of Clinical Nutrition 2007;86(1) 7-13.

[2] Tucci P. Caloric Restriction: Is Mammalian Life Extension Linked to p53? Aging (Albany NY) 2012;4(8) 525-534.

[3] Speakman JR, Mitchell SE. Caloric Restriction. Molecular Aspects of Medicine 2011;32(3) 159-221.

[4] Fasting and obesity. British Medical Journal 1978;1(6114) 673.

[5] Tuomilehto J, Lindström J, Eriksson JG, Valle TT, Hämäläinen H, Ilanne-Parikka P, Keinänen-Kiukaanniemi S, Laakso M, Louheranta A, Rastas M, Salminen V, Uusitupa M; Finnish Diabetes Prevention Study Group. Prevention of Type 2 Diabetes Mellitus by Changes in Lifestyle among Subjects with Impaired Glucose Tolerance. New England Journal of Medicine 2011;344(18) 1343-1350.

[6] Knowler WC, Barrett-Connor E, Fowler SE, Hamman RF, Lachin JM, Walker EA, Nathan DM; Diabetes Prevention Program Research Group. Reduction in the Incidence of Type 2 Diabetes with Lifestyle Intervention or Metformin. New England Journal Medicine 2002;346(6) 393-403.

[7] Kume S, Uzu T, Kashiwagi A, Koya D. SIRT1, a Calorie Restriction Mimetic, in a New Therapeutic Approach for Type 2 Diabetes Mellitus and Diabetic Vascular Complications. Endocrine, Metabolic & Immune Disorders-Drug Targets 2010;10(1) 16-24.

[8] Anderson JW, Kendall CW, Jenkins DJ. Importance of Weight Management in Type 2 Diabetes: Review with Meta-Analysis of Clinical Studies. Journal of The American College of Nutrition 2003;22(12) 331-339.

[9] Capstick F, Brooks BA, Burns CM, et al. Very Low Calorie Diet (VLCD): A Useful Alternative in The Treatment of The Obese NIDDM Patient. Diabetes Research & Clinical Practice 1997;36(2) 105-110.

[10] Lim EL, Hollingsworth KG, Aribisala BS, et al. Reversal of Type 2 Diabetes: Normalisation of Beta Cell Function in Association with Decreased Pancreas and Liver Triacylglycerol. Diabetologia 2011;54(10) 2506-2514.

[11] Amatruda JM, Richeson JF, Welle SL, et al. The Safety and Efficacy of A Controlled Low-Energy ('Very-Low-Calorie') Diet in The Treatment of Non-Insulin-Dependent Diabetes and Obesity. Archives Internal Medicine 1988;148(4) 873-877.

[12] Henry RR, Gumbiner B. Benefits and Limitations of Very-Low-Calorie Diet Therapy in Obese NIDDM. Diabetes Care 1991;14(9) 802-823.

[13] Uusitupa MI, Laakso M, Sarlund H, et al. Effects of A Very-Low-Calorie Diet on Metabolic Control and Cardiovascular Risk Factors in The Treatment of Obese Non-Insulin-Dependent Diabetics. American Journal of Clinical Nutrition 1990;51(5) 768-773.

[14] Unick JL, Beavers D, Bond DS, et al. The Long-Term Effectiveness of A Lifestyle Intervention in Severely Obese Individuals. American Journal of Medicine 2013;126(3) 236-242.

[15] Dhindsa P, Scott AR, Donnelly R. Metabolic and Cardiovascular Effects of Very-Low-Calorie Diet Therapy in Obese Patients with Type 2 Diabetes in Secondary Failure: Outcomes After 1 Year. Diabetic Medicine 2003;20(4) 319-324.

[16] Jazet IM, de Craen AJ, van Schie EM, et al. Sustained Beneficial Metabolic Effects 18 Months After A 30-Day Very Low Calorie Diet in Severely Obese, Insulin-Treated Patients with Type 2 Diabetes. Diabetes Research & Clinical Practice 2007;77(1) 70-76.

[17] Willi SM, Martin K, Datko FM, et al. Treatment of Type 2 Diabetes in Childhood Using A Very-Low-Calorie Diet. Diabetes Care 2004;27(2) 348-353.

[18] Espeland MA, Rejeski WJ, West DS, et al. Intensive Weight Loss Intervention in Older Individuals: Results From The Action for Health in Diabetes Type 2 Diabetes Mellitus Trial. Journal of American Geriatrics Society 2013;61(6) 912-922.

[19] Malandrucco I, Pasqualetti P, Giordani I, et al. Very-Low-Calorie Diet: A Quick Therapeutic Tool to Improve Beta Cell Function in Morbidly Obese Patients with Type 2 Diabetes. American Journal of clinical nutrition 2012;95(3) 609.

[20] Bergman BC, Cornier MA, Horton TJ, et al. Effects of Fasting on Insulin Action and Glucose Kinetics in Lean and Obese Men and Women. American Journal of Physiology-Endocrinology & Metabolism 2007;293(4) 1103-1111.

[21] Sumithran P, Proietto J. Ketogenic Diets: A Review of Their Principles, Safety and Efficacy. Obesity Research & Clinical Practice 2008;2(1) I-II.

[22] Svendsen PF, Jensen FK, Holst JJ, et al. The Effect of A Very Low Calorie Diet on Insulin Sensitivity, Beta Cell Function, Insulin Clearance, Incretin Hormone Secretion, Androgen Levels and Body Composition in Obese Young Women. Scandinavian Journal of Clinical & Laboratory Investigation 2012;72(5) 410-419.

[23] Yki-Järvinen H. Nutritional Modulation of Nonalcoholic Fatty Liver Disease and Insulin Resistance: Human Data. Current Opinion in Clinical Nutrition & Metabolic Care 2010;13(6) 709-714.

[24] Mulholland Y, Nicokavoura E, Broom J, et al. Very-Low-Energy Diets and Morbidity: A Systematic Review of Longer-Term Evidence. British Journal of Nutrition 2012;108(5) 832-51.

[25] Varady KA, Hellerstein MK. Alternate-Day Fasting and Chronic Disease Prevention: A Review of Human and Animal Trials. American Journal of Clinical Nutrition 2007;86(1) 7-13.

[26] Speakman JR, Mitchell SE. Caloric restriction. Mol Aspects Med. 2011, 32(3): 159-221.

[27] Qiao L, Lee B, Kinney B, et al. Energy Intake and Adiponectin Gene Expression. American Journal of Physiology-Endocrinology & Metabolism 2011;300(5) E809-816.

[28] Avenell A, Brown TJ, McGee MA, et al. What Are The Long-Term Benefits of Weight Reducing Diets in Adults? A Systematic Review of Randomized Controlled Trials. Journal of Human Nutrition & Dietetics 2004;17(4) 317-335.

[29] Sumithran P, Proietto J. Ketogenic diets: a review of their principles, safety and efficacy. Obes. Res. Clin, 2008, 2:1-13.

[30] Seim HC, Mitchell JE, Pomeroy C, et al. Electrocardiographic findings associated with very low calorie dieting. Int J Obes Relat Metab Disord, 1995, 19 (11): 817-819.

[31] Baker S, Jerums G, Proietto J, et al. Effects and Clinical Potential of Very-Low-Calorie Diets (VLCDs) in Type 2 Diabetes. Diabetes Research & Clinical Practice 2009;85(3) 235-242.

Chapter 8

Current Recommendations for Surgical Treatment of Diabetes

Anca Elena Sirbu, Aura Reghina, Carmen Barbu and Simona Fica

Additional information is available at the end of the chapter

http://dx.doi.org/10.5772/59182

1. Introduction

The incidence of type 2 diabetes mellitus continues to rise worldwide and it is now estimated that diabetes affects more than 382 million people worldwide [1]). In the United States, the prevalence of diabetes ranges from 5.8 to 12.9 percent [2], but one of the most bothersome finding is the continuous increase in its prevalence; both community-based Framingham Heart Study and the National Health and Nutrition Examination Survey (NHANES) reported nearly doubling in the incidence of type 2 diabetes over the past decades [3] [4]

Obesity is one of the most important clinical risk factor for diabetes. In Nurses' Health Study, there was an approximately 100-fold increased risk of incident diabetes over 14 years in individuals whose baseline BMI was >35 kg/m^2 compared with those with BMI <22 [5]. While the relationship between BMI and the risk of type 2 diabetes seems to be curvilinear, there is also an additional risk brought by the weight gain. In the same study, a weight gain of 8.0 to 10.9 kg after 18 years was associated with a relative risk for diabetes of 8.0 to 10.9 kg compared with those with minimal weight gain [5].

Sustained weight loss, on the other hand, can substantially improve glycemic control in patients with type 2 diabetes, by providing a partial correction of the two major metabolic abnormalities in type 2 diabetes: insulin resistance and impaired insulin secretion. A weight reduction of only 5 to 10 percent of initial body weight in overweight individuals can have a lasting beneficial impact on serum glucose, dyslipidemia, and hypertension [6]. However, the amount of weight loss required to achieve an ideal glycemic response may depend on the initial glucose level, as shown by the UKPDS study, with higher goals needed for those with non-controlled diabetes [7].

While the benefits of weight loss for obese patients with diabetes are indubitable, there are several strategies for achieving weight loss, with physical activity and intensive lifestyle modification being important components of almost all programs. The Look AHEAD Study, the largest and longest randomized controlled trial of a behavioral intervention for weight loss in patients with diabetes, showed a mean body weight reduction of 8.5% at year one; over the next four years, a gradual regaining of weight was observed, followed by the maintenance of losses of approximately 4-5% in subsequent years [8]. This quite poor maintenance of weight loss, associated with the trial's negative finding with regard to its cardiovascular endpoints [9] sustains the need, at least in some diabetic patients, for more aggressive approaches in order to obtain substantial and durable weight loss.

2. History of bariatric surgery and its use in treating diabetes

The first report of a surgical procedure aiming for weight loss is said to be the Talmud. There it is said that Rabbi Eleazor, who was morbidly obese, underwent an operation after being given a soporific potion wherein his abdomen, or abdominal wall, was opened and a number of "baskets of fat were removed" [10]. However, the first bariatric surgery intervention performed in modern time dates back to 1953, when Varco from Minessota University performed a bypass of small intestine in an obese patient, with bowel reconstruction by an jejunoileostomy [11]. This jejuno-ileal by-pass caused excellent and lasting weight loss but proved to be associated with extensive complications due to short bowel syndrome and bacterial overgrowth. In 1966, Edward Mason, who is considered the father of bariatric surgery, published the landmark paper on gastric bypass [12], while in 1977 Griffen and his colleagues performed the first gastric bypass with a Roux-en-Y gastrojejunostomy (RYGB). The popularity of this intervention rapidly rose, as it proved to be efficient and quite safe, with reduced request for revisional surgery. From the beginning of the 70's gastroplasty was introduced as an important bariatric procedure, firstly as a partial horizontal gastric transection, than as a vertical banded gastroplasty. The following years brought into attention other innovative techniques, such as bilio pancreatic diversion (BPD), laparoscopic adjusted gastric banding (LAGB), sleeve gastrectomy (SG) or gastric plication, designed to improve the main outcome: weight loss and metabolic improvement, but also to reduce the incidence of complications.

The Greek word "baros" means weight and the term bariatric came into use in 1965, defining a branch of medicine dealing with causes, prevention, and treatment of obesity. At the beginning, interventions performed in order to obtain weight loss were mechanistically defined as purely restrictive of food intake (e.g., vertical banded gastroplasty, laparoscopic adjustable gastric banding), restrictive/malabsorptive (e.g., gastric bypass), and primarily malabsorptive (e.g.,biliopancreatic diversion/duodenal switch). It was lately clear that these anatomical descriptions did not provide the mechanism of action and the mechanical explanation of weight loss was subsequently challenged. More than that, the consequences of these procedures go far beyond weight loss, as, in addition to solving mechanical problems of gastroesophageal reflux disease, obstructive sleep apnea, and back and joint pain, they

http://dx.doi.org/10.5772/59182

improve or even cure metabolic diseases (e.g., type 2 diabetes, hyperlipidemia, hypertension, polycystic ovary syndrome, nonalcoholic steatohepatitis, possibly cancer).

Metabolic surgery was defined in 1978 by Henry Buchwald and Richard Varco as "the operative manipulation of a normal organ or organ system to achieve a biological result for a potential health gain" [13]. The practice of metabolic surgery goes, however, way before this timeline; examples are the procedures of gastrectomy or vagotomy for duodenal ulcers, procedures that don't touch the actual lesion, or splenectomy for idiopathic thrombocytopenic purpura. In the late 80's, The Program on the Surgical Control of the Hyperlipidemias (POSCH) showed that a surgical procedure (partial ileal by-pass) could dramatically improve total cholesterol and low-density lipoprotein cholesterol levels, as well as atherosclerotic coronary heart disease mortality and recurrent nonfatal myocardial infarction as well as overall mortality, the incidence of coronary artery bypass grafting and percutaneous transluminal coronary angioplasty, and the development of peripheral vascular disease [14].

Nicola Scopinaro and Walter Pories were among the first who stated the effectiveness of gastrointestinal surgery procedures in correcting or even curing type 2 diabetes; they showed normalization of blood glucose levels after biliopancreatic diversion [15] and gastric by-pass, respectively [16]. In a milestone publication entitled *"Who would have thought it? An operation proves to be the most effective therapy for adult-onset diabetes mellitus"*, Pories underlined the importance of hormonal mechanisms in the process of improving or even curing type 2 diabetes mellitus, independent of weight loss. Bariatric surgery is beyond doubt metabolic surgery, as it causes dramatic improvement of type 2 diabetes and can effectively prevent progression from impaired glucose tolerance to diabetes in severely obese individuals, but it also resolves or mitigates some other important complications of obesity, such as dyslipidemia, hypertension, insulin resistance, sleep apnea [17].

3. Short description of the main bariatric surgery procedures used in diabetic patients

Currently accepted bariatric procedures for the treatment of type 2 diabetic patients are Roux-en-Y gastric by-pass (RYGB), laparoscopic adjusted gastric banding (LAGB), bilio-pancreatic diversion (BPD) and duodenal switch variant (BPD-SD), and sleeve gastrectomy (SG) [18]

The Roux-en-Y gastric bypass (Figure 1) is one of the most commonly performed bariatric procedures worldwide. It developed in the late 60's from the observation that patients with partial gastrectomy suffer a significant and persistent weight loss. After successive changes and optimizations, it is now considered the gold-standard in bariatric surgery. The intervention has several components: in the first step, a 30 milliliters stomach pouch is created by dividing the top of the stomach from the rest of it. Next, the first portion of the small intestine is divided, and the bottom end of the divided small intestine is connected to the newly created stomach pouch. In the final step, the top portion of the divided small intestine is connected to the small intestine further down so that the stomach acids and digestive enzymes from the bypassed stomach and first portion of small intestine will eventually mix with the food [19].

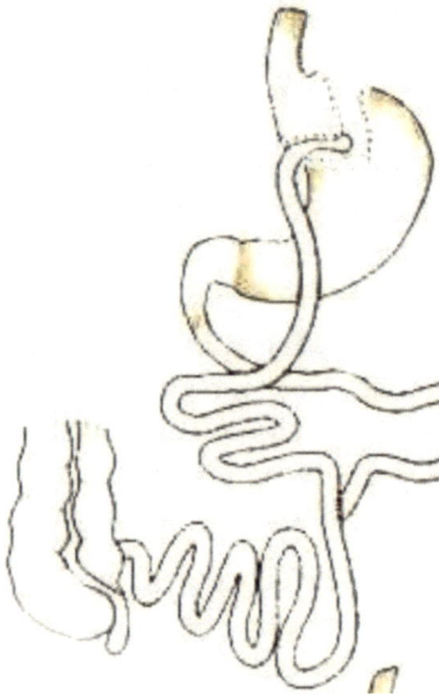

Figure 1. Roux-en-Y gastric bypass

Laparoscopic adjusted gastric banding (Figure 2) involves surgical insertion of an adjustable inflatable band that is placed around the upper part of the stomach to create a smaller stomach pouch. This slows and limits the amount of food that can be consumed at one time, but it does not decrease gastric emptying time. The size of the stomach opening can be adjusted by filling the band with sterile saline, which is injected through a port placed under the skin.

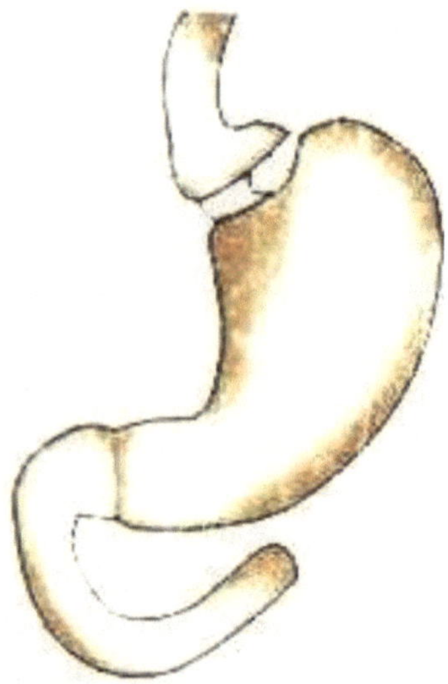

Figure 2. Laparoscopic adjusted gastric banding

http://dx.doi.org/10.5772/59182

Sleeve Gastrectomy (SG) is a procedure that involves removing the lateral part of the great gastric curvature, with stomach resection along the little curvature, from Hiss angle to the antrum [20] – Figure 3. The intervention was initially used as the first part of a two-stage procedure for super-obese patients (BMI > 60kg/m^2), who were considered poor surgical candidates and who would not tolerate a prolonged or more involved procedure. The aim of the procedure was to allow the patients an opportunity to achieve some weight loss before being converted to the more complex gastric bypass or biliopancreatic diversion with duodenal switch (BPD-DS) [21]. It was, however, rapidly proved that weight loss and metabolic benefits were significant and nowadays it is used as a definitive weight loss procedure, with the advantage of the technical simplicity and the lower risk for complications [22]. The most recent guideline of the American Society for Metabolic and Bariatric Surgery also endorsed by the American Association of Clinical Endocrinology does not include this procedure among the investigational ones but considers it consecrated [23]

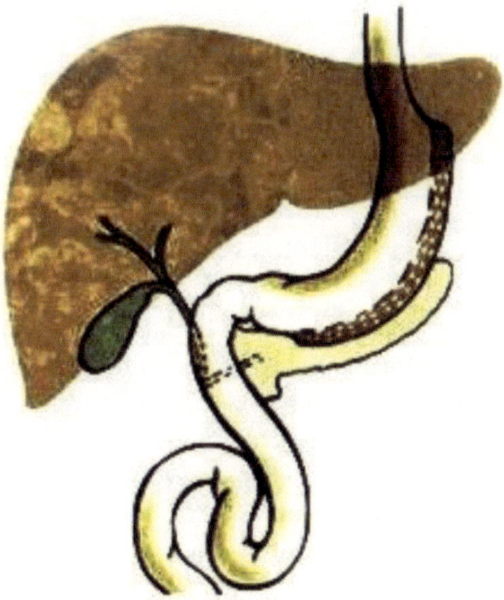

Figure 3. Sleeve gastrectomy

Biliopancreatic diversion with duodenal switch (Figure 4) is a weight loss surgery intervention that is composed of two procedures: in the first one, a smaller, tubular stomach pouch is created by removing a portion of the stomach, and afterwards, a large portion of the small intestine is bypassed. After dividing duodenum just past the outlet of the stomach, a segment of the distal small intestine is then brought up and connected to the outlet of the newly created stomach; in this way, approximately three-fourth of the small intestine in by-passes by food. The bypassed small intestine, which carries the bile and pancreatic enzymes, is reconnected to the last portion of the small intestine [19]

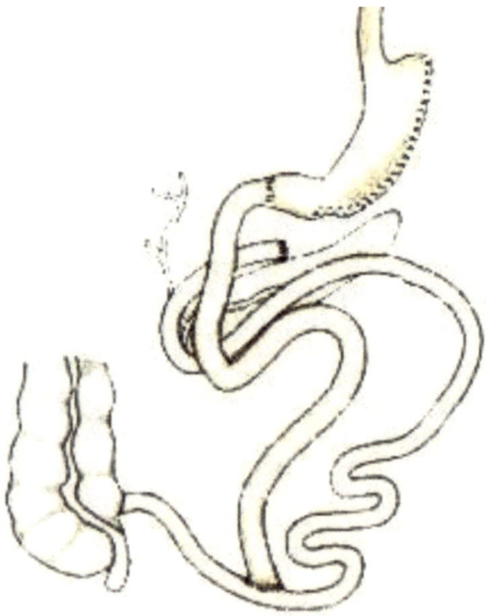

Figure 4. Biliopancreatic diversion with duodenal switch

4. Mechanisms involved in diabetes control or remission

It is very clear that weight loss has a profound impact on diabetes control and much of the effects of bariatric surgery on glucose homeostasis were attributed to its impact on weight. However, several investigators demonstrated the very rapidly normalisation in glucose metabolism (in a few days), way before the weight loss becomes significant [24]. This suggests that diabetes remission may be due to mechanisms involving the surgical technique, aside from weight loss. The most common hypothesis are:

4.1. Caloric restriction hypothesis

It is well-known that very low calories diets may significantly and early improve glycemic control in diabetes patients [25], as caloric restriction can improve hyperglycemia through regulation of hepatic glucose production [26]. Considering the level of caloric absorption from the intestinal tract, all bariatric procedures are restrictive; caloric intake can be restricted by the inhibition of eating, as in AGB, SG or RYGB, or by the insufficient intestinal surface, as in BPD or other so-called "malabsorbtive" procedures.

In a recent study, Jackness et al compared the effect of a very low–calorie diet (VLCD) (500 kcal/day) and RYGB on β-cell function in type 2 diabetic patients during the first 3 weeks after intervention and reported similar degrees of weight loss and no significant differences in β-cell function between the groups [27]. Similar results were presented by Plourde et al in a study regarding the improvement of insulin sensitivity and β-cell function following bilio-pancreatic diversion with duodenal switch (BPD-DS) [28]. Both groups concluded that caloric restriction was primarily responsible for the early effects of bariatric surgery procedures on glucose metabolism. However, this theory doesn't explain the long term differences in efficiency between the different bariatric procedures, despite the similar caloric restriction.

4.2. The neural networks hypothesis

The intestinal tract has important parasympathetic and sympathetic innervations. Vagally mediated reflexes are critical to the control, regulation and organization of appropriate GI functions, including hunger, appetite and satiety. Several studies have demonstrated that the behavior, activity and responsiveness of vagal afferents are altered by diet and obesity [29]. As shown by Browning et al [30], RYGB reversed some of the alteration of dorsal motor nucleus of the vagus neurons induced by high fat diet and improved vagal neuronal health in the brain. Sympathetic gut innervation, on the other hand, is involved in glucose production and release, inhibition of peristalsis and inhibition of gastrointestinal enzyme secretion. Weight loss induced by bariatric surgery may trigger profound sympathoinhibitory effects [31]

4.3. The hindgut hypothesis

This is probably the most accepted hypothesis that focuses on the expedited delivery of nutrients to the ileum after most of the bariatric procedures, which results in the accentuated production of peptides produced by L cells in the distal small intestine, including glucagon-like peptide (GLP)-1, peptide YY (PYY), and oxyntomodulin [32]. GLP-1 and PYY are both secreted by the L cells located in the distal gastrointestinal tract in response to nutrient ingestion and elicit almost the same metabolic responses. Together with GIP, they are responsible for the incretin effect, which consists in the greater insulin response after oral ingestion of glucose as compared with the insulin response after intravenous infusion of glucose when plasma glucose concentrations are the same [33].

It was shown that GLP-1 amplifies important steps in insulin synthesis and transcription, stimulates beta cell proliferation, reduces appetite and gastrointestinal motility [34]. It has been shown that GLP-1 is reduced in patients with type 2 diabetes and this have resulted in the development of t two drug classes currently approved for the treatment of T2DM: the long-acting analogues of GLP-1, and the inhibitors of dipeptidyl peptidase 4 (the enzyme responsible for the rapid degradation of GLP-1) [33]. After RYGB, postprandial secretion of GLP-1 increases approximately 20 times [32]; this effect has been demonstrated as early as one week after surgery and persists for at least 10 years thereafter [35]. The improvement in incretin levels is not dependent on weight loss and, in diabetic patients, it has been paralleled by improved glucose tolerance [33]. An increased of postprandial GLP-1 levels has also been reported following gastric sleeve, apparently comparable to that obtained after RYGB, in the short and in the long term [36]. However, several recent studies suggest that the dramatic increase in GLP-1 secretion observed in the long term after RYGB surgery contributes to improved beta-cell function but does not appear to be the key determinant for the resolution of T2DM following this type of surgery [36]. Likewise, data from a rodent model have shown that blocking the action of GLP-1 does not influence the dramatic improvement in glucose tolerance observed after sleeve gastrectomy and therefore that GLP-1 receptor activity is not necessary for the beneficial metabolic effects of SG [37].

4.4. The foregut hypothesis

This theory suggests that the bypass of the duodenum and proximal jejunum after RYGB, or the lack of food exposure to these areas of the small intestine, might determine the decrease in secretion of an unknown duodenal factor (an antiincretin) influencing glucose homeostasis. The anti-incretin hypothesis, embraced by Rubino [38], postulates that, in addition to the well-known incretin effect, nutrient passage in the bowel can also cause activation of negative feedback mechanisms (anti-incretins) to balance the effects of incretins and other postprandial glucose-lowering mechanisms. Supporters of this theory suggest the physiologic necessity of these control mechanisms to prevent the risk for postprandial hyperinsulinemic hypoglycemia and uncontrolled beta cell proliferation induced by incretins. Excess of anti-incretin signals, perhaps stimulated by macronutrient composition or chemical additives of modern diets, might cause insulin resistance, reduced insulin secretion, and beta cell depletion, leading to type 2 diabetes [38]. On the other hand, bariatric surgery, by resecting or excluding parts of the small bowel from nutrients transit, changes the incretins/anti-incretins balance; this might explain the improvement or even the cure of type 2 diabetes, but also the postprandial hyperinsulinemic hypoglycaemia that can complicate RYGB [39]

4.5. Other theories

4.5.1. Bile acids hypothesis

Among the changes to intestinal physiology that occur after bariatric surgery is the altered enterohepatic circulation of bile acids. Bile acids are now recognized to be involved in the regulation of various metabolic processes including lipids, glucose, and energy homeostasis. Their binding to a nuclear receptor (farsenoid-X-receptor or FXR) produces alterations in hepatic glucose production and intestinal glucose absorption influences on peripheral insulin sensitivity and incretin effects [40]. After RYGB, fasting and postprandial serum concentrations of bile acids increase. Gerhard et al reported that patients with postoperative remission of diabetes after RYGB showed larger increases in fasting bile acids than did patients who did not achieve diabetes remission or who did not have diabetes preoperatively [41]. A recent study published by Karen Ryan and colleagues from the University of Cincinnati showed that VSG is associated with increased circulating bile acids and that, in the absence of FXR, the ability of VSG to reduce body weight and improve glucose tolerance is substantially reduced. These results point to bile acids and FXR signaling as an important molecular underpinning for the beneficial effects of bariatric surgery [42].

4.5.2. Gut microbiota hypothesis

The gut microbiota is recognized to have an important role in energy storage and the subsequent development of obesity. It is well-known that obese individuals have an increased ratio

http://dx.doi.org/10.5772/59182

of Firmicutes to Bacteroidetes bacteria and decreased bacterial diversity compared with lean controls—differences that disappear in response to weight loss, whether surgical or dietary intervention [43]. Recent studies proved the change in gut flora after RYGB; in addition to the standard decrease in the Firmicutes to Bacteroidetes ratio that accompanies weight loss, a major finding from microbial sequencing analyses after RYGB is the comparative overabundance of the phylum Proteobacteria in the distal gut microbiome [44]. In a murine bariatric model changes in gut microbiota were similar to those seen in humans after RYGB, and transfer of the surgically altered microbial species to non-operated, germ-free mice resulted in weight loss; this suggests that changes in gut microbiota might contribute to the beneficial effect of RYGB [45].

5. Trials proving the efficacy of bariatric surgery in diabetes control

Obesity and type 2 diabetes mellitus are both major health problems due to growing incidence and increasing costs of care [46]. Type 2 diabetes mellitus closely follow incidence and prevalence of obesity and the evolution of the disease is marked by several complications such as retinopathy and blindness, neuropathy and lower limb amputations, end stage renal disease, myocardial infarction and stroke if the disease is not well controlled. Despite of tremendous progressions which have been made in type 2 diabetes mellitus treatment, more than fifty percent of patients do not reach their glycemic control targets [47].

There are a number of **observational trials** and published meta-analyses that demonstrate consistent improvement of type 2 diabetes after metabolic surgery. In an observational controlled study from Norway, morbidly obese patients with mean BMI 45.1 kg/m^2 were treated with either Roux-en-Y gastric bypass or intensive medical therapy. At one year weight loss was 30% in surgery group compared with 8% in lifestyle group and diabetes remission rate was 70% versus 33%. [48]

A meta-analysis of studies on type 2 diabetes obese patients who underwent different types of bariatric procedures showed at baseline the mean age 40.2 years, body mass index was 47.9 kg/m^2, 80% were female, weight loss overall was 38.5 kg or 55.9% excess body weight loss and an overall rate of remission of diabetes of 78%. [49] Remission of diabetes occurred in half of patients who underwent laparoscopic adjustable gastric bypass, 80% of patients who underwent Roux-en-Y gastric bypass, and 95% of those who underwent biliopancreatic diversion. [49]

The key results from the Swedish Obese Subjects (SOS) study have been published in a review. This is a long term, prospective, controlled trial on 2010 obese subjects who underwent metabolic surgery (13% gastric bypass, 19% banding and 68% vertical banded gastroplasty) and 2037 matched obese control subjects receiving usual care. [50] The diabetes remission rate was increased several fold at 2 years (adjusted OR=8.42) and 10 years (adjusted OR=3.45). After 2 years of follow-up, 72% of SOS patients with type 2 diabetes mellitus at baseline were in remission in the surgery group. But amongst patients who underwent surgery with remission of diabetes at 2 years, 50% had relapsed after 10 years. [50]

The outcomes of bariatric surgery are analyzed in a retrospective case-matched study comparing medical treatment, duodenal switch, and laparoscopic adjustable gastric band to Roux-en-Y gastric bypass for treatment of obese type 2 diabetes. [51] At one year of follow-up the Roux-en-Y gastric bypass produced greater weight loss, A1c improvement, and higher diabetes medication score reduction than medical therapy and laparoscopic adjustable gastric bypass but duodenal switch produced greater reduction in A1c and diabetic medication score than Roux-en-Y gastric bypass. [51]

Recently more and more evidences come from **randomized controlled trials**. These studies are difficult to be compared because of different inclusions criteria regarding the mean age, duration of diabetes, mean BMI and different primary endpoints and also lack of homogenous definition of diabetes remission. The first randomized controlled trial conducted on a small group compared conventional diabetes therapy consisting on weight loss by lifestyle changes versus laparoscopic adjustable gastric banding associated to diet on 60 obese patients (BMI >30 and <40) with recently diagnosed type 2 diabetes [52]. After two years of follow-up, remission of type 2 diabetes defined by fasting glucose level <126 mg/dl and glycated hemoglobin value <6.2% without glycemic therapy, was achieved by 73% in surgical group and by 13% in the conventional group. [52] As the authors recognized, this study has several limitations: relatively small number of patients, limited time of follow-up thus the results cannot be extrapolated for a longer period, lack of hard end points such as mortality and cardiovascular events [52].

A higher number of patients, 150 were included in Surgical Treatment and Medications Potentially Eradicate Diabetes Efficiently trial (STAMPEDE trial) and were randomly assigned to intensive medical therapy alone or intensive medical therapy plus either Roux-en-Y gastric bypass or sleeve gastrectomy. [53] These patients had a longer duration of diabetes, >8 years and mean BMI was 36 and glycated hemoglobin at baseline range from 8.9% to 9.5%. At 12 months of follow-up the target glycated hemoglobin level <6% was achieved by 12% in the intensive medical therapy alone group versus 42% in the gastric-bypass group and 37% in the sleeve-gastrectomy group, without significant differences between surgical groups. [53] Glycated hemoglobin and fasting plasma glucose improved significantly faster and at a great magnitude at three months in surgical groups compared with medical therapy group with a lower use of antidiabetic agents and this improvement was sustained over the entire follow-up period. [53] Type 2 diabetes mellitus control was significantly improved after both bariatric surgery procedures with a reduction of glycated hemoglobin by 2.9 percentage points. The average number of diabetes medications per patient per day increased in intensive medical therapy from 2.8 at baseline to 3 at one year and decreased in surgical groups from 2.6 (Roux-en-Y bypass group) and 2.4 (Sleeve gastrectomy group) to 0.3 and 0.9 respectively. [53] Insulin treatment at 12 months of follow-up was more prevalent among patients on intensive medical therapy group 38% versus gastric by-pass group 4% and sleeve-gastrectomy group 8%. [53] Not only glycemic control was improved secondly bariatric surgery but also HOMA-IR index, CRP level, lipid profile, with significantly decreased of triglycerides and increased of high-density lipoprotein (HDL) cholesterol. The main limitation of this study, short duration of follow-up is overcome by another study with a follow-up period of two years, performed on

60 obese (BMI over 35), type 2 diabetic patients randomized on medical therapy, laparoscopic gastric bypass and biliopancreatic diversion. [54] In this study remission of diabetes was defined by fasting plasma glucose level of less than 100 mg/dl (5.6 mmol/l) and glycated hemoglobin level of less than 6.5% for at least one year without antidiabetic agents. At two years of follow-up the remission of diabetes occurred in 75% of patients in gastric bypass group, 95% of patients in biliopancreatic diversion group and none of patients in medical therapy group. [54] The relative risk of diabetes remission was 7.5 in the gastric-bypass group and 9.5 in the biliopancreatic-diversion group as compared with the medical-therapy group. [54] The average time to the normalization of fasting glucose and glycated hemoglobin was 10 months for gastric bypass versus 4 months for biliopancreatic diversion, differences being significant. [54] Biliopancreatic diversion and gastric bypass are much more effective in controlling glycemia in type 2 obese diabetes patients than medical therapy. [54] The Diabetes Surgery Study compared Roux-en-Y gastric bypass versus medical therapy in achieving a composite endpoint consisting in cardiovascular risk factors, glycated hemoglobin under 7%, LDL cholesterol under 100 mg/dl and systolic blood pressure under 130 mg/dl. [55] At 12 months, 19% in the medical group and 49% in the gastric bypass group achieved the primary composite endpoint. [55]

Glycated hemoglobin was significantly improved at follow-up visit in all groups who underwent a surgical procedure compared with medical group. In the Diabetes Surgery Study the mean A1c at 1 year after gastric bypass was 6.3%, in the Schauer et al study A1c was 6.4% after Roux-en-Y gastric bypass and in the Mingrone et al study A1c was 6.3% after laparoscopic gastric bypass or biopancreatic diversion. [53-55]

Very recently a systematic review and meta-analysis focused on medium term outcomes (five years) after banded Roux-en-Y gastric bypass showed that diabetes remission occurred in 82.2%. [56]

5.1. Lipid profile

Total cholesterol, LDL cholesterol and triglycerides were significantly lower in patients undergoing biliopancreatic diversion than among those receiving medical therapy but there were no significantly differences between medical therapy and gastric bypass. [54] The mean LDL cholesterol at follow-up was 83 mg/dl among patients who underwent gastric bypass versus 89 mg/dl in medical therapy groups. [54, 55] But triglycerides were significantly lower after one year in gastric bypass group versus medical group. [55] HDL cholesterol increased significantly in all three groups (medical therapy, gastric bypass and biliopancreatic diversion) but much more among patients undergoing gastric bypass. [54, 55]

5.2. Blood pressure

Systolic and diastolic blood pressures were significantly improved by gastric bypass and biliopancreatic diversion. [54, 55] No improvement of systolic and diastolic blood pressures was found in another study after Roux-en-Y gastric bypass or sleeve gastrectomy. [53]

Almost all studies showed that all metabolic improvements in the lifestyle-medical group were realized in the first 6 months of follow-up with subsequent decrease of the benefits by 12 months. In contrast improvement continues to increase in the bariatric surgery groups throughout the entire period of follow-up. [52-55]

The most recently published meta-analysis on observational and randomized clinical trial included 6131 patients: 3076 underwent bariatric surgery and 3055 underwent conventional therapy. [57] The mean age of patients included in this meta-analytic research was 47.8 years, ranging from 35.8 to 62.0 years. In the observational studies, the mean A1c in surgery groups was 7.6% versus 7.2% in conventional groups and at follow-up the mean A1c was 6.1% in surgery group versus 7% in conventional group. In the randomized trials, the mean A1c in surgery group was 8.9% versus 8.7% in conventional group and at follow-up the mean A1c was 6.1% in surgery group versus 7.6% in conventional group. In this meta-analysis the remission rate of type 2 diabetes ranged from 38% to 100% in surgery group versus 0% to 46.7% in conventional group. The odds of bariatric surgery patients reaching T2DM remission ranged from 9.8 to 15.8 times the odds of patients treated with conventional therapy. [57]

5.3. Safety and adverse events

The 30-day mortality associated with bariatric surgery is low, estimated at 0.1-0.3%, a rate similar to that for laparoscopic cholecystectomy. [58]

Biliopancreatic diversion and gastric by-pass are relatively safe and adverse events were rare including: incisional hernia, intestinal occlusion. [54, 55] Postoperative complications after gastric bypass consist on anastomotic and staple-line leaks (3.1%), wound infection (2.3%), pulmonary events (2.2%) and wound hematoma (1.7%) and late surgical complications consist on stricture, bleeding anastomotic ulcer, gastritis proximal pouch and small bowel obstruction but no mortality. [55, 59] Rare but often severe hypoglycemia form insulin hypersecretion could occur. [60] Patients in the gastric bypass group experienced 50% more serious and 55% more nonserious adverse events than did those in the lifestyle-medical group. [55] The most serious complication, anastomotic leakage, has decreased in incidence from 5% to 0.8%. [61, 62] A study performed by the US Agency for Healthcare Research and Quality reported a 21% decline in complications after bariatric surgery between 2002 and 2006. [63] The prevalence of postsurgical infections decreased by 58% and abdominal hernias, staple leakage, respiratory failure and pneumonia rates decreased by 29-50%.

Nutritional deficiencies such as: iron-deficiency anemia, hypoalbuminemia, vitamin B deficiency, vitamin D deficiency, osteopenia were more frequent in patients who underwent Roux-en-Y gastric bypass or biliopancreatic diversion despite monitoring of laboratory values and prescription of nutritional supplements. [54, 55, 60]

Some patients and surgery procedures factors related to higher risk have been identified until now. Patients' factors are: older age, increasing BMI, male gender, hypertension, obstructive sleep apnoea, high risk of pulmonary thromboembolism, limited physical mobility. Surgery procedures factors are: surgeon inexperience, low volume centre or surgeon performing surgery occasionally, morbidity and mortality increase with the complexity of the procedure, open compared with laparoscopic procedures, revisional surgery. [60, 64, 65] The presence of type 2 diabetes has not been found to be associated with increased risk for bariatric surgery.

5.4. Conclusions

Up to date, all randomized controlled studies proving effects of bariatric surgery among obese type 2 diabetic subjects have been short-term and have been conducted on relatively small number of patients. Until now only the Swedish Obese Subjects (SOS) study provides evidence of cardiovascular benefits and prolonged improvement in glycemia but this is a non randomized trial. [66, 67] Lager multicenter randomized controlled studies will be required in order to confirm these results. Furthermore is mandatory that studies designed for cardiovascular safety to be performed. More studies are needed especially studies that may provide a better prediction and duration of the remission of diabetes and long-term complications. The success of different bariatric surgery procedures suggests that they should not be seen as a last treatment. Such procedures have to be taken into account earlier in the treatment of type 2 diabetes obese patients.

6. Factors predicting the outcome of surgery in diabetic patients

Most obese type 2 diabetes subjects who underwent bariatric surgery show an important improvement of metabolic features but not every patient has diabetes remission after surgery, suggesting that some clinical characteristics could predict which patient is best suitable for a particular metabolic surgery procedure. Furthermore it is important to identify patients who will not respond to metabolic surgery, so that these patients not to be exposed to an unnecessary surgical procedure that could be without clear benefits. Clinical studies showed that the main factors that contribute to the control of diabetes and eventually to the remission of the diseases are as follows:

a. **Age**: A younger age at the moment of bariatric surgery increased the chance of diabetes remission. [68] In a study on 154 Chinese patients who underwent gastric bypass, younger age was associated with remission of diabetes at 12 months [69]. However, in other studies age was not a predictor of diabetes remission one year after Roux-en-Y gastric bypass or sleeve gastrectomy [53], or at two years of follow-up after gastric by-pass and biliopancreatic diversion. [54]

b. **Diabetes duration**: As an estimation of diabetes severity, the longer the duration, the lower the chances of remission [70]. An analysis of 161 patients showed that duration of diabetes below 4 years was a predictive factor of diseases remission [71]. The duration of diabetes strongly and independently influenced remission at 1 year after gastric bypass [69]. On the other hand at two years of follow-up after gastric by-pass and biliopancreatic diversion diabetes duration was not a predictor of diabetes remission [54].

c. **Insulin treatment** Frequently insulin treatment is used in type 2 diabetes as ad on therapy after oral antidiabetic agents have failed because of the progressive nature of the disease characterized by continuous decrease of beta cell function. Absence of insulin treatment was a predictive factor for remission of diabetes after bariatric surgery. [68, 71] The insulin use was associated with lower remission rates compared with oral medication (13.5 versus 53.8%). [72]

d. **Weight loss**. The amount of weight loss seems to be of major importance in the improvement of glucose control after laparoscopic adjustable gastric banding. [52] Also percentage weight loss at 1 year over 25% independently influenced remission of diabetes after gastric bypass. [69] But no correlation between normalization of fasting glucose levels and weight loss after gastric bypass and biliopancreatic diversion was observed in another study. [54] Weight changes after these former surgical procedures were not significant predictors of diabetes remission at 2 years or of normalization of glycated hemoglobin. [54] But in the Diabetes Surgery Study weight loss explains most of the benefit on glycemic control of gastric bypass. [55] A baseline BMI under 50 kg/m^2 and a one year BMI under 35 kg/m^2 were predictive factors for diabetes remission whatever the procedures. [71]

e. **Initial level of C peptide:** Fasting C-peptide concentration is correlated with beta cell mass and insulin secretion. Very low C-peptide levels could be useful in identifying type 1 diabetes and latent autoimmune diabetes in adults that could have as comorbidity obesity. C-peptide levels are increased as response to insulin resistance in obese type 2 diabetes subjects and are correlated with BMI but decreased with duration of diabetes. [69] A high level of C-peptide before metabolic surgery increased the chance of a good outcome. The cut-off value of C-peptide ≥2.9ng/ml at baseline predicts the remission of diabetes after gastric bypass. [69] Also in another study the diabetes remission rates strongly correlate with the level of C-peptide: 55.3% for those with preoperative C-peptide <3ng/ml, 82% for C-peptide 3-6ng/ml, and 90.3% for C-peptide >6ng/ml. [73] Another study showed that 90% of type 2 diabetes patients with preoperative fasting C-peptide levels over 1 nmol/l had mean A1c <6.5% after Roux-en-Y gastric bypass and 74% had complete resolution of diabetes. But none of the patients with fasting C-peptide level less than 1 nmol/l before surgery experienced diabetes remission. The authors of this study recommend fasting C-peptide levels to be measured in order to a better prediction of diabetes remission after surgery. [74]

f. **Type of surgical procedures** Preoperative data of patients could be of greater importance in the resolution of diabetes than the choice of bariatric surgery procedures. There are several studies that analysed the efficiency of different types of surgical procedures, reporting remission rates of 7-70% for gastric banding, 38-98% for gastric by-pass, 33-85% for sleeve gastrectomy and 52-100% for biliopancreatic diversion. [75] Weight loss and diabetes resolution were greatest for patients undergoing biliopancreatic diversion/ duodenal switch, followed by gastric bypass, and least for banding procedures. [49]

The combination of these factors has an increased power in prediction of the outcomes. If a score of 1 is assigned to duration of diabetes <4years, percentage weight loss at 1 year >25%, and C-peptide ≥2.9ng/ml at baseline, a cumulative score of 2 or 3 was associated with a remission rate of 92%, and a score of 0 or 1 was associated with a remission rate of 27%. [69]

In a retrospective cohort study on 690 patients was developed a score, DiaRem, to predict probability of diabetes remission within five years after Roux-en-Y gastric bypass surgery. Four preoperative clinical variables were identifying of importance in this score: insulin use (no use 0, use of insulin 10 points), age (<40 years 0, 40-49 years 1 point, 50-59 years 2 points, >60 years 3 points), glycated hemoglobin (<6.5% 0, 6.5-6.9% 2 points, 7-8.9% 4 points, >9% 6 points), and type of antidiabetic drugs (no sulfonylureas or insulin-sensitising agents other than metformin 0, sulfonylureas and insulin-sensitising agents other than metformin 3 points). [68] The DiaRem score ranges from 0 to 22. [68] The study showed that 88% of patients who scored 0-2, 64% of those who scored 3-7, 23% of those who scored 8-12, 11% of those who scored 13-17, and 2% of those who scored 18-22 achieved remission (partial or complete) according ADA definition. [68]

7. Actual guidelines for surgical treatment in diabetic patients

Obesity and type 2 diabetes mellitus are chronic, multifactorial and complex disorders with serious outcomes on health and requires multidisciplinary approach in order to improve prognostic.

Several international society have launched their guidelines, position statement and recommendations on type 2 diabetes mellitus and metabolic surgery based on growing evidences form observational, randomized controlled studies and metaanalysis. [60, 76-79] These guidelines and position statement are needed because the global prevalence of type 2 diabetes is rising dramatically as a consequence of obesity epidemic and environmental changes including high calorie food abundance and lack of physical activity. Type 2 diabetes and obesity are associated with premature morbidity and mortality and are major public health threats of the 21st century. There is increasing evidence that prognostic of patients with type 2 diabetes mellitus and obesity is dramatically improved by bariatric surgery that produces important weight loss, substantially decreases of glycated hemoglobin, improvement of lipid profile and reduces the cardiovascular risk and it even can produces remission of diabetes. [60] Bariatric surgery for severe obesity associated with diabetes mellitus is cost-effective. [60]

8. Indications for bariatric surgery in adults with type 2 diabetes mellitus

Bariatric surgery is clearly indicated in type 2 diabetes mellitus patients with BMI >35kg/m^2 (evidence level A) especially if diabetes or associated comorbidities are difficult to control with lifestyle and pharmacological therapy. In these patients surgery can contribute to beta cell function improvement and diabetes remission. For patients with type 2 diabetes mellitus and BMI ranged between 30 and 35 kg/m^2 surgery may be considered on an individual basis (evidence level A, B, C and D). [77] In patients with type 2 diabetes and BMI >30 kg/m^2 and <35 kg/m^2, bariatric surgery may be considered if HbA1c >7.5% despite fully optimized conventional therapy, especially weight is increasing, or other weight responsive co-morbidities not achieving targets on conventional therapies (blood pressure, dyslipidaemia, and obstructive sleep apnea). [60] There are insufficient data to generally recommend surgery in patients with BMI under 35 kg/m^2 outside of a research protocol. [76] Table 1 summarized indications of bariatric surgery in type 2 diabetes mellitus according different international organizations.

9. Indications for bariatric surgery in adolescents

Surgery should be considered if adolescents had BMI >40 kg/m^2, or >35 kg/m^2 with severe co-morbidities, including type 2 diabetes mellitus, aged >15 years, with Tanner pubertal stage 4 or 5 and skeletal maturity, and could provide informed consent and patients have failed a lifestyle and pharmacotherapy for six months [80]. International Diabetes Federation position statement advised that only two procedures Roux-en-Y gastric bypass and laparoscopic adjustable gastric banding are currently conventional bariatric surgical procedures for adolescents [60].

	Type 2 diabetes mellitus and BMI >35kg/m^2	Type 2 diabetes mellitus and BMI >30, <35 kg/m^2	Type 2 diabetes mellitus and BMI <30 kg/m^2
IDF 2011 [60]	Yes	May be considered on individual basis	Research only
ADA 2014 [76]	Yes	May be considered on individual basis	Research only
AACE 2013 [79]	Yes	May be considered on individual basis	Research only
EASO/IFSO EC 2013 [77]	Yes	May be considered on individual basis	Research only
AHA/ACC/TOS 2013 [78]	Yes	No recommendation for or against	

Table 1. Current recommendations for surgical treatment in type 2 diabetes

Contraindications for bariatric surgery in the treatment of type 2 diabetes mellitus are: secondary diabetes, pancreatic autoantibodies (anti glutamic acid decarboxilasis, islet cells antibodies) positivity, C-peptide < 1ng/ml or unresponsive to mixed meal challenge.

Which surgical procedures are indicated for obese type 2 diabetes patients? Nowadays there is no evidence in favor of any particular procedure but the impact on weight loss, lipid profile, glycated hemoglobin and diabetes remission is increasing according to the surgical procedures as follows: adjustable gastric banding, sleeve gastrectomy, Roux-en-Y gastric bypass, bilio-pancreatic diversion with duodenal switch, biliopancreatic diversion. A laparoscopic technique should be considered as the preferable approach to the operation. Some pre-operative factors specific to type 2 diabetes mellitus could influence the choice of surgical procedures: duration of diabetes, pre-operative level of glycated hemoglobin, number of antidiabetic drugs used, and fasting C-peptide levels. [60, 77]

The assessment of bariatric surgery outcomes in type 2 diabetes and factors indicating the beneficial effects of bariatric surgery in diabetes: There is not an international consensus regarding definition of success of bariatric surgery in diabetes mellitus.

Partial remission of diabetes is characterized by: HbA1c >6% but <6.5%, fasting plasma glucose 100-125 mg/dl, at least 1 year duration, no active pharmacological therapy or ongoing procedures. Complete remission of diabetes is characterized by: HbA1c <6%, fasting plasma glucose <100 mg/dl, at least 1 year duration, no active pharmacological therapy or ongoing procedures. Prolonged remission is characterized by complete remission of at least 5 years duration. [60, 76, 77]

According IDF optimization of the metabolic state may be defined as: HbA1c ≤ 42 mmol/mol (6%); no hypoglycaemia; total cholesterol < 4mmol/l; LDL cholesterol <2 mmol/l; triglycerides <2.2mmol/l; blood pressure < 135/85 mmHg; >15% weight loss; with reduced medication from the pre-operated state or without other medications. A substantial improvement in the metabolic state may be defined as: lowering of HbA1c by >20%; LDL cholesterol <2.3 mmol/l; blood pressure <135/85 mmHg with reduced medication from the pre-operated state. [60]

Adverse events: The morbidity and mortality associated with bariatric surgery is generally low and similar to that of well-accepted procedures such as elective gall bladder or gallstone surgery. [60] There are patients and surgical procedures factors that can modify the risk of operation. The surgical complexity and potential surgical risks of procedures decrease in following order: biliopancreatic diversion, biliopancreatic diversion with duodenal switch, Roux-en-Y gastric bypass, laparoscopic sleeve gastrectomy, adjustable gastric bypass. [77]

Follow-up should be provided to all patients who underwent bariatric surgery in interdisciplinary (medical and surgery) joint clinics. Generally the follow-up starts at 1 month after surgery and after that every 3 months in the first year, every 6 months for the second year and annually thereafter. Patients with type 2 diabetes who underwent to metabolic surgery need lifelong nutritional support and medical monitoring. The nutritional support consists in: adequate protein intake (minimum advised protein intake of approximately 90 g/day after biliopancreatic diversion) in order to prevent excessive lean body mass loss, avoidance of ingestion of concentrated sweets to prevent dumping syndrome, vitamin and other micronutrients supplementations according to the type of surgical procedures. Medication for diabetes and insulin should be adjusted immediately after surgery in order to decrease the risk of hypoglycaemia. After biliopancreatic diversion procedure, proton pump inhibitors/histamine 2 receptor antagonists for the entire first post-operative year are recommended. [60, 77, 78]

It is necessary to perform more research (larger, well-designed, randomized control trial with longer-term follow-up) in order to bring up evidence for guidelines in the following areas: which type 2 diabetes patients are most likely to benefit from and least likely to have adverse events of bariatric surgery and which surgical procedures are best fitted to different populations.

Author details

Anca Elena Sirbu*, Aura Reghina, Carmen Barbu and Simona Fica

*Address all correspondence to: ancaelenasirbu@yahoo.com

Carol Davila University of Medicine and Pharmacy, Endocrinology Department, Bucharest, Romania

References

[1] *Diabetes Atlas 6th Edition http://www.idf.org/diabetesatlas.*

[2] *National Diabetes Statistics Report, 2014 http://www.cdc.gov/diabetes/pubs/statsreport14/national-diabetes-report-web.pdfv.*

[3] Fox, C.S., et al., *Trends in the incidence of type 2 diabetes mellitus from the 1970s to the 1990s: the Framingham Heart Study.* Circulation, 2006. 113(25): p. 2914-8.

[4] Selvin, E., et al., *Trends in prevalence and control of diabetes in the United States, 1988-1994 and 1999-2010.* Ann Intern Med, 2014. 160(8): p. 517-25.

[5] Colditz, G.A., et al., *Weight gain as a risk factor for clinical diabetes mellitus in women.* Ann Intern Med, 1995. 122(7): p. 481-6.

[6] Pasanisi, F., et al., *Benefits of sustained moderate weight loss in obesity.* Nutr Metab Cardiovasc Dis, 2001. 11(6): p. 401-6.

[7] *UK Prospective Diabetes Study 7: response of fasting plasma glucose to diet therapy in newly presenting type II diabetic patients, UKPDS Group.* Metabolism, 1990. 39(9): p. 905-12.

[8] Look, A.R.G., *Eight-year weight losses with an intensive lifestyle intervention: the look AHEAD study.* Obesity (Silver Spring), 2014. 22(1): p. 5-13.

[9] Look, A.R.G., et al., *Cardiovascular effects of intensive lifestyle intervention in type 2 diabetes.* N Engl J Med, 2013. 369(2): p. 145-54.

[10] Buchwald, H., *The Evolution of Metabolic/Bariatric Surgery.* Obes Surg, 2014.

[11] Buchwald, H. and J.N. Buchwald, *Evolution of operative procedures for the management of morbid obesity 1950-2000.* Obes Surg, 2002. 12(5): p. 705-17.

[12] Mason, E.E. and C. Ito, *Gastric bypass in obesity.* Surg Clin North Am, 1967. 47(6): p. 1345-51.

[13] Buchwald, H. and R.L. Varco, *Metabolic surgery.* Modern surgical monographs1978, New York: Grune & Stratton. xii, 317 p.

[14] Buchwald, H., et al., *Plasma lipids and cardiovascular risk: a POSCH report. Program on the Surgical Control of the Hyperlipidemias.* Atherosclerosis, 2001. 154(1): p. 221-7.

[15] Scopinaro, N., *Biliopancreatic diversion: mechanisms of action and long-term results.* Obes Surg, 2006. 16(6): p. 683-9.

[16] Pories, W.J., et al., *Who would have thought it? An operation proves to be the most effective therapy for adult-onset diabetes mellitus.* Ann Surg, 1995. 222(3): p. 339-50; discussion 350-2.

[17] Buchwald, H., et al., *Bariatric surgery: a systematic review and meta-analysis.* JAMA, 2004. 292(14): p. 1724-37.

[18] Buchwald, H. and D.M. Oien, *Metabolic/bariatric surgery Worldwide 2008.* Obes Surg, 2009. 19(12): p. 1605-11.

[19] *https://asmbs.org/patients/bariatric-surgery-procedures.* [cited 2014 august].

[20] Copaescu, C., *[Laparoscopic sleeve gastrectomy for morbid obesity].* Chirurgia (Bucur), 2009. 104(1): p. 79-85.

[21] Almogy, G., P.F. Crookes, and G.J. Anthone, *Longitudinal gastrectomy as a treatment for the high-risk super-obese patient.* Obes Surg, 2004. 14(4): p. 492-7.

[22] Felberbauer, F.X., et al., *Laparoscopic sleeve gastrectomy as an isolated bariatric procedure: intermediate-term results from a large series in three Austrian centers.* Obes Surg, 2008. 18(7): p. 814-8.

[23] Mechanick, J.I., et al., *Clinical practice guidelines for the perioperative nutritional, metabolic, and nonsurgical support of the bariatric surgery patient-2013 update: cosponsored by american association of clinical endocrinologists, the obesity society, and american society for metabolic & bariatric surgery.* Endocr Pract, 2013. 19(2): p. 337-72.

[24] Schauer, P.R., et al., *Effect of laparoscopic Roux-en Y gastric bypass on type 2 diabetes mellitus.* Ann Surg, 2003. 238(4): p. 467-84; discussion 84-5.

[25] Henry, R.R. and B. Gumbiner, *Benefits and limitations of very-low-calorie diet therapy in obese NIDDM.* Diabetes Care, 1991. 14(9): p. 802-23.

[26] Kelley, D.E., et al., *Relative effects of calorie restriction and weight loss in noninsulin-dependent diabetes mellitus.* J Clin Endocrinol Metab, 1993. 77(5): p. 1287-93.

[27] Jackness, C., et al., *Very low-calorie diet mimics the early beneficial effect of Roux-en-Y gastric bypass on insulin sensitivity and beta-cell Function in type 2 diabetic patients.* Diabetes, 2013. 62(9): p. 3027-32.

[28] Plourde, C.E., et al., *Biliopancreatic diversion with duodenal switch improves insulin sensitivity and secretion through caloric restriction.* Obesity (Silver Spring), 2014. 22(8): p. 1838-46.

[29] Little, T.J., M. Horowitz, and C. Feinle-Bisset, *Modulation by high-fat diets of gastrointestinal function and hormones associated with the regulation of energy intake: implications for the pathophysiology of obesity.* Am J Clin Nutr, 2007. 86(3): p. 531-41.

[30] Browning, K.N., S.R. Fortna, and A. Hajnal, *Roux-en-Y gastric bypass reverses the effects of diet-induced obesity to inhibit the responsiveness of central vagal motoneurones.* J Physiol, 2013. 591(Pt 9): p. 2357-72.

[31] Seravalle, G., et al., *Long-term sympathoinhibitory effects of surgically induced weight loss in severe obese patients.* Hypertension, 2014. 64(2): p. 431-7.

[32] Dirksen, C., et al., *Mechanisms of improved glycaemic control after Roux-en-Y gastric bypass.* Diabetologia, 2012. 55(7): p. 1890-901.

[33] Vidal, J. and A. Jimenez, *Diabetes remission following metabolic surgery: is GLP-1 the culprit?* Curr Atheroscler Rep, 2013. 15(10): p. 357.

[34] Holst, J.J., *The physiology of glucagon-like peptide 1.* Physiol Rev, 2007. 87(4): p. 1409-39.

[35] Dar, M.S., et al., *GLP-1 response to a mixed meal: what happens 10 years after Roux-en-Y gastric bypass (RYGB)?* Obes Surg, 2012. 22(7): p. 1077-83.

[36] Jimenez, A., et al., *Long-term effects of sleeve gastrectomy and Roux-en-Y gastric bypass surgery on type 2 diabetes mellitus in morbidly obese subjects.* Ann Surg, 2012. 256(6): p. 1023-9.

[37] Wilson-Perez, H.E., et al., *Vertical sleeve gastrectomy is effective in two genetic mouse models of glucagon-like Peptide 1 receptor deficiency.* Diabetes, 2013. 62(7): p. 2380-5.

[38] Rubino, F. and S.A. Amiel, *Is the gut the "sweet spot" for the treatment of diabetes?* Diabetes, 2014. 63(7): p. 2225-8.

[39] Patti, M.E. and A.B. Goldfine, *Hypoglycemia after gastric bypass: the dark side of GLP-1.* Gastroenterology, 2014. 146(3): p. 605-8.

[40] Staels, B. and V.A. Fonseca, *Bile acids and metabolic regulation: mechanisms and clinical responses to bile acid sequestration.* Diabetes Care, 2009. 32 Suppl 2: p. S237-45.

[41] Gerhard, G.S., et al., *A role for fibroblast growth factor 19 and bile acids in diabetes remission after Roux-en-Y gastric bypass.* Diabetes Care, 2013. 36(7): p. 1859-64.

[42] Ryan, K.K., et al., *FXR is a molecular target for the effects of vertical sleeve gastrectomy.* Nature, 2014. 509(7499): p. 183-8.

[43] Aron-Wisnewsky, J., J. Dore, and K. Clement, *The importance of the gut microbiota after bariatric surgery.* Nat Rev Gastroenterol Hepatol, 2012. 9(10): p. 590-8.

[44] Sweeney, T.E. and J.M. Morton, *The human gut microbiome: a review of the effect of obesity and surgically induced weight loss.* JAMA Surg, 2013. 148(6): p. 563-9.

[45] Liou, A.P., et al., *Conserved shifts in the gut microbiota due to gastric bypass reduce host weight and adiposity.* Sci Transl Med, 2013. 5(178): p. 178ra41.

[46] Danaei, G., et al. *National, regional, and global trends in fasting plasma glucose and diabetes prevalence since 1980: systematic analysis of health examination surveys and epidemiological studies with 370 country-years and 2.7 million participants.* Lancet, 2011. 378, 31-40 DOI: 10.1016/S0140-6736(11)60679-X.

[47] Ali, M.K., et al., *Achievement of goals in U.S. diabetes care, 1999-2010.* N Engl J Med, 2013. 368(17): p. 1613-24.

[48] Hofso, D., et al., *Obesity-related cardiovascular risk factors after weight loss: a clinical trial comparing gastric bypass surgery and intensive lifestyle intervention.* Eur J Endocrinol, 2010. 163(5): p. 735-45.

[49] Buchwald, H., et al., *Weight and type 2 diabetes after bariatric surgery: systematic review and meta-analysis.* Am J Med, 2009. 122(3): p. 248-256 e5.

[50] Sjostrom, L., *Review of the key results from the Swedish Obese Subjects (SOS) trial-a prospective controlled intervention study of bariatric surgery.* J Intern Med, 2013. 273(3): p. 219-34.

[51] Dorman, R.B., et al., *Case-matched outcomes in bariatric surgery for treatment of type 2 diabetes in the morbidly obese patient.* Ann Surg, 2012. 255(2): p. 287-93.

[52] Dixon, J.B., et al., *Adjustable gastric banding and conventional therapy for type 2 diabetes: a randomized controlled trial.* JAMA, 2008. 299(3): p. 316-23.

[53] Schauer, P.R., et al., *Bariatric surgery versus intensive medical therapy in obese patients with diabetes.* N Engl J Med, 2012. 366(17): p. 1567-76.

[54] Mingrone, G., et al., *Bariatric surgery versus conventional medical therapy for type 2 diabetes.* N Engl J Med, 2012. 366(17): p. 1577-85.

[55] Ikramuddin, S., et al., *Roux-en-Y gastric bypass vs intensive medical management for the control of type 2 diabetes, hypertension, and hyperlipidemia: the Diabetes Surgery Study randomized clinical trial.* JAMA, 2013. 309(21): p. 2240-9.

[56] Buchwald, H., J.N. Buchwald, and T.W. McGlennon, *Systematic Review and Meta-analysis of Medium-Term Outcomes After Banded Roux-en-Y Gastric Bypass.* Obes Surg, 2014.

[57] Ribaric, G., J.N. Buchwald, and T.W. McGlennon, *Diabetes and weight in comparative studies of bariatric surgery vs conventional medical therapy: a systematic review and meta-analysis.* Obes Surg, 2014. 24(3): p. 437-55.

[58] Buchwald, H., et al., *Trends in mortality in bariatric surgery: a systematic review and meta-analysis.* Surgery, 2007. 142(4): p. 621-32; discussion 632-5.

[59] Nguyen, N.T., et al., *Use and outcomes of laparoscopic versus open gastric bypass at academic medical centers.* J Am Coll Surg, 2007. 205(2): p. 248-55.

[60] Dixon, J.B., et al., *Bariatric surgery: an IDF statement for obese Type 2 diabetes.* Diabet Med, 2011. 28(6): p. 628-42.

[61] DeMaria, E.J., et al., *Results of 281 consecutive total laparoscopic Roux-en-Y gastric bypasses to treat morbid obesity.* Ann Surg, 2002. 235(5): p. 640-5; discussion 645-7.

[62] Hutter, M.M., et al., *First report from the American College of Surgeons Bariatric Surgery Center Network: laparoscopic sleeve gastrectomy has morbidity and effectiveness positioned between the band and the bypass.* Ann Surg, 2011. 254(3): p. 410-20; discussion 420-2.

[63] Encinosa, W.E., et al., *Recent improvements in bariatric surgery outcomes.* Med Care, 2009. 47(5): p. 531-5.

[64] DeMaria, E.J., D. Portenier, and L. Wolfe, *Obesity surgery mortality risk score: proposal for a clinically useful score to predict mortality risk in patients undergoing gastric bypass.* Surg Obes Relat Dis, 2007. 3(2): p. 134-40.

[65] Longitudinal Assessment of Bariatric Surgery, C., et al., *Perioperative safety in the longitudinal assessment of bariatric surgery.* N Engl J Med, 2009. 361(5): p. 445-54.

[66] Sjostrom, L., et al., *Lifestyle, diabetes, and cardiovascular risk factors 10 years after bariatric surgery.* N Engl J Med, 2004. 351(26): p. 2683-93.

[67] Sjostrom, L., et al., *Bariatric surgery and long-term cardiovascular events.* JAMA, 2012. 307(1): p. 56-65.

[68] Still, C.D., et al., *Preoperative prediction of type 2 diabetes remission after Roux-en-Y gastric bypass surgery: a retrospective cohort study.* Lancet Diabetes Endocrinol, 2014. 2(1): p. 38-45.

[69] Dixon, J.B., et al., *Predicting the glycemic response to gastric bypass surgery in patients with type 2 diabetes.* Diabetes Care, 2013. 36(1): p. 20-6.

[70] Ramos-Levi, A.M., et al., *Which criteria should be used to define type 2 diabetes remission after bariatric surgery?* BMC Surg, 2013. 13: p. 8.

[71] Robert, M., et al., *Predictive factors of type 2 diabetes remission 1 year after bariatric surgery: impact of surgical techniques.* Obes Surg, 2013. 23(6): p. 770-5.

[72] Blackstone, R., et al., *Type 2 diabetes after gastric bypass: remission in five models using HbA1c, fasting blood glucose, and medication status.* Surg Obes Relat Dis, 2012. 8(5): p. 548-55.

[73] Lee, W.J., et al., *C-peptide predicts the remission of type 2 diabetes after bariatric surgery.* Obes Surg, 2012. 22(2): p. 293-8.

[74] Aarts, E.O., et al., *Preoperative fasting plasma C-peptide level may help to predict diabetes outcome after gastric bypass surgery.* Obes Surg, 2013. 23(7): p. 867-73.

[75] Ramos-Levi, A.M. and M.A. Rubio Herrera, *Metabolic surgery: quo vadis?* Endocrinol Nutr, 2014. 61(1): p. 35-46.

[76] American Diabetes, A., *Standards of medical care in diabetes--2014*. Diabetes Care, 2014. 37 Suppl 1: p. S14-80.

[77] Fried, M., et al., *Interdisciplinary European guidelines on metabolic and bariatric surgery*. Obes Surg, 2014. 24(1): p. 42-55.

[78] Jensen, M.D., et al., *2013 AHA/ACC/TOS Guideline for the Management of Overweight and Obesity in Adults: A Report of the American College of Cardiology/American Heart Association Task Force on Practice Guidelines and The Obesity Society*. J Am Coll Cardiol, 2014. 63(25 Pt B): p. 2985-3023.

[79] Mechanick, J.I., et al., *Clinical practice guidelines for the perioperative nutritional, metabolic, and nonsurgical support of the bariatric surgery patient--2013 update: cosponsored by American Association of Clinical Endocrinologists, the Obesity Society, and American Society for Metabolic & Bariatric Surgery*. Endocr Pract, 2013. 19(2): p. 337-72.

[80] Baur, L.A. and D.A. Fitzgerald, *Recommendations for bariatric surgery in adolescents in Australia and New Zealand*. J Paediatr Child Health, 2010. 46(12): p. 704-7.

Chapter 9

The Involvement of Environmental Endocrine-Disrupting Chemicals in Type 2 Diabetes Mellitus Development

Carmen Purdel, Mihaela Ilie and Denisa Margina

Additional information is available at the end of the chapter

http://dx.doi.org/10.5772/59110

1. Introduction

The incidence of diabetes and associated metabolic disorders has tripled over recent decades and continues to rise at an alarming rate. Currently, 382 million individuals worldwide are estimated to have diabetes and this number is believed to increase to 592 million by 2035 [1]; the vast majority of the cases is type 2 diabetes mellitus (T2DM).

Taking into account the number of patients impacted by T2DM and its long-term consequences in terms of morbidity, mortality and economic costs, there is considerable interest in understanding the contribution of non-traditional risk factors to the diabetes epidemic, especially concerning environmental chemicals and particularly endocrine-disrupting chemicals (EDCs).

Researches addressing the role of environmental chemicals in the development of metabolic disorders, like obesity and T2DM, have rapidly expanded. Epidemiological and experimental evidence suggest an association between exposure to EDCs and T2DM, especially since the exposure to chemicals increased massively in the last decade.

In this chapter we tried to elucidate the following issues: (1) the concept of EDCs; (2) human exposure to EDCs; (3) particular concepts related to EDCs; (4) mechanisms of EDCs action involved in the development of T2DM; (5) evidence of T2DM in animal models; (6) epidemiological data linking EDCs exposure to T2DM and (7) challenges in EDCs research.

2. The concept of EDCs

Originally articulated in the early 1990s by Colbron [2], the theory of *endocrine disruption* referes to exogenous chemicals present in the environment and/or diet that interfere and disrupt physiological hormonal systems, inducing adverse effects on human and wildlife health. The term "endocrine disruptor" was first used at the Wingspread Conference in Wisconsin, USA in 1991 for those EDCs, which may lead to an adverse health effect [3]. Initially the term focused on chemicals with estrogenic activity that would alter reproductive function, commonly referred to as environmental estrogens or xenoestrogens; it has expanded to compounds with androgenic activity, as well as thyroid-active chemicals [4]. Consequently, different variable terms appeared, e.g. endocrine disrupter or endocrine disruptor, hormone mimics, hormone inhibitors or endocrine modulators [5]. Today, these compounds are commonly referred to as EDCs.

Various attempts to set up a scientific definition of an EDC have been made. Today is generally wide acceptance of using the WHO definition [6], which is similar with the EU definition [7]: *„An endcorine disruptor is an exogenous substance or mixture that alters function(s) of the endocrine system and consequently causes adverse health effects in an intact organism, or its progeny, or (sub)populations".*

EDCs interfere and disrupt physiological hormonal balance inducing adverse effects on human health through different mechanisms including direct interaction with hormone receptors, competition on binding and transport proteins or interference with hormone metabolism (blocking or inducing the synthesis of the hormones). Starting from this definition there are clearly two requirements for a substance to be defined as an EDCs, namely the demonstration of an adverse effect and an endocrine disruption mode-of-action. Additionally, the definition implies proof of causality between the observed adverse effect and the endocrine disruption mode-of-action.

It is important to underline that the definition of EDC includes the term "adverse" which was considered as a key criterion to differentiate a genuine EDC from a mere endocrine modulator (that elicits an adaptative reversible response in endocrine homeostasis). According to WHO the term "adversity" means: "*a change in morphology, physiology, growth, reproduction, development or lifespan of an organism which results in impairment of functional capacity or impairment of capacity to compensate for additional stress or increased susceptibility to the harmful effects of other environmental influences.*" [8].

This definition is not covering the potential or indicates EDC. A potential (or suspected) EDC may alter function(s) of the endocrine system and consequently may cause adverse health effects, while a substance with indication of endocrine disrupting properties (called indicated EDC) might be expected to lead to endocrine disruption in an intact organism, or its progeny, or (sub)populations.

The need for an expansion of the general term to potential EDCs is reflected on the new Guidance document on Standardised Test Guidelines for Evaluating Chemicals for Endocrine Disruption (OECD 2011) [9]: "*A possible endocrine disrupter is a chemical that is able to alter the*

http://dx.doi.org/10.5772/59110

functioning of the endocrine system but for which information about possible adverse consequences of that alteration in an intact organism is uncertain".

Recently, the Endocrine Society published a statement of principles on endocrine disruptors [10] in which another definition of an EDC has been proposed: *"An EDC is an exogenous chemical, or mixture of chemicals, that interferes with any aspect of hormone action."* This definition emphasizes that the ability of a chemical to interfere with hormone action is of itself a reliable predictor for adverse outcomes.

A wide variety of chemicals act as EDCs. The Endocrine Disruption Exchange List (TEDX) to date lists almost 1000 endocrine disruptors [11]. The group of EDCs is highly heterogeneous and includes synthetic chemicals used as industrial solvents/lubricants and their by-products (persistent organic pollutants – POPs, dioxins like 2,3,7,8-tetrachlorodibenzo-p-dioxin – TCDD), plastics (bisphenol A – BPA), pesticides (as dichlorodiphenyltrichloroethane – DDT), plasticizers (phthalates like diethylhexyl phthalate – DEHP), heavy metals (arsenic, cadmium), tributyl tin (TBT), fungicides (vinclozolin) and pharmaceutical agents (diethylstilbestrol – DES). POPs comprise a broad class of organohalides, including polychlorinated biphenyls (PCBs), polybrominated biphenyls (PBBs) and organochlorine pesticides.

However, one should keep in mind that there is also a large number of EDCs of natural origin occurring in plants consumed as food and also some secondary metabolites from fungi that may contaminate food. Examples of EDCs with oestrogenic activity are present in soy (e.g. genistein and daidzein), mycotoxins in cereals (e.g. zearalenone), goitrogens in cabbage (with the potential to inhibit iodine uptake) and glycirrhizine in liquorice (with the potential to disturb the mineralocorticoid system) [12].

EDCs are widely dispersed in the environment. Some are persistent, having long half-lives [13], while others are rapidly degraded in the environment or human body or may be present for only short periods of time but at critical periods of development, considered windows of susceptibility.

The effects of EDCs are observed especially on sensitive groups (foetus and child), based on their susceptibility to hormonal effects [14]. Therefore, for these groups the adverse effects may occur at concentrations that are far below levels that would be considered harmful in the adult [15]

Of a special concern are EDCs such as phthalates [16], PBBs [17] and BPA, detected in pregnant women, fetuses and newborns, taking into account that exposure occuring early in pregnancy can have short-term health effects, while exposure later or during early childhood may induce cognitive and developmental deficiencies [18].

Published studies illustrate that *in utero* developmental period is a critically sensitive window of vulnerability. Disruptions during this time-frame can lead to subtle functional changes that may not emerge until later in life [19] or even later to the next generation.

Actually, is considered that *in utero* and early postnatal exposures play an important role in the development of reproductive defects, obesity and metabolic syndrome as a result of inheritable chemical-induced epigenetic changes [20, 21, 22]. As an example of epigenetic change involved in reproductive defects one can note the developmental exposure to vinclozolin causing an increase in spermatogenic cell apoptosis in the adult rats [23]. This spermatogenic defect was found to be transgenerational at least to F4 generation due to a permanent altered DNA methylation of the male germ-line [21].

Criteria	Available data – according to OECD Conceptual Framework [29,30]
Category 1: EDCs	
• *in vivo data* (mode of action clearly linked to adverse effects)	• *In vivo* assays providing data on effects clearly linked to endocrine mechanisms (OECD, conceptual Framework (CF) level 5) • On a case-by-case basis, *in vivo* assays providing data about single or multiple endocrine mechanisms and effects (OECD, CF levels 3 & 4), combined with other relevant information • In special cases, categorization or QSAR approaches may provide the necessary data in combination with *in vivo* ADME information and *in vitro* data • Reliable and good quality evidence from human cases or epidemiological studies
Category 2a: Suspected EDCs	
• *in vivo data* (mode of action suspected to be linked to adverse effects) or • *in vitro* mode of action combined with toxicokinetic *in vivo* data	• *In vivo* assays providing data on effects linked to endocrine or other mechanisms (OECD, CF level 5), but where ED mode of action is suspected • *In vivo* assays providing data about single or multiple endocrine mechanisms and effects (OECD, CF levels 3 & 4) • In some cases, read across, chemical categorization and/or QSAR approaches may provide the necessary data in combination with *in vivo* ADME information and *in vitro* data • Good quality epidemiological studies showing associations between exposure and adverse human health effects related to endocrine systems.
Category 2b: Indicated EDCs	
• *Some in vitro/in silico* evidence	• *In vitro* assays providing mechanistic data (OECD, CF level 2) • QSAR, read-across, chemical categorization, ADME information (OECD, CF level 2) • System biology methods indicating associations between the substance and adverse human health effects related to endocrine systems.

Table 1. Classification of EDCs based on Danish criteria

Many other chemicals have also been implicated in promoting toxicity for multiple generations, including BPA [24] or pesticides [25], but in these cases the multigenerational effects involved direct exposures, therefore are not considered transgenerational because they are not transmitted solely through the germ cells. Only effects appearing in the F3 generation are considered to be truly transgenerational [26].

There are multiple classifications of EDCs, based on their mechanisms of action (on enzymes, transport proteins or receptors), the pathways modulated (e.g., xenoestrogens/antiestrogens,

http://dx.doi.org/10.5772/59110

xenoandrogens/antiandrogens), or the biological outcomes (simulation or inhibition) [27]. However, the best classification is the Danish criteria, based on available data (*in vitro, in vivo* and epidemiological studies), which is scientifically legitimated by Hass et al. [28]. Using this approach, EDCs are divided into 3 categories: *category 1,* for substances known to produce endocrine disrupting adverse effects in humans or animal species, *category 2a* for suspected EDCs, and *category 2b* for indicated EDC. Details regarding classification criteria are included in Table 1.

3. Human exposure to EDCs

Environmental human exposure occurs through a variety of routes and varies widely around the world. Food ingestion represents the major route by which people are exposed to EDCs. For example, diet is thought to account for up to 90% of a person's POPs body burden [31]. Taking into account that these pollutants are accumulated particularly in highly rank predators, like fish, in Sweden, consumption of fatty fish from the Baltic Sea is the major source of POPs, but also dairy products and meat contain these pollutants [32]. Also contaminated ground water is a major exposure source to inorganic arsenic in the general adult population in several regions, notably Bangladesh and India [33,34].

Regarding BPA exposure, small amounts of BPA can migrate from polymers to food or water, especially when heated. The human consumption of BPA from epoxy-lined food cans alone is estimated to be about 6.6 μg per person per day [35]. BPA has been found in concentrations of 1–10 ng/ml in serum of pregnant women, in the amniotic fluid of their fetus, and in cord serum taken at birth [36]. Moreover, BPA concentrations up to 100 ng/g were reported in placenta [37], but also in breast adipose tissue, taking into account its lipophilicity.

With the increase in household products containing pollutants and the decrease in the quality of building ventilation, indoor air has become a significant source of EDCs exposure, via inhalation [38]. Published studies [39,40] suggest that contaminated house dust may be the major source of PBBs body burden (up to 82%).

Other routes of exposure include the dermal contact (e.g. parabens or triclosan), via lactation or infants fed formula (especially for phytoestrogens as genistein or BHA). A published study [41] reported that urinary concentrations of genistein and daidzein were about 500-fold higher in infants fed with soy formula compared with those fed cow's milk formula.

4. Particular concepts related with EDCs

For decades, two major interrelated concepts are particularly addressed regarding EDCs: the low dose effect and non-monotonous dose–response relationships (e.g. "inverted U-shapes" of the dose–response curve).

Like hormones, some of EDCs act at low or very low doses, other variable, therefore their blood levels are not reflecting the real activity [42].

The traditional toxicological endpoints are not sufficient to preclude the adverse outcome. Therefore for the endocrine-sensitive endpoints it was suggested to set the NOAEL (no observed adverse effect level) or the LOAEL (lowest observed adverse effect level) from traditional toxicological studies or even below the range of human exposures, as the highest dose in experiments designed to test EDCs. For example, low-dose effects of BPA should be investigated in rodents exposed to 400 μg/kg bw/day BPA or lower, because this concentration produces levels of unconjugated BPA in the range of human blood concentrations [43]; this level is incomparable lower with the classical developmental studies, where LOAEL corresponds to 50 mg/kg bw/day [44]. Actually, most effects were seen at doses below 50 μg/kg [43], so even lower concentration than those normally detected in humans may induce adverse effects.

The effect of EDCs also depends on the type of tissue and the expression of hormone receptors on those cells, therefore the effect is considered to be tissue specific. Taking into account that some EDCs can exhibit different potencies on different receptors isoforms (e.g ERα or ERβ), the effect is also receptor-selective.

A well-known example is related to methyl-and propylparaben. *In vitro*, both parabens are binding to estrogen receptors (ERα and β), but methylparaben exhibits a weak estrogenic activity, while for propylparaben the estrogenic potential is a stronger [45,46]; *in vivo* parabens estrogenic potencies are comparable [46]. The relative activity of parabens compared with estradiol (E_2) is 1000 times lower [47]. Interesting, the estrogenic effects of parabens are not modulated only by estrogen receptors, but are also related to the inhibition of sulfotransferases in skin, elevating the local level of free estrogens [48].

By comparison with native hormones, EDCs exhibits lower affinity for hormone receptors, with some exceptions, such as TBT, which is the most potent agonist of retinoid-X-receptor and PPARγ (peroxisome proliferator activating receptor subtype gamma) in the low nanomolar range [49].

The shape of the dose-response curve for EDCs does not follow the usual dose-response curve. The curve can have a sigmoidal shape (relationship between dose and effect occure based on the saturability of the receptors), but in general EDCs do act via a non-monotonic dose-response relationship [43]. In this case, the slope of the curve changes sign somewhere within the range of the examined doses. In other words, some effects can be seen at very low doses, while slightly higher doses can show no effects and then, at high doses, some different types of effects may be found.

For example, hypoglycaemic or hyperglycaemic effects of TCDD (tetrachlorodibenzo-p-dioxin) observed in animal models are dose-dependent. Repeated low-dose of TCDD (500 ng/kg p.o.) reduced glucokinase gene expression in mice [50], while higher dosage (12.8 μg/kg TCDD p.o) induced a significantly reduction of serum glucose levels [51]. Moreover, a higher dose of TCDD (116 μg/kg i.p.) impaired insulin-stimulated glucose uptake in mice [52].

http://dx.doi.org/10.5772/59110

Another example is BPA. On isolated pancreatic islets of Langerhans BPA induced an increase of insulin content following an inverted U-shape dose response curve, with a significant effect observed at 1 nM and 10 nM BPA compared to vehicle. Higher concentrations of BPA (1 μM) produced no increase in insulin content [53].

A similar non-monotonic behaviour is exhibited by BPA in animal studies where treatment with high dosage (BPA 100 μg/kg bw/day) twice per day for 4 days increased pancreatic insulin content, produced hyperinsulinemia, and induced insulin resistance in adult male mice [54] while sustained exposure of pregnant mouse dams to lower levels of BPA (10 μg/kg bw/day) from gestation day 9–16 impaired glucose tolerance, increased plasma insulin, triglycerides and leptin concentrations, thus revealing the ability of BPA to alter pancreatic function and metabolic parameters [55].

Also PBBs, especially PBDE-153 (polybrominated diphenyl ether) showed an inverted U-shaped association with metabolic syndrome in epidemiological study in humans [56].

So, the most important effects of EDCs observed in animal models are those that occur at low doses, similar with the level of human environmental exposure, therefore only these toxicological data should be corroborated with epidemiological studies.

We also should note that for the assessment of EDCs effects, the assumption of an experimental threshold (like a NOAEL) is questionable. A first reason is related to the lack of adversity for some endpoints investigated (e.g., uterotrophic assay). A second reason is connected with the difficulties to establish it. According to Blair et al. [57], a threshold could be established in the absence of endogenous hormone at some life stage, if the endogenous hormone induces no adverse effect or if there is effective homeostatic control. Even if a threshold does exist, for a certain endpoint, taking into account the population variability and the connection with already ongoing biological process (EDCs exhibit additive effects), the threshold will not be observable.

5. Mechanisms of action involved in development of T2DM

In addition to the classical pathway modulated by EDCs (as interaction with aryl hydrocarbon receptor (AhR) or nuclear hormone receptors, in particular estrogens, androgens and thyroid receptors), it was observed that EDCs exhibit the capacity to modulate signalling pathways involved in energy regulation, in general, and glucose homeostasis in particular. EDCs can decrease insulin sensitivity, impair β-cell insulin production, impair cellular insulin action or alter the intermediary metabolism. All these mechanisms contribute to the pathogenesis of T2DM. Experimental data revealed that one EDC acts on different levels and receptors, therefore the ultimate effect on insulin action may be the result of all pathways involved (Table 2).

Compound	Mechanisms of action	Primary effects
BPA	(+)ERα via ERK1/2	↑ β-cell insulin content ↓ GLUT4
	(+) ER-GPR30	↑ β-cell insulin content
	↑ CREB phosphorylation	↑ $[Ca^{2+}]i$
	↑ Akt phosphorylation ↑ PI3-kinase activity	↓ IRS activity
	Potent antagonist of PPARγ (-) PDI	↑ TNF-α, IL-6; ↓ adiponectin release ↓ IR phosphorylation
PCBs **(especially PCB-77)**	(+) AhR	↑ TNF-α, IL-6; ↑ MCP-1 ↓ PEPCK
	(+) MAPK1/2 (+) CaMK2	↑ [Ca]i (-) IRS-1 phosphorylation
	(-)Akt phosphorilation	Insulin resistance
	↑ oxidative stress	↑ β-cell death

Legend: (+) activate; (-) inhibit; ↑ increase; ↓ decrease; ER-estrogenic receptors; ERK1/2 extracellular regulated kinase1/2; GLUT4 – glucose transporter type4; ER-GPR30-membrane G protein related estrogen-receptor; CREB-cAMP response element-binding protein; $[Ca^{2+}]i$ - intracellular calcium ion levels; IRS – insulin receptor substrate 1; PI3 - phosphatidylinositol-4,5-bisphosphate 3-kinase; PPARγ - peroxisome proliferator-activated receptor gamma; TNF-α - tumor necrosis factor-α; IL-6 interleukin-6; PDI - protein disulfide isomerase; IR – insulin receptor; AhR -aryl hydrocarbon receptor; MCP-1- monocyte chemoattractantprotein-1;PEPCK- phosphoenolpyruvate carboxykinase; MAPK1/2 - mitogen-activated protein kinase 1/2; CaMK2 - Ca^{2+}/calmodulin-dependent kinase II

Table 2. Example of EDC that acts on multiple pathways

Interestingly, some EDCs such as TCDD [58], PCBs [59], inorganic arsenic [60] or cadmium [61] that modulate β-cell function, may also play a role in type 1 diabetes mellitus, as a result of β-cell destruction or dysfunction as well as promotion of β-cell death.

The following mechanisms of action can explain the development of T2DM: (1) activation of aryl hydrocarbon receptor (AhR) or interaction with estrogenic receptors (ERs); (2) β-cell dysfunction and impairment of insulin secretion; (3) impairment of cellular insulin action and (4) alteration of the intermediary metabolism.

5.1. Activation of AhR or interaction with ERs

EDCs can exhibit their metabolic effects through the classical pathways, such as the activation of AhR or the interaction with ERs. It is well known that AhRs are involved in the glucose homeostasis [50], therefore activation of AhR or its heterodimerization partner, called ARNT (AhR nuclear translocator) by EDCs could interfere with glucose uptake. Gunton et al. [62] revealed that abnormal ARNT expression causes impaired insulin release in human islets, but it is unclear if this effect is a cause or a consequence of T2DM.

PCBs [63] or PBDE [64] reduce primary hepatocyte glycogen levels and impair gluconeogenesis due to a specific down regulation of phosphoenolpyruvate carboxykinase (PEPCK) expression, a central regulator of gluconeogenesis. The alteration of PEPCK expression was proportional to activation of the AhR, suggesting a direct correlation between AhR activation and perturbation in intermediary metabolism.

PCBs (especially PCB-77) also impaired glucose homeostasis through another AhR-dependent mechanism, associated with an adipose-specific increase in TNF-α (tumor necrosis factor-α) expression and interleukin-6 (IL-6) levels [65, 66]. In addition to its effects on TNF-α and IL-6, PCB-77 also increases expression of MCP-1 (monocyte chemoattractant protein-1), an adipocyte-secreted molecule with inflammatory function that contributes to global insulin sensitivity [67].

The implication of estrogenic receptors (especially ERα) in the pancreatic β-cell insulin content is confirmed by BPA studies. At physiologically relevant doses, BPA increases pancreatic β-cell insulin content, the effect being mediated by ERα activation via extracellular regulated kinase1/2 (ERK1/2) [53]. ERα is also implicated in β-cell survival [68], regulates the glucose transporter (GLUT4) in skeletal muscle [69] and insulin sensitivity in the liver [70]

Also the non-classical membrane G protein related estrogen-receptor (ER-GPR30), expressed in pancreatic islets is involved in the effects of estrogens on glucose metabolism, its deficiency inducing hyperglycemia, impaired glucose tolerance, and elevated blood pressure [71]. GPR30 activation by several EDCs, e.g. BPA could partly contribute to the increase of insulin after BPA exposure [72]

5.2. Beta-cell dysfunction and impairment of insulin secretion

Taking into account their reduced capacity to fight against chronic oxidative stress and the lack of detoxification mechanisms, β-cells are the perfect target for EDCs that disrupt their structure and function or promote death.

Oxidative stress is the mechanism implicated in T2DM induced by exposure to inorganic arsenic. At relatively low concentrations arsenic-induced oxidative stress produces impairment of glucose-stimulated insulin secretion [73], while exposure to high concentrations results in irreversible damage (including oxidative damage) to β-cells followed by apoptosis or necrosis [74]. Actually, the mechanism behind arsenic-induced oxidative stress is more complex. Chronic exposure to relative low concentration of arsenite (1–2 μM) produced an adaptive response, activating the transcription factor NF-E2–related factor 2 (Nrf2). Even if Nrf2 is generally considered a protective cellular component that induces antioxidant / detoxification enzymes [73], in this case Nrf2 activation that diminishes the reactive oxygen species (ROS) have a negative impact on insulin secretion. In normal cells, ROS signals produced during glucose metabolism increase the insulin secretion [75], thefore arsenic Nrf2-mediated response appears to play an important role in reduced glucose-stimulated insulin secretion. Inorganic arsenic also promotes β-cell apoptosis via induction of endoplasmic reticulum stress, but this mechanism is poorly studied and necessitates further investigations [76].

Regarding the interference and impairment of insulin secretion, different examples can be provided, especially taking into account that insulin secretion is a calcium-dependent process. On isolated pancreatic β-cells BPA at low concentration (10^{-9} M) increases the phosphorylation of CREB (transcription factor cyclic adenosine monophosphate-response element-binding protein) via an alternative mechanism, involving a non-classical membrane estrogen receptor [77], which provokes the closure of K^+/ATP channels. As a result the plasma membrane depolarizes, opening the L-type voltage-dependent calcium channels and increasing intracellular calcium ion levels [Ca^{2+}]i and triggering insulin secretion [78].

Also abnormal levels of [Ca^{2+}]i and the impairment of insulin secretion were observed on isolated islet cells exposed to TBT and are associated with the disruption of protein-kinase A activity [79].

PCB treatment of RINm5F cells resulted in a rapid increase of [Ca^{2+}]i as a result of Ca^{2+}/calmodulin-dependent kinase II (CaMK2) and mitogen-activated protein kinase 1 and 2 (MAPK 1 and 2) activation [80]. In addition, RINm5F cells exposed to inorganic arsenic (III) exhibited a reduction of insulin secretion as a result of decreased calcium-dependent calpain-10 activity, a pathway that triggers insulin exocytosis [81]. Arsenic also reduces the β-cell line proliferation in a dose-dependent manner, as an indirect consequence of the decrease in insulin secretion.

5.3. Impairment of cellular insulin action

Taking into account that insulin signalling mechanisms are described in detail elsewhere [82], we present only a short analysis of the insulin signalling cascade in order to provide some insights into how EDCs might modulate insulin action.

Insulin acts on target cells and stimulates glucose uptake via membrane –bound tertrametric insulin receptor (IR) with tyrosine kinase activity. Binding to extracellular α-subunits of IR leads to activation of tyrosine kinase. Once the tyrosine kinase of IR is activated, it promotes autophosphorylation of the β subunit, where phosphorylation of three tyrosine residues (Tyr-1158, Tyr-1162, and Tyr-1163) is required for amplification of the kinase activity. Then tyrosine kinase phosphorylates the insulin receptor substrate proteins (IRS 1 and 2) and phosphotyrosine residues on IRS proteins become targets for the p85 regulatory subunit of phosphatidylinositol 3-kinase (PI3-kinase).

The activated PI3-kinase generates higher levels of phosphotidylinositides, such as phosphatidyl-inositol-3,4-bisphosphate (PIP2) and phosphatidyl-inositol-3,4,5-trisphosphate (PIP3), which bind to the phosphoinositidedependent kinase-1 (PDK1). PDK1 can directly phosphorylate all protein kinase C (PKCs).

Downstream from PI3-kinase, activation of Akt (protein kinase B) produces its effects, including those on gene transcription as well as glucose uptake through the translocation of facilitative glucose transporter 4 (GLUT4) to the cell membrane.

Each step in this signaling cascade is a potential target for EDCs. EDCs interact and impair the cellular insulin effect acting at different levels: on IRS, PI3-kinase, Akt, PDK or PKC or through associated mechanisms. Some examples are included in figure 1.

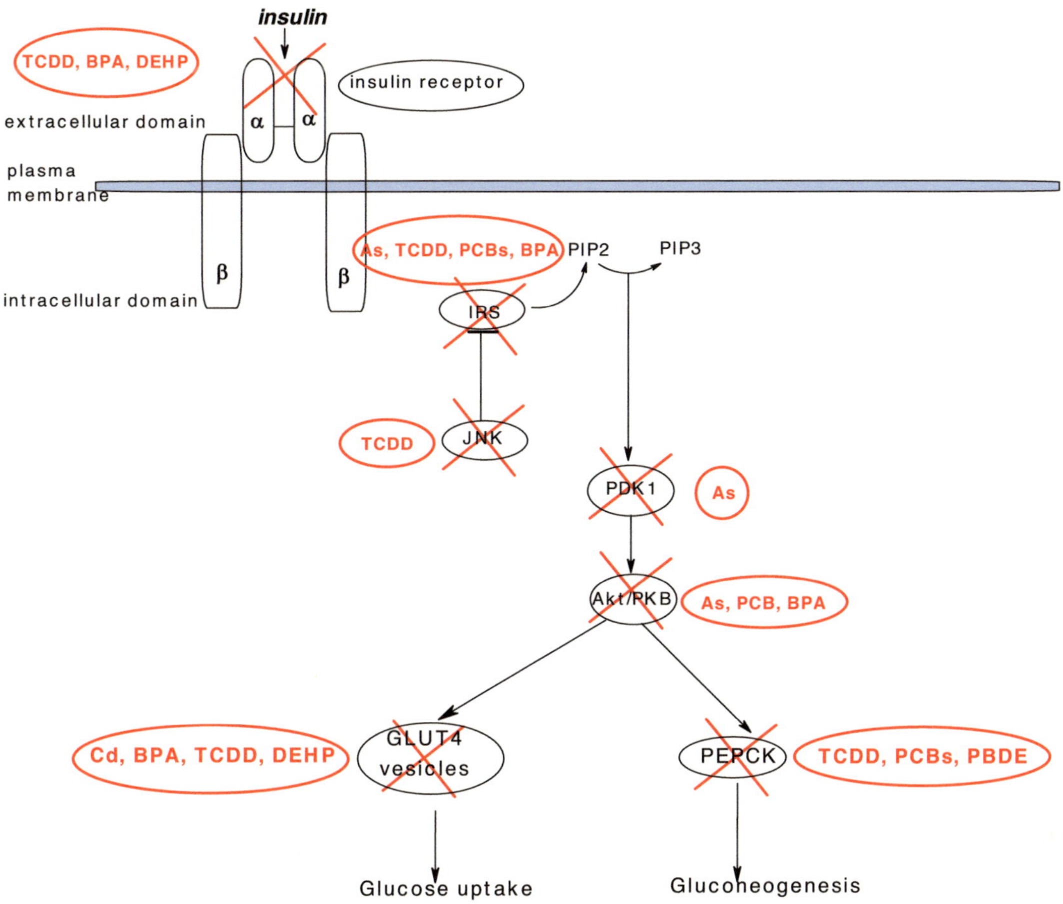

Figure 1. A schematic illustration of EDCs interference on insulin signaling pathways. Arrows represent an activation process; X represent an inhibition process

For example, TCDD, arsenic or PCB alter IRS activity (especially IRS-1 phosphorylation) through different mechanisms: TCDD increasing MAPK (mitogen-activated protein kinase) activity and JNK (c-Jun N-terminal kinase) activity [83], arsenic decreasing p70-S6-kinase activity [84] and PCBs increasing CaMK2 and MAPK 1 and 2 activity [80].

Other EDCs act on insulin-stimulated Akt phosphorylation. Akt phosphorylation is attenuated by PCB-77 [65] or BPA [55]. Arsenic (III) exposure was also associated with suppression of AkT phosphorylation and glucose uptake in 3T3-L1 adipocytes, causing an insulin resistant phenotype [85,86].

BPA acts not only on Akt phosphorylation, but also stimulates tyrosine phosphorylation via PI3-kinase, the global effect being the impairment of IRS activity [87].

Additional studies have demonstrated that TCDD [83], BPA [88] or DEHP [89] are modulating the insulin signalling cascade by down-regulation of the insulin receptors or acting on plasma membrane GLUT4 level and antagonizing insulin action [90].

Also, cadmium induces impaired glucose tolerance by down-regulating GLUT4 expression in adipocytes [91].

Inorganic arsenic (III) inhibits PDK-1 activity, thus suppressing PDK-1-catalyzed phosphorylation of PKB/Akt and p-PKB/Akt–mediated translocation of GLUT4 transporters to the plasma membrane [85,92].

5.4. Alteration of the intermediary metabolism

In addition to direct effects on the insulin signalling cascade, EDCs alter the intermediary metabolism, mainly the gluconeogenesis. TCDD [63], or PCBs [93] have been shown to down-regulate the expression of phosphoenolpyruvate carboxykinase (PEPCK), reducing its activity and inducing hypoglicemia. In the case of PCBs, the suppression of hepatic PEPCK expression was proportional to activation of the AhR, suggesting a direct correlation between AhR activation and perturbation of the intermediary metabolism.

Alternative mechanisms are implicated in the development of T2DM, such as inflammation or oxidative stress. For example, PCB-77 has been shown to promote expression of IL-6 and TNF-α, leading to impaired insulin signalling in endothelial cells [64]. In addition to its effects on TNF-α and IL-6, PCB-77 also increases expression of MCP-1, adipocyte-secreted molecule that contributes to global insulin sensitivity [66].

BPA augments secretion of IL-6 and TNF-α, but simultaneously inhibits the release of adiponectin in human adipose tissue explants [94]. The suppression of adiponectin release could promote insulin resistance and increase the risk of developing the metabolic syndrome. The same outcome is expected based on elevated IL-6 levels.

We should highlight the strong correlation between increased TNFα production and insulin resistance [95]. TNFα affects insulin resistance by downregulating the glucose transporter, interfering with IR phosphorylation and signaling, and by inhibiting transcription factors that affect insulin sensitivity.

Some EDCs are acting on other nuclear receptors involved in fat metabolism and regulation of glucose uptake, like PPARs (peroxisome proliferator-activated receptors), especially on PPARγ which are involved in the regulation of adipocyte differentiation, production of adipokines or insulin responsiveness [96]. By antagonizing PPARγ, EDCs significantly inhibit the release of adiponectin that has insulin-sensitizing effects, as it enhances inhibition of hepatic glucose output as well as glucose uptake and utilization in fat and muscle tissues. So, adiponectin levels are correlated with insulin sensitivity, therefore supressing its biological effects affects glucose homeostasis.

For example, BPA at 0.1 and 1 nM doses is a potent antagonist of PPARγ, which suppresses adiponectin release in human adipose tissue explants [97]. In the same time, BPA influences adiponectin level via another mechanism that implies binding to protein disulfide isomerase (PDI), a critical player in the retention of adiponectin in cells [98]

Interestingly, *in vitro* it was observed that ERβ can act as a negative regulator of PPARγ, decreasing ligand-induced PPARγ and PPARγ induced adipogenesis [99], therefore it is obvious that PPARγ function is affected by EDCs directly interacting with the receptor, but also by EDCs that modulate ERβ activity. Also, TCDD inhibits adipogenesis through a suppression of PPARγ [100].

Other EDCs such as phthalates (DEHP) act as potent agonists of PPARα or PPARγ. In rodent models, PPARα appears to mediate high-dose DEHP-induced body weight loss [101], but these effects can not be extrapolated to humans, taking into account that the levels required to activate human PPARα are almost three times higher than the concentrations required to activate mouse PPARα, and the maximum-fold induction is less for human PPARα than for mouse PPARα [102].

In conclusion, the investigation of insulin signaling pathways may explain how EDCs modulate insulin action, especially in the case of exposure to singular compound; however, in the context of accidental or occupational exposures, humans are exposed to mixtures of compounds and this complicates understanding the global biological effects. For example, if different compounds are acting through the same pathway, but at different points, co-exposure is likely to have additive or synergistic effects that promote the development of insulin resistance and T2DM. Moreover, points of pathway convergence (e.g., IRS) might be the perfect target of drug intervention to treat environmentally-mediated diabetes.

6. Evidence of T2DM in animal models after EDC exposure

There are enough published data in animal models that investigated the correlation between EDCs exposure and T2DM. This correlation between exposure in the animal models and alterations in glucose homeostasis, including hyperglycemia and glucose intolerance is crucial, taking into account that epidemiological studies fail to establish a causality.

A number of examples are given below.

Repeated low dose of TCDD (500 ng/kg bw), administered orally, reduced glucokinase gene expression, predicting a rise in blood glucose levels on C57BL/6 mice [103], while in diabetic rats, a higher dose of 12.8 μg/kg bw TCDD had significantly reduced serum glucose levels by day 8 of treatment [51]. Moreover, a single but high dose of TCDD (116 μg/kg bw i.p.) impaired insulin-stimulated glucose uptake in C57BL/6 and DBA/2J mice [52].

Administration of 75 μg/kg bw DEHP for 14 days reduced insulin levels and raised serum glucose levels in exposed female Wistar Kyoto rats [104]. Almost similar results were obtained on male rats treated for a longer period (21 days) with diet supplemented with 2% (w/w) of DEHP [105].

Male mice treated orally with 0.5-50 μg/kg bw TBT for 45 days demonstrated hepatic steatosis, hyperinsulinemia, hyperleptinemia and a reduction in hepatic adiponectin levels, in a dose-dependent fashion, confirming PPARγ stimulation observed *in vitro* [106].

Similar results were obtained in adult Sprague-Dawley rats exposed for 28 days to crude salmon oil containing POPs [107]. The animals developed insulin resistance syndrome, abdominal obesity and hepatosteatosis, the contribution of POPs to insulin resistance being confirmed also by the same authors in cultured adipocytes. These findings are important since POPs are accumulating in the lipid fraction of fish, and fish consumption represents the main source of POP exposure to humans.

Also coplanar PCBs (e.g. PCB-77 and PCB-126), at dosage of 50 mg/kg orally, impaired glucose homeostasis in lean C57BL/6 mice and mitigate beneficial effects of weight loss on glucose homeostasis in obese mice [66], while inorganic arsenic (III) administered in the drinking water for 20 weeks, at doses of 25 or 50 ppm As/kg bw/day, impaired glucose tolerance in C57BL/6 mice in a dose-dependent manner [108].

In the animal studies mentioned before, not just blood glucose levels were investigated, but other markers of insulin regulation, such as HOMA-IR, pancreatic production of NO, SOD and CAT activity, in order to reflect the magnitude of the global disturbance. While most studies have demonstrated perturbations in insulin action, some of them have shown improved glucose tolerance or even hypoglycaemia. Acute exposure of adult male mice to high dosage of BPA (100 μg/kg bw/day) produced a rapid hyperinsulinemia based on significant increase in β-cell insulin content, as a direct result of BPA estrogenic properties [109], while sustained exposure to lower dosage (10 μg /kg bw/day) impaired glucose tolerance and reduced the hypoglycaemic effect of insulin, through a compensatory peripheral insulin resistance [54]. These results are easily correlated with non-monotonic dose response curve exhibited *in vitro* by BPA.

Taking into account that EDCs alter glucose homeostasis and endocrine pancreatic function not just in adult animals but also during pregnancy or in offspring, these effects were also investigated in pregnant animals. For example, prenatal exposure to high dosage of diisobutyl phthalate (600 mg/kg bw/day) from gestation Day 7 to Day 21 reduced plasma leptin and insulin levels in male and female offspring, complementary to sexual distrurbance [110]. Maternal glucose intolerance was observed in pregnant mice exposed to inorganic arsenic (V) at dosage of 9.6 mg/kg bw, this explaining the neural tube defects induced by arsenate [111].

In conclusion, all these examples regarding *in vivo* effects in animal models are highly suggestive, taking into account that the experimental exposure is very close or even similar with environmental human exposure. However, data on co-exposure are lacking, therefore new studies should focus on this issue, in order to reveal possible additive, synergistic or antagonistic effects exhibited by the mixtures.

http://dx.doi.org/10.5772/59110

7. Epidemiological data linking EDCs exposure to T2DM

There is growing concern in the scientific community that EDCs may be contributing to the high incidence of diabetes, particularly in young people.

Epidemiological studies (as occupational or population-based studies) but also disasters tried to link, at least partially, the environmental exposure to EDCs with the development of T2DM.

We collected and compiled from a comprehensive scientific literature the most relevant epidemiological studies concerning the T2DM and exposure to EDCs like TCDD, arsenic, phthalates or BPA.

Disasters such as Seveso accident or exposure of military personnel during the Vietnam War and follow-up studies have suggested a link between TCDD exposure and a higher incidence of diabetes [112, 113, 114]. Other cross-sectional studies [115, 116] did not revealed such correlation, while longitudinal studies that have been conducted are inconsistent [117].

Some poisoning cases reported during late 1970s have involved contaminated rice oil with PCBs. PCB exposure was associated with an increased prevalence of diabetes in women [118]. Other prospective studies on PCB153 showed a positive association with T2DM, but taking into account the variation across studies, it did not allow a metaanalysis. For example, five studies used different diagnostic strategies and several approaches to address serum lipid levels [119]. In addition, the age varied between cohorts from 18 to 30 years [119] to 70 years [120] while gender was also inconsistent, exclusively female in one study [121], exclusively male in another [119] and mixed in the remaining studies [120; 122, 123]. The temporal and geographic variation among the studies induced significant differences in the exposure assessment especially on duration of exposures or on the composition of the mixtures. However, other variables must be considered in the interpretation of PCBs studies, such as the use of PCB153 as a surrogate for total PCBs or the lack of data regarding kinetics of different PCBs (especially on accumulation) that influence their current serum levels.

A closer evaluation of the cohorts described before revealed the non-monotonic exposure-response relationships exhibited by PCBs: the risk of diabetes was significantly increased with small increases within the lower ranges of PCBs concentrations, but only slightly increased with significant increases in concentrations of PCBs. This non-monotonic relationship exhibited by PCBs in cohorts was also observed in brominated flame retardants studies, like those conducted on PBDE-153 [124], but not in BPA cohorts, where BPA urinary levels were associated with diabetes incidence in a dose-dependent manner [125].

Evaluation of studies conducted on EDCs (PCBs or TCDD) reveal that many of them focused specific populations (e.g. occupational studies or exposure through industrial accidents or disasters), so they might not reflect the actual risk of the general population. However, recent investigations were done on representative sampling of the US population, using data from the National Health and Nutrition Examination Survey (NHANES). For example, Lee et al. [126] reported strong and highly significant associations, among participants in the NAHNES study, between serum concentrations of POPs and the HOMA-IR insulin resistance values, after correction for age, sex, BMI, and waist circumference.

Study design	Diagnosis	Findings (95% CI)	As in drinking water (μg/L)	Exposure	Ref.
		Low-to-moderate exposures (< 150 μg/L drinking water)			
Cross-sectional [male 225 nonsmokers 209 smokers]	Self-report	Increased urinary As in nonsmoking diabetics	n.r.	Nonsmokers: 5.59 (diabetics) vs. 4.7 (nondiabetics) μg As/L Smokers: 7.27 (diabetics) vs. 5.41 (nondiabetics) μg As/L (urine)	127
Cross-sectional [n=11,319]	Self-report prior to baseline	adjOR=1.24 (0.82- 1.87)	0.1–864	41–92 (Q3) vs. 0.1–8 (Q1) μg As/L drinking water, CEI	128
Case–control [n=144 female]	Fasting blood glucose, OGTT	Increased As in urine from diabetics	n.r.	4.13 (diabetics) vs. 1.48 (nondiabetics) μg As/L in urine	129
Retrospective [41,282male 38,722 female]	Death certificate	Male SMR =1.28 (1.18-1.37) Female SMR =1.27 (1.19- 1.35)	1.27–11.98	6 counties vs. state μg As/L (drinking water)	130
Case–control [n=87]	Not reported	RR=0.87 (0.5- 1.53)	n.r.	75th vs. 25th percentile μg As/L (urine)	131
Retrospective [n=1,074 deaths]	Death certificate	RR=1.6 (0.36- 7.16)	n.r.	Residence time within 1.6 km (1 mi): ≥ 10 years vs. < 1 year	132
Cross-sectional [n=235]	Hospital records	RR=1.098 (0.98- 1.231)	16–272	21–272 (range) vs. 16–38 (range) μg As/L (drinking water)	133
Case–control [n=117]	Not reported	RR=1.09 (0.79- 1.49)	n.r.	75th vs. 25th percentile μg As/mL (plasma)	134
Cross-sectional [n=1,185]	Self-report	adjOR=1.02 (0.49 - 2.15)	0–2,389	> 10 vs. < 2 μg As/L (well-water)	135
Cross-sectional [n=788]	Fasting blood glucose, self-report, medication	adjOR=3.58 (1.18- 10.83)	-	18 (≥ 80th) vs. 3.5 (≤ 20th percentile) μg As/L (urine)	136
Cross-sectional [n=1,279]	Fasting blood glucose, self-report, medication	adjOR=2.60 (1.12 - 6.03)	-	7.4 (80th) vs. 1.6 (20th percentile) μg As/L (urine)	137
Cross-sectional [n=795]	Fasting blood glucose, self-report, medication	adjOR=1.15 (0.53 - 2.50)	-	12 (≥ 80th) vs. 2.7 (≤ 20th percentile) μg As/L (urine, not adjusted for creatinine)	138
Study design	**Diagnosis**	**Findings (95% CI)**	**As in drinking water (μg/L)**	**Exposure**	**Ref.**
		High exposure (≥ 150 μg/L drinking water)			
Cross-sectional [n=11,319]	Self-report prior to baseline	adjOR=1.11 (0.73- 1.69)	0.1–864	176.2–864 (Q5) vs. 0.1–8 (Q1) μg As/L drinking water, CEI	134

http://dx.doi.org/10.5772/59110

Study design	Diagnosis	Findings (95% CI)	As in drinking water (μg/L)	Exposure	Ref.
Cross-sectional [n=891]	Self-report, OGTT, treatment history	adjOR=10.05 (1.3-77.9)	700–930	≥ 15 vs. 0 ppm-year drinking water, CEI	141
Case–control [n=235]	Glucose, blood	OR=2.95 (0.954, - 9.279)	3–875	218.1 μg As/L vs. 11.3 μg As/L(mean)	140
Cross-sectional [n=1,107]	Self-report, OGTT, glucosuria	adjPR=5.2 (2.5- 10.5)	10–2,100	Keratosis vs. non-keratosis	141
Retrospective [n=19,536]	Death certificate	SMR=1.46 (1.28- 1.67)	250–1,140	Blackfoot endemic region vs. national reference	142
Prospective [n=446]	Fasting blood glucose, OGTT	RR=2.1 (1.1- 4.2)	700–930	≥ 17 vs. < 17 mg/L-year As (drinking water, CEI)	143
Cross-sectional [n=706,314]	Insurance claims	adjOR=2.69 (2.65- 2.73)	350–1,140	Endemic vs. non-endemic region	144

Abbreviations: 95% CI – confidence interval 95%; adjOR-adjusted odds ratio; adjPR-adjusted prevalence ratio; As-arsenic; CEI, cumulative exposure index; OGTT-oral glucose tolerance test; Q-quintile; RR-relative risk; SMR-standardized mortality ratios; n.r. – not reported

Table 3. Association between arsenic and diabetes

The correlation between the level of arsenic in drinking water and the incidence of T2DM was extensively investigated. The published cohorts were categorized based on the level of exposure (table 3) in order to identify the correlation between exposure and critical endpoints. In addition to diabetes, epidemiological studies have associated exposure to arsenic with other measures of disturbed glucose homeostasis, such as glucose tolerance or metabolic syndrome.

Preliminary analysis on the existing human data provide limited support for an association between arsenic and diabetes in populations exposed to relatively high levels (≥ 150 μg As/L in drinking water), but the evidence is insufficient to conclude that exposure to low to moderate level is associated with diabetes. However, a major gap is obvious. The measurement of arsenic in drinking water supplies, which was often used to assess arsenic exposure, is not appropriate to calculate the internal dose, taking into account individual variation in arsenic uptake and metabolism. Also, individual information on the duration and timing of exposure, which is critical, especially for estimating cumulative exposure, are missing.

Regarding phthalates, cohort studies were mainly focused on correlation between exposure and obesity and less on T2DM. However, those found were done on representative sampling of the US population, using data from NHANES. For example, Stahlhut et al. [145] investigated 1,292 adult US male participants in the NHANES 1999–2002 and revealed that urinary concentrations of three phthalate metabolites (mono-n-butyl phthalate, monobenzyl phthalate and monoethylphthalate) were associated with increased insulin resistance, assessed by HOMA-IR. In addition, phthalates levels were associated with increased waist circumference. A similar association between urinary phthalate metabolite concentrations, body mass index and waist circumference was found in another cross-sectional study of NHANES data [146]. However, considering the methodological limitations of the existing data, there is no sufficient evidence to conclude there is a correlation between phthalates and diabetes or obesity.

The epidemiological data on BPA and T2DM is less consistent compared with POPs, but is growing. There are two cross-sectional analyses of NHANES data 2003-2008 that reported a positive associations of BPA exposure (median 2.5 and 1.8 μg/l) with self-reported diagnosis of diabetes [125, 147]. However, these analyses have an important weakness that limits their value: the use of a single spot urine sample collected concurrent with the information on diagnosis of diabetes. The single spot sample reflects only recent BPA exposure, so cannot be extrapolated to longer period (like years or decades) which is relevant for the development of diabetes. Other large cross-sectional studies on BPA in China provide conflicting data [148,149].

A closer evaluation of all epidemiological studies on EDCs reveals some weaknesses, such as the assessment of one compound as a surrogate for total mixture (in case of PCBs), the lack of data regarding kinetics, especially on accumulation in lipid-rich tissues (in case of POPs), limited type of biological material used for direct measurement EDCs (serum or urine) or environmental measurement which is not appropriate to calculate the internal dose (in case of As). Other caveats must be considered in the interpretation of studies, such as heterogeneity in the definition of diabetes or insulin resistance.

8. Challenges in EDCs research

There are a number of challenges limiting our understanding of the impact of EDCs on T2DM related to the physical properties of EDCs: the selection of experimental models to assess effects on glucose homeostasis or coexisting risk factors on the exposed individuals included in the epidemiological studies.

The thousands of chemicals released into the environment create the real scenario of human co-exposure and an enormous analytical challenge in the assessment. Sometimes the physical properties of EDCs such as lipophilicity contribute to their accumulation and persistence in human tissues, even after the exposure has terminated. In this case biomonitoring is the key for the assessment of EDCs. Regarding the types of sample used in analysis, these must be expanded beyond urine and serum to lipid-rich organs (e.g., POPs are accumulated in brain and adipose tissue) as well as tissues relevant to *in utero* and early postnatal stages of exposure (e.g., human breast milk). Also the development of clinical biomarkers it will be useful to identify chemically exposed population.

Although environmental and tissue levels of certain EDCs (e.g., PCBs) have declined in some countries in response to EU regulations, they remain of concern in other countries, and uncertainty still exists regarding future trends.

http://dx.doi.org/10.5772/59110

Another important challenge is related with the lack of clear structure-function relationships that excludes a possible *in silico* prediction of endocrine disrupting effects and demands the use of bioassays to characterize the physiological effects of the exposure.

The experimental design is further complicated by non-monotonic dose response correlation, multiple mechanisms of action for a single compound, potential additive, synergistic or antagonistic effects observed during co-exposure or the lack of adversity for some endpoints defined in OECD guideline (e.g. uterotrophic assay).

The main gaps of epidemiological studies were already addressed. Still other factors like geographic and temporal variation among the studies can induce differences in the exposure assessment, especially on the composition of chemical mixtures (especially for POPs) and duration of exposure.

Also inter-individual variation, transgenerational effects or predisposing factors (such as obesity or a family history of diabetes) may influence the metabolic effects observed in the epidemiological studies.

9. Conclusion

More studies are necessary to establish the exact mechanisms through which EDCs determine impairments of glucose homeostasis; these studies are imperatively important in order to impose international guidelines that will lead to a reduction of the incidence of T2DM cases induced by chemical exposure.

Acknowledgements

The work has been performed under the Young Investigator Grant (28344/04.11.2013) supported by UMF Carol Davila

Author details

Carmen Purdel[1], Mihaela Ilie[1] and Denisa Margina[2*]

*Address all correspondence to: denisa.margina@gmail.com

1 Carol Davila University of Medicine and Pharmacy, Faculty of Pharmacy, Department of Toxicology, Bucharest, Romania

2 Carol Davila University of Medicine and Pharmacy, Faculty of Pharmacy, Department of Biochemistry, Bucharest, Romania

References

[1] International Diabetes Federation: Diabetes atlas. Available from: http://www.idf.org/diabetesatlas (accessed 14 June 2014).

[2] Colborn T, vom Saal FS., Soto AM. Developmental effects of endocrine disrupting chemicals in wildlife and humans. Environ Health Perspect 1993;101(5):378–384

[3] Colborn T, Corlie C., editor. Chemically-induced alterations in sexual and functional development: The wildlife/human connection. Princeton Scientific Publishing Co. Inc.; NJ. 1992.

[4] Rhomberg L., Seeley M. Environmental Hormone Disruptors, In: P. Wexler (ed.), Encyclopedia of Toxicology. Elsevier Press; 2005. pp. 205-208.

[5] Jobling S.. Natural and anthropogenic environmental oestrogens: the scientific basis for risk assessment. Review of suggested testing methods for endocrine-disrupting chemicals. IUPAC Pure and Applied Chemistry 1998; Vol. 70(9): 1805-1827.

[6] Damstra T, Barlow S, Bergman A, Kavlock R, Van Der Kraak G. Global assessment of the state-of-the-science of endocrine disruptors. WHO/PCS/EDC/02.2. Geneva: World Health Organisation, 2002. http://www.who.int/pcs/emerg_site/edc/global_edc_TOC.htm (accessed 17 June 2014)

[7] Endocrine disrupters website: http://ec.europa.eu/environment/endocrine/definitions/endodis_en.html (accessed 14 June 2014)

[8] IPCS (International Programme on Chemical Safety). Risk Assessment Terminology. World Health Organization, Geneva, 2004. http://www.who.int/ipcs/methods (accessed 8 June 2014)

[9] OECD (Organisation for Economic Cooperation and Development). Draft Guidance Document on the Assessment of Chemicals for Endocrine Disruption Version 10 march 2011. Paris. http://www.oecd.org/(accessed 8 June 2014)

[10] Zoeller RT, Brown TR, Doan LL, Gore AC, Skakkebaek NE, Soto AM, Woodruff TJ, Vom Saal FS. Endocrine-disrupting chemicals and public health protection: a statement of principles from The Endocrine Society. Endocrinology 2012; 153(9): 4097-4110. doi: 10.1210/en.2012-1422.

[11] TEDX List of Potential Endocrine Disruptors. http://endocrinedisrution.org/ (accessed 8 June 2014)

[12] EFSA Scientific Committee; Scientific Opinion on the hazard assessment of endocrine disruptors: scientific criteria for identification of endocrine disruptors and appropriateness of existing test methods for assessing effects mediated by these substances on human health and the environment. EFSA Journal 2013;11(3):3132. www.efsa.europa.eu/efsajournal (accessed 14 June 2014)

[13] Stahlhut RW, Welshons WV, Swan SH. Bisphenol A data in NHANES suggest longer than expected half-life, substantial non-food exposure, or both. Environ Health Perspect 2009; 117(5):784–789. doi: 10.1289/ehp.0800376.

[14] Skinner MK, Manikkam M, Guerrero-Bosagna C. Epigenetic transgenerational actions of environmental factors in disease etiology. Trends Endocrinol Metab 2010; 21(4):214-222.doi: 10.1016/j.tem.2009.12.007.

[15] Newbold RR, Padilla-Banks E, Jefferson WN. Adverse effects of the model environmental estrogen diethylstilbestrol are transmitted to subsequent generations. Endocrinology 2006; 147(6 Suppl):S11–17.

[16] Wolff MS, Engel SM, Berkowitz GS, Ye X, Silva MJ, Zhu C, Wetmur J, Calafat AM. Prenatal phenol and phthalate exposures and birth outcomes. Environ Health Perspect. 2008; 116(8):1092– 1097. doi: 10.1289/ehp.11007.

[17] Apelberg BJ, Goldman LR, Calafat AM, Herbstman JB, Kuklenyik Z, Heidler J, Needham LL, Halden RU, Witter FR. Determinants of fetal exposure to polyfluoroalkyl compounds in Baltimore, Maryland. Environ Sci Technol. 2007; 41(11):3891–3897.

[18] Lovasi GS, Quinn JW, Rauh VA, Perera FP, Andrews HF, Garfinkel R, Hoepner L, Whyatt R, Rundle A. Chlorpyrifos exposure and urban residential environment characteristics as determinants of early childhood neurodevelopment. Am J Public Health. 2011; 101(1):63–70.

[19] Grandjean P, Heindel JJ. In utero and early-life conditions and adult health and disease. N Engl J Med. 2008; 359(14):1523.

[20] Anway MD, Cupp AS, Uzumcu M, Skinner MK. Epigenetic transgenerational actions of endocrine disruptors and male fertility. Science 2005;308(5727):1466–1469

[21] Anway MD, Leathers C, Skinner MK. Endocrine disruptor vinclozolin induced epigenetic transgenerational adult-onset disease. Endocrinology 2006; 147(12):5515-5523.

[22] Newbold RR, Padilla-Banks E, Jefferson WN, Heindel JJ. Effects of endocrine disruptors on obesity. Int J Androl 2008; 31(2):201-208.

[23] Uzumcu M, Suzuki H, Skinner MK. Effect of the anti-androgenic endocrine disruptor vinclozolin on embryonic testis cord formation and postnatal testis development and function. Reprod Toxicol 2004; 18(6):765-774.

[24] Dolinoy DC, Huang D, Jirtle RL. Maternal nutrient supplementation counteracts bisphenol A induced DNA hypomethylation in early development. Proc. Natl. Acad. Sci. 2007; 104(32): 13056–13061.

[25] Andersen HR, Schmidt IM, Grandjean P, Jensen TK, Budtz-Jorgensen E, Kjaerstad MB, et al.. Impaired reproductive development in sons of women occupationally exposed to pesticides during pregnancy. Environ Health Perspect. 2008; 116(4): 566–572.

[26] Skinner MK. Role of epigenetics in developmental biology and transgenerational inheritance. Birth Defects Res C Embryo Today. 2011; 93(1):51–55.

[27] Diamanti-Kandarakis E, Bourguignon JP, Giudice LC, Hauser R, Prins GS, Soto AM, Zoeller RT, Gore AC. Endocrine-disrupting chemicals: an Endocrine Society scientific statement. Endocr Rev. 2009; 30(4):293–342.

[28] Ulla Hass, Sofie Christiansen, Julie Boberg, Anne Marie Vinggaard, Anna-Maria Andersson, Niels Erik Skakkebæk, Katrine Bay, Henrik Holbech and Poul Bjerregaard Report on Criteria for Endocrine disrupters, Danish Centre on Endocrine Disrupters, May 2011. http://www.cend.dk/litteraturs%C3%B8gninger/EDC_criteria_report.pdf (accessed 8 June 2014)

[29] OECD (Organisation for Economic Co-operation and Development). Series on Testing and Assessment: No 150: Guidance Document on Standardised Test Guidelines for Evaluating Chemicals for Endocrine Disruption. 2012; ENV/JM/MONO(2012)22. http://www.oecd.org/officialdocuments/publicdisplaydocumentpdf/?cote=env/jm/mono(2012) (accessed 8 June 2014)

[30] OECD (Organisation for Economic Co-operation and Development). Series on Testing and Assessment: No 178: Detailed Review Paper on the State of the Science on Novel *In vitro* and *In vivo* Screening and Testing Methods and Endpoints for Evaluating Endocrine Disruptors. 2012; ENV/JM/MONO(2012)23.. http://www.oecd.org/officialdocuments/publicdisplaydocumentpdf/?cote=env/jm/mono(2012) (accessed 8 June 2014)

[31] Fürst P. Dioxins, polychlorinated biphenyls and other organohalogen compounds in human milk. Levels, correlations, trends and exposure through breastfeeding. Mol Nutr Food Res. 2006; 50(10): 922–933..

[32] Darnerud PO, Atuma S, Aune M, Bjerselius R, Glynn A et al, Dietary intake estimations of organohalogen contaminants(dioxins, PCB, PBDE and chlorinated pesticides, e.g. DDT) based on Swedish market basket data. Food Chem. Toxicol, 2006, 44(9): 1597-1606.

[33] Bhattacharya P, Welch AH, Stollenwerk KG, McLaughlin MJ, Bundschuh J, Panaullah G. Arsenic in the environment: Biology and chemistry. Science of the Total Environment,2007; 379(2-3):109-120.

[34] Smith AH, Lingas EO, Rahman M. Contamination of drinkingwater by arsenic in Bangladesh: A public health emergency. Bulletin of the World Health Organization, 2000, 78(9):1093-1103.

[35] Howe S, Borodinsky L, Lyon R. 1998 Potential exposure to bisphenol A from food-contact use of epoxy coated cans. Journal of Coatings Technology 70 (877): 69-74.

[36] Ikezuki Y, Tsutsumi O, Takai Y, Kamei Y, Taketani Y. Determination of bisphenol A concentrations in human biological fluids reveals significant early prenatal exposure. Hum Reprod 2002;17(11):2839–2841.

[37] Schönfelder G, Wittfoht W, Hopp H, Talsness CE, Paul M, Chahoud I. Parent bisphenol A accumulation in the human maternal-fetal-placental unit. Environ Health Perspect 2002;110(11):A703–A707.

[38] Weschler CJ. Changes in indoor pollutants since the 1950s. Atmospheric Environment 2009;43 (1): 153–169.

[39] Lorber M. Exposure of Americans to polybrominated diphenyl ethers. J Expo Sci Environ Epidemiol 2008;18(1): 2–19.

[40] Morland KB, Landrigan PJ, Sjödin A, Gobeille AK, Jones RS, McGahee EE, Needham LL, Patterson DG Body burdens of polybrominated diphenyl ethers among urban anglers. Environ. Health Perspect. 2005; 113 (12): 1689–92.

[41] Cao Y, Calafat AM, Doerge DR, Umbach DM, Bernbaum JC, Twaddle NC, Ye X, Rogan WJ. Isoflavones in urine, saliva and blood of infants—data from a pilot study on the estrogenic activity of soy formula. J Expo Sci Environ Epidemiol 2009;19(2):223–234.

[42] Vandenberg LN., Colborn T, Hayes TB, Heindel JJ, Jacobs Jr DR, Lee DH,,Shioda T, et al. Hormones and endocrine-disrupting chemicals: low-dose effects and nonmonotonic dose responses. Endocrine Reviews 2012; 33(3): 378–455.

[43] Vandenberg LN, Hauser R, Marcus M, Olea N, Welshons WV. Human exposure to bisphenol A (BPA). Reprod Toxicol 2007; 24(2):139–177.

[44] Welshons WV, Thayer KA, Judy BM, Taylor JA, Curran EM, vom Saal FS. Large effects from small exposures: I. Mechanisms for endocrine-disrupting chemicals with estrogenic activity. Environ Health Perspect 2003;111(8):994–1006.

[45] Vo TT, Jeung EB. An evaluation of estrogenic activity of parabens using uterine calbindin-D9k gene in an immature rat model. Reprod Toxicol. 2010; 29(3): 306–316.

[46] Lemini C, Jaimez R, Avila ME, Franco Y, Larrea F, Lemus AE. In vivo and in vitro estrogen bioactivities of alkyl parabens. Toxicol Ind Health 2003;19(2-6):69-79.

[47] Morohoshi K., Yamamoto H, Kamata R, Shiraishi F, Koda T, Morita M.Estrogenic activity of 35 components of commercial sunscreen lotions evaluated by in vitro assays. Toxicol. In Vitro 2005; 19(4): 457-469.

[48] Prusakiewicz JJ, Harville HM, Zhang Y, Ackermann C, Voorman RL.Parabens inhibit human skin estrogen sulfotransferase activity: possible link to paraben estrogenic effects. Toxicology 2007; 232(3):248-56.

[49] Grun F, Blumberg BEnvironmental obesogens: organotins and endocrine disruption via nuclear receptor signaling. Endocrinology, 2006; 147(6 Suppl):S50-55.

[50] Sato S, Shirakawa H, Tomita S, Ohsaki Y, Haketa K, Tooi O, et al. Low-dose dioxins alter gene expression related to cholesterol biosynthesis, lipogenesis, and glucose metabolism through the aryl hydrocarbon receptor-mediated pathway in mouse liver. Toxicology and Applied Pharmacology 2008;229(1): 10–19

[51] Fried KW, Guo GL, Esterly N, Kong B, Rozman KK. 2,3,7,8-tetrachlorodibenzop-dioxin (TCDD) reverses hyperglycemia in a type II diabetes mellitus rat model by a mechanism unrelated to PPAR gamma. Drug Chem Toxicol 2010;33(3):261–268 doi: 10.3109/01480540903390026

[52] Liu PC, Matsumura F. Differential effects of 2,3,7,8-tetrachlorodibenzop-dioxin on the "adipose-type" and "brain-type" glucose transporters in mice. Mol Pharmacol 1995;47(1) :65–73

[53] Alonso-Magdalena P, Ropero AB, CarreraMP, Cederroth CR, BaquieM, Gauthier BR, Nef S, Stefani E & Nadal A 2008 Pancreatic insulin content regulation by the estrogen receptor ER alpha. PLoS ONE 3(4): e2069

[54] Alonso-Magdalena P., S. Morimoto, C. Ripoll, E. Fuentes, A. Nadal, The estrogenic effect of bisphenol A disrupts pancreatic beta-cell function in vivo and induces insulin resistance, Environ. Health Perspect. 2006; 114(1): 106–112.

[55] Alonso-Magdalena P, Vieira E, Soriano S, Menes L, Burks D, Quesada I, Nadal A. Bisphenol A exposure during pregnancy disrupts glucose homeostasis in mothers and adult male offspring, Environ. Health Perspect. 2010; 118(9):1243–1250.

[56] Lim JS, Lee DH, Jacobs DR Jr. Association of brominated flame retardants with diabetes and metabolic syndrome in the U.S. population, 2003-2004. Diabetes Care. 2008;31(9):1802–1807

[57] Blair RM, Fang H, Gaylor D, Sheehan D.M. Threshold analysis of selected dose-response data for endocrine active chemicals. APMIS 2001; 109(3):198-208.

[58] Piaggi S, Novelli M, Martino L, Masini M, Raggi C, Orciuolo E, et al.. Cell death and impairment of glucose-stimulated insulin secretion induced by 2,3,7,8-tetrachlorodibenzo-p-dioxin (TCDD) in the beta-cell line INS-1E. Toxicol Appl Pharmacol 2007;220(3):333-340.

[59] Wassermann D, Wassermann M, Lemesch C. Ultrastructure of beta-cells of the endocrine pancreas in rats receiving polychlorinated biphenyls. Environ Physiol Biochem 1975;5(5):322-340.

[60] Douillet C, Currier J, Saunders J, Bodnar WM, Matousek T, Styblo M. Methylated trivalent arsenicals are potent inhibitors of glucose stimulated insulin secretion by murine pancreatic islets. Toxicol Appl Pharmacol2013;267(1):11-15.

[61] El Muayed M, Raja MR, Zhang X, MacRenaris KW, Bhatt S, Chen X, Urbanek M, O'Halloran TV, Lowe WL Jr. Accumulation of cadmium in insulin-producing β cells. Islets 2012;4(6):405-416.

[62] Gunton JE, Kulkarni RN, Yim S, Okada T, Hawthorne WJ, Tseng YH, et al. Loss of ARNT/HIF1beta mediates altered gene expression and pancreatic-islet dysfunction in human type 2 diabetes. Cell 2005;122(3): 337–349.

[63] Zhang W, Sargis RM, Volden PA, Carmean CM, Sun XJ, Brady MJ. PCB 126 and other dioxin-like PCBs specifically suppress hepatic PEPCK expression via the aryl hydrocarbon receptor. PLoS One 2012;7 (5): :e37103.

[64] Nash JT, Szabo DT, Carey GB. Polybrominated diphenyl ethers alter hepatic phosphoenolpyruvate carboxykinase enzyme kinetics in male Wistar rats: implications for lipid and glucose metabolism. J Toxicol Environ Health A 2013;76(2):142-56.

[65] Wang J, Lv X, Du Y. Inflammatory response and insulin signaling alteration induced by PCB77. J Environ Sci (China) 2010;22(7):1086-90.

[66] Baker NA, Karounos M, English V, Fang J, Wei Y, Stromberg A, Sunkara M, Morris AJ, Swanson HI, Cassis LA. Coplanar polychlorinated biphenyls impair glucose homeostasis in lean C57BL/6 mice and mitigate beneficial effects of weight loss on glucose homeostasis in obese mice. Environ Health Perspect 2013;121 (1):105-110. doi: 10.1289/ehp.1205421.

[67] Arsenescu V, Arsenescu RI, King V, Swanson H, Cassis LA. Polychlorinated biphenyl-77 induces adipocyte differentiation and proinflammatory adipokines and promotes obesity and atherosclerosis. Environ Health Perspect 2008;116(6):761-768.

[68] Le May C, Chu K, Hu M, Ortega CS, Simpson ER, et al. (2006) Estrogens protect pancreatic beta-cells from apoptosis and prevent insulin-deficient diabetes mellitus in mice. Proc Natl Acad Sci U S A 103(24): 9232–9237.

[69] Barros RP, Machado UF, Warner M, Gustafsson JA.Muscle GLUT4 regulation by estrogen receptors ERbeta and ERalpha. Proc Natl Acad Sci U S A 2006; 103(5): 1605–1608.

[70] Bryzgalova G, Gao H, Ahren B, Zierath JR, Galuska D, et al. Evidence that oestrogen receptor-alpha plays an important role in the regulation of glucose homeostasis in mice: insulin sensitivity in the liver. Diabetologia 2006; 49(3): 588–597.

[71] Martensson UE, Salehi SA, Windahl S, Gomez MF, Sward K, Daszkiewicz-Nilsson J, et al. Deletion of the G protein-coupled receptor GPR30 impairs glucose tolerance, reduces bone growth, increases blood pressure, and eliminates estradiol-stimulated insulin release in female mice. Endocrinology 2008;150(2): 687–698.

[72] Thomas P, Dong J, Binding and activation of the seven-transmembrane estrogen receptor GPR30 by environmental estrogens: a potential novel mechanism of endocrine disruption. Journal of Steroid Biochemistry and Molecular Biology 2006;102(1-5):175–179.

[73] Fu J, Woods CG, Yehuda-Shnaidman E, Zhang Q, Wong V, Collins S, et al. Low-level arsenic impairs glucose-stimulated insulin secretion in pancreatic beta cells: involve-

ment of cellular adaptive response to oxidative stress. Environ Health Perspect 2010; 118(6):684–870.

[74] Ortsater H, Liss P, Akerman KE, Bergsten P. Contribution of glycolytic and mitochondrial pathways in glucose-induced changes in islet respiration and insulin secretion. Pflugers Arch 2002; 444(4):506–512.

[75] Leloup C, Tourrel-Cuzin C, Magnan C, Karaca M, Castel J, et al. Mitochondrial reactive oxygen species are obligatory signals for glucose-induced insulin secretion. Diabetes 2009; 58(3):673–681.

[76] Lu TH, Su CC, Chen YW, Yang CY, Wu CC, et al. Arsenic induces pancreatic beta-cell apoptosis via the oxidative stress-regulated mitochondria-dependent and endoplasmic reticulum stress-triggered signaling pathways. Toxicol Lett 2011;201(1):15–26 doi: 10.1016/j.toxlet.2010.11.019.

[77] Quesada I, Fuentes E, Viso-Leon MC, Soria B, Ripoll C, Nadal A. Low doses of the endocrine disruptor bisphenol-A and the native hormone 17-beta-estradiol rapidly activate transcription factor CREB. FASEB J 2002;16(12):1671-1673.

[78] Prentki M, Matschinsky FM. Ca2+, cAMP, and phospholipid-derived messengers in coupling mechanisms of insulin secretion. Physiol. Rev.1987; 67(4):1185-1248.

[79] Miura Y, Matsui H. Triphenyltin impairs a protein kinase A (PKA)-dependent increase of cytosolic Na+and Ca2+and PKA-independent increase of cytosolic Ca2+associated with insulin secretion in hamster pancreatic beta-cells. Toxicol Appl Pharmacol 2006;216(3):363-72.

[80] Fischer LJ, Wagner MA, Madhukar BV. Potential involvement of calcium, CaM kinase II, and MAP kinases in PCB-stimulated insulin release from RINm5F cells. Toxicol Appl Pharmacol 1999;159(3):194-203.

[81] Diaz-Villasenor A, Burns AL, Salazar AM, Sordo M, Hiriart M, Cebrian ME, Ostrosky-Wegman P. Arsenite reduces insulin secretion in rat pancreatic beta-cells by decreasing the calcium-dependent calpain-10 proteolysis of SNAP-25. Toxicol Appl Pharmacol 2008;231(3):291-9.

[82] Rhodes C J, White MF. Molecular insights into insulin action and secretion European Journal of Clinical Investigation 2002; 32 (Suppl. 3): 3–13

[83] Nishiumi S, Yoshida M, Azuma T, Yoshida K, Ashida H. 2,3,7,8-tetrachlorodibenzo-p-dioxin impairs an insulin signaling pathway through the induction of tumor necrosis factor-alpha in adipocytes. Toxicol Sci 2010;115(2):482-91.

[84] Yen YP, Tsai KS, Chen YW, Huang CF, Yang RS, Liu SH. Arsenic inhibits myogenic differentiation and muscle regeneration. Environ Health Perspect 2010;118(7): 949-956. doi: 10.1289/ehp.0901525

[85] Xue P, Hou Y, Zhang Q, Woods CG, Yarborough K, Liu H, Sun G, Andersen ME, Pi J. Prolonged inorganic arsenite exposure suppresses insulin-stimulated AKT S473

phosphorylation and glucose uptake in 3T3-L1 adipocytes: involvement of the adaptive antioxidant response. Biochem Biophys Res Commun 2011;407(2):360-5. doi: 10.1016/j.bbrc.2011.03.024.

[86] Paul DS, Harmon AW, Devesa V, Thomas DJ, Styblo M. Molecular mechanisms of the diabetogenic effects of arsenic: inhibition of insulin signaling by arsenite and methylarsonous acid. Environ Health Perspect 2007;115(5):734-742.

[87] Masuno H, Iwanami J, Kidani T, Sakayama K, Honda K. Bisphenol A accelerates terminal differentiation of 3T3-L1 cells into adipocytes through the phosphatidylinositol 3-kinase pathway. Toxicol Sci 2005;84(2):319-27.

[88] Indumathi D, Jayashree S, Selvaraj J, Sathish S, Mayilvanan C, Akilavalli N, Balasubramanian K. Effect of bisphenol-A on insulin signal transduction and glucose oxidation in skeletal muscle of adult male albino rat. Hum Exp Toxicol 2013;32(9):960-71 doi: 10.1177/0960327112470273.

[89] Rengarajan S, Parthasarathy C, Anitha M, Balasubramanian K. Diethylhexyl phthalate impairs insulin binding and glucose oxidation in Chang liver cells. Toxicol In Vitro 2007;21(1):99-102.

[90] Rajesh P, Sathish S, Srinivasan C, Selvaraj J, Balasubramanian K. Phthalate is associated with insulin resistance in adipose tissue of male rat: role of antioxidant vitamins. J Cell Biochem 2013;114(3):558-69.

[91] Han JC, Park SY, Hah BG, Choi GH, Kim YK, et al. Cadmium induces impaired glucose tolerance in rat by down-regulating GLUT4 expression in adipocytes. Arch Biochem Biophys 2003;413(2):213-220.

[92] Walton FS, Harmon AW, Paul DS, Drobna Z, Patel YM, Styblo M. Inhibition of insulin-dependent glucose uptake by trivalent arsenicals: possible mechanism of arsenic induced diabetes. Toxicol Appl Pharmacol 2004; 198(3):424–433

[93] Viluksela M, Unkila M, Pohjanvirta R, Tuomisto JT, Stahl BU, et al. Effects of 2,3,7,8-tetrachlorodibenzo-p-dioxin (TCDD) on liver phosphoenolpyruvate carboxykinase (PEPCK) activity, glucose homeostasis and plasma amino acid concentrations in the most TCDD-susceptible and the most TCDD-resistant rat strains. Arch Toxicol 1999;73(6):323-36.

[94] Ben-Jonathan N, Hugo ER, Brandebourg TD. Effects of bisphenol A on adipokine release from human adipose tissue: Implications for the metabolic syndrome. Mol Cell Endocrinol 2009;304(1-2):49–54

[95] Ryden M, Arner P. Tumour necrosis factor-alpha in human adipose tissue-from signalling mechanisms to clinical implications. J Intern Med 2007;262(4):431–438.

[96] Janesick A, Blumberg B. Minireview: PPARI3 as the target of obesogens. J Steroid Biochem Mol Biol 2011; 127(1–2):4–8.

[97] Hugo ER, Brandebourg T D, Woo JG, Loftus J, J. Alexander W,Ben-Jonathan N. Bisphenol A at Environmentally Relevant Doses Inhibits Adiponectin Release from Human Adipose Tissue Explants and Adipocytes, Environmental Health Perspectives, 2008, 116(12): 1642-1647.

[98] Trujillo ME, Scherer PE. Adiponectin—journey from an adipocyte secretory protein to biomarker of the metabolic syndrome. J Intern Med 2005; 257 (2):167–175.

[99] Foryst-Ludwig A, Clemenz M, Hohmann S, Hartge M, Sprang C, et al. Metabolic actions of estrogen receptor beta (ERbeta) are mediated by a negative cross-talk with PPARgamma. PLoS Genetics 2008;4(6):e1000108. doi: 10.1371/journal.pgen.1000108

[100] Hanlon PR, Ganem LG, Cho YC, Yamamoto M, Jefcoate CR. AhR-and ERK-dependent pathways function synergistically to mediate 2,3,7,8-tetrachlorodibenzo-p-dioxin suppression of peroxisome proliferator-activated receptor-gamma1 expression and subsequent adipocyte differentiation. Toxicol Appl Pharmacol 2003;189 (1):11–27

[101] Itsuki-Yoneda A, Kimoto M, Tsuji H, Hiemori M, Yamashita H.. Effect of a hypolipidemic drug, di (2-ethylhexyl) phthalate, on mRNA-expression associated fatty acid and acetate metabolism in rat tissues. Biosci Biotechnol Biochem 2007; 71(2):414–420.

[102] Bility MT, Thompson JT, McKee RH, David RM, Butala JH, Vanden Heuvel JP, et al. Activation of mouse and human peroxisome proliferator-activated receptors (PPARs) by phthalate monoesters. Toxicol Sci 2004; 82(1):170–182.

[103] Sato S, Shirakawa H, Tomita S, Ohsaki Y, Haketa K, et al. Low-dose dioxins alter gene expression related to cholesterol biosynthesis, lipogenesis, and glucose metabolism through the aryl hydrocarbon receptor-mediated pathway in mouse liver. Toxicol Appl Pharmacol 2008;229(1):10–19 doi: 10.1016/j.taap.2007.12.029.

[104] Gayathri NS, Dhanya CR, Indu AR, Kurup PA. Changes in some hormones by low doses of di (2-ethyl hexyl) phthalate (DEHP), a commonly used plasticizer in PVC blood storage bags & medical tubing. Indian J Med Res 2004;119 (4):139–144

[105] Martinelli MI, Mocchiutti NO, Bernal CA. Dietary di(2-ethylhexyl)phthalate impaired glucose metabolism in experimental animals. Hum Exp Toxicol 2006;25(9): 531-538.

[106] Zuo Z, Chen S, Wu T, Zhang J, Su Y, et al. Tributyltin causes obesity and hepatic steatosis in male mice. Environ Toxicol 2011;26(1):79–85

[107] Ruzzin J, Petersen R, Meugnier E, Madsen L, Lock E-J, et al. Persistent organic pollutant exposure leads to insulin resistance syndrome. Environ Health Perspect 2010;118 (4):465–471

[108] Paul DS, Walton FS, Saunders RJ, Styblo M. Characterization of the impaired glucose homeostasis produced in C57BL/6 mice by chronic exposure to arsenic and high-fat diet. Environ Health Perspect 2011;119 (8):1104-9. doi: 10.1289/ehp.1003324

[109] Alonso-Magdalena P, Morimoto S, Ripoll C, Fuentes E, Nadal A. The estrogenic effect of bisphenol A disrupts pancreatic beta-cell function in vivo and induces insulin resistance, Environ. Health Perspect. 2006; 114 (1): 106–112.

[110] Boberg J Metzdorff S, Wortziger R, Axelstad M, Brokken L, et al.. Impact of diisobutyl phthalate and other PPAR agonists on steroidogenesis and plasma insulin and leptin levels in fetal rats. Toxicology. 2008; 250(2-3):75-81. doi: 10.1016/j.tox. 2008.05.020.

[111] Hill D, Wlodarczyk B, Mitchell L, Finnell R. Arsenate-induced maternal glucose intolerance and neural tune defects in a mouse model *Toxicol Appl Pharmacol*. 2009; 239(1): 29–36.' doi:10.1016/j.taap.2009.05.009.

[112] Bertazzi PA, Bernucci I, Brambilla G, Consonni D, Pesatori AC. The Seveso studies on early and long-term effects of dioxin exposure: a review. Environ Health Perspect 1998;106 (suppl 2):625–633

[113] Michalek JE, Akhtar FZ, Kiel JL. Serum dioxin, insulin, fasting glucose, and sex hormone-binding globulin in veterans of Operation Ranch Hand. J Clin Endocrinol Metab 1999; 84(5):1540–1543

[114] Warner M, Mocarelli P, Brambilla P, Wesselink A, Samuels S, et al. Metabolic Syndrome, and Obesity in Relation to Serum Dioxin Concentrations: The Seveso Women's Health Study Environ Health Perspect 2013;121:906–911 http://dx.doi.org/10.1289/ehp.1206113

[115] Zober A, Ott MG, Messerer P. Morbidity follow up study of BASF employees exposed to 2,3,7,8-tetrachlorodibenzo-*p*dioxin (TCDD) after a 1953 chemical reactor incident. Occup Environ Med 1994; 51:479–486

[116] Calvert GM, Sweeney MH, Deddens J, Wall DK. Evaluation of diabetes mellitus, serum glucose, and thyroid function among United States workers exposed to 2,3,7,8-tetrachlorodibenzo-*p*-dioxin. Occup Environ Med 1999; 56(4):270–276

[117] Cranmer M, Louie S, Kennedy RH, Kern PA, Fonseca VA. Exposure to 2,3,7,8-tetrachlorodibenzo-*p*-dioxin (TCDD) is associated with hyperinsulinemia and insulin resistance. Toxicol Sci 2000; 56:431–436.

[118] Wang SL, Tsai PC, Yang CY, Leon Guo Y. Increased risk of diabetes and polychlorinated biphenyls and dioxins: a 24-year follow-up study of the Yucheng cohort. Diabetes Care 2008;31:1574–1579

[119] Lee DH, Steffes MW, Sjödin A, Jones RS, Needham LL, Jacobs DR Jr.. Low dose of some persistent organic pollutants predicts type 2 diabetes: a nested case–control study. Environ Health Perspect 2010; 118:1235–1242

[120] Lee DH, Lind PM, Jacobs DR Jr, Salihovic S, van Bavel B, Lind L. Polychlorinated biphenyls and organochlorine pesticides in plasma predict development of type 2 dia-

betes in the elderly: the Prospective Investigation of the Vasculature in Uppsala Seniors (PIVUS) study. Diabetes Care 2011; 34(8):1778–1784.

[121] Rignell-Hydbom A, Lidfeldt J, Kiviranta H, Rantakokko P, Samsioe G, et al. Exposure to p,p′-DDE: a risk factor for type 2 diabetes. PLoS One 2009; 4(10):e7503;

[122] Turyk M, Anderson H, Knobeloch L, Imm P, Persky V. Organochlorine exposure and incidence of diabetes in a cohort of Great Lakes sport fish consumers. Environ Health Perspect 2009;117(7):1076–1082

[123] Vasiliu O, Cameron L, Gardiner J, Deguire P, Karmaus W. Polybrominated biphenyls, polychlorinated biphenyls, body weight, and incidence of adult-onset diabetes mellitus. Epidemiology 2006; 17(4):352–359.

[124] Lim JS, Lee DH, Jacobs DR. Association of brominated flame retardants with diabetes and metabolic syndrome in the U.S. population, 2003–2004, Diabetes Care, 2008; 31(9): 1802–1807.

[125] Lang I., Galloway TS, Scarlett A, Henley WE, Depledge M, et al. Association of urinary bisphenol A concentration with medical disorders and laboratory abnormalities in adults. JAMA 2008; 300(11): 1303-1310.

[126] Lee DH, Lee I K, Song K, et al. A strong dose-response relation between serum concentrations of persistent organic pollutants and diabetes: results from the National Health and Examination Survey 1999–2002. Diabetes Care 2006; 29(7): 1638–1644.

[127] Afridi HI, Kazi TG, Kazi N, et al. Evaluation of status of toxic metals in biological samples of diabetes mellitus patients. Diabetes Res Clin Pract 2008; 80(2):280–288

[128] Chen Y, Ahsan H, Slavkovich V, Peltier GL, Gluskin RT, et al. No association between arsenic exposure from drinking water and diabetes mellitus: a cross-sectional study in Bangladesh. Environ Health Perspect 2010; 118(9):1299–1305.

[129] Kolachi NF, Kazi TG, Afridi HI, et al. Status of toxic metals in biological samples of diabetic mothers and their neonates. Biol Trace Elem Res 2010; 143(1):196–212.

[130] Meliker JR, Wahl RL, Cameron LL, Nriagu JO. Arsenic in drinking water and cerebrovascular disease, diabetes mellitus, and kidney disease in Michigan: a standardized mortality ratio analysis. Environ Health 2007;6:4.

[131] Ruiz-Navarro ML, Navarro-Alarcón M, Lopez González-de la Serrana H, Pérez-Valero V, López-Martinez MC. Urine arsenic concentrations in healthy adults as indicators of environmental contamination: relation with some pathologies. Sci Total Environ 1998; 216(1–2):55–61.

[132] Tollestrup K, Frost FJ, Harter LC, McMillan GP. Mortality among children residing near the American Smelting and Refining Company (ASARCO) copper smelter in Ruston, Washington. Arch Environ Health 2003; 58(11):683–691.

[133] Wang JP, Wang SL, Lin Q, Zhang L, Huang D, Ng JC. Association of arsenic and kidney dysfunction in people with diabetes and validation of its effects in rats. Environ Int 2009; 35(3):507–511.

[134] Ward NI, Pim B. Trace element concentrations in blood plasma from diabetic patients and normal individuals. Biol Trace Elem Res. 1984; 6 (6):469–487

[135] Zierold KM, Knobeloch L, Anderson H. Prevalence of chronic diseases in adults exposed to arsenic-contaminated drinking water. Am J Public Health 2004; 94(11):1936–1937.

[136] Navas-Acien A, Silbergeld EK, Pastor-Barriuso R, Guallar E. Arsenic exposure and prevalence of type 2 diabetes in US adults. JAMA 2008; 300(7):814–822.

[137] Navas-Acien A, Silbergeld EK, Pastor-Barriuso R, Guallar E. Arsenic exposure and prevalence of type 2 diabetes: updated findings from the National Health Nutrition and Examination Survey, 2003–2006. Epidemiology 2009;20(6):816–820.

[138] Steinmaus C, Yuan Y, Liaw J, Smith AH. Low-level population exposure to inorganic arsenic in the United States and diabetes mellitus: a reanalysis. Epidemiology 2009;20(6):807–815.

[139] Lai MS, Hsueh YM, Chen CJ, et al. Ingested inorganic arsenic and prevalence of diabetes mellitus. Am J Epidemiol 1994;139(5):484–492

[140] Nabi AH, Rahman MM, Islam LN. Evaluation of biochemical changes in chronic arsenic poisoning among Bangladeshi patients. Int J Environ Res Public Health. 2005; 2(3–4):385–393

[141] Rahman M, Tondel M, Ahmad SA, Axelson O. Diabetes mellitus associated with arsenic exposure in Bangladesh. Am J Epidemiol 1998; 148(2):198–203.

[142] Tsai SM, Wang TN, Ko YC. Mortality for certain diseases in areas with high levels of arsenic in drinking water. Arch Environ Health 1999; 54(3):186–193.

[143] Tseng CH, Tai TY, Chong CK, Tseng CP, Lai MS, et al. Long-term arsenic exposure and incidence of noninsulin-dependent diabetes mellitus: a cohort study in arseniasis-hyperendemic villages in Taiwan. Environ Health Perspect 2000; 108(9):847–851

[144] Wang SL, Chiou JM, Chen CJ, Tseng CH, Chou WL et al. Prevalence of non-insulin-dependent diabetes mellitus and related vascular diseases in southwestern arseniasis-endemic and nonendemic areas in Taiwan. Environ Health Perspect 2003. 111(2): 155–159.

[145] Stahlhut RW, van Wijngaarden E, Dye TD, Cook S, Swan SH. Concentrations of urinary phthalate metabolites are associated with increased waist circumference and insulin resistance in adult U.S. males Environmental Health Perspectives, 2007; 115 (6): 876–882.

[146] Hatch EE, Nelson JW, Qureshi MM, Weinberg J, Moore LL, Singer M, Webster TF. Association of urinary phthalate metabolite concentrations with body mass index

and waist circumference: a cross-sectional study of NHANES data, 1999–2002. Environ Health 2008; 7:27. http://www.ehjournal.net/content/7/1/27

[147] Melzer D, Galloway TS. Bisphenol A and adult disease: making sense of fragmentary data and competing inferences. Annals of internal medicine 2011;155(6):392-394.

[148] Ning G, Yufang Bi, Wang T, Xu M, Xu Y, et al.Relationship of urinary bisphenol A concentration to risk for prevalent type 2 diabetes in Chinese adults: a cross-sectional analysis. Annals of internal medicine 2011;155(6):368-74

[149] Wang T, et al. Urinary bisphenol A (BPA) concentration associates with obesity and insulin resistance. J Clin Endocrinol Metab.2012;97(2):E223-227. doi: 10.1210/jc. 2011-1989.

Chapter 10

Statins in Type 2 Diabetes

Kazuko Masuo

Additional information is available at the end of the chapter

http://dx.doi.org/10.5772/59862

1. Introduction

Cardiovascular disease (CVD) is one of the foremost causes of mortality and is a major contributor to morbidity for individuals with diabetes. Lipids abnormalities play an important role in raising the cardiovascular risk in diabetic and obese individuals. The main components of dyslipidemia in diabetes and metabolic syndrome is documented as small, dense low-density lipoprotein (LDL-cholesterol), the elevation in remnant triglyceride-rich lipoprotein particles, and the low high-density lipoprotein (HDL-cholesterol), which have very powerful atherogenic components.

Diabetes and chronic diseases such as chronic kidney diseases (CKD) were assessed as high-risk for cardiovascular risks by JNC-7, JSH-2009, the Adult Treatment Program III (ATP III)., therefore those conditions require more aggressive control of hypertension and dyslipidemia. [1, 2, 3, 4]. The American Heart Association (AHA) and the American College of Cardiology (ACC) recommended the following four groups of patients should be treated by statins; (1) patients with cardiovascular disease including angina, a previous heart attack or stroke, or other related condition; (2) patients with an LDL cholesterol ≥190 mg/dL; (3) patients with type 2 diabetes aged between 40 and 75 years. They reported that (4) patients with an estimated 10-year risk of cardiovascular diseases including a heart attack or stroke or developing other form of cardiovascular disease of ≥7.5% aged between 40 and 75 years. In addition, both Adult Treatment Program (ATP III) [3] and the American Diabetes Association (ADA) [4] guidelines have identified low-density lipoprotein cholesterol and the first priority of lipid lowering. There is strong evidence from landmark secondary prevention studies, that LDL cholesterol lowering in patients with diabetes leads to significant clinical benefits. Therefore, the benefit of statins on type 2 diabetes has been confirmed. [5]

Assellberg *et al.* [6] found 4 polymorphisms for HDL-cholesterol, 6 polymorphisms of LDL-cholesterol, 10 for total cholesterol, and 4 polymorphisms for triglycerides might be responsible for these lipids' parameters phenotypes in the investigation using 2,000 genes.Genome-wide association studies (GWASs) have shown strong relationships between genetic polymorphisms and lipids levels. Dyslipidemia may have, at least partly, determined genetic backgrounds, and understanding the heritability of dyslipidemia may help to control dyslipidemia.

Dyslipidemia is known as one of the important causes for the atherogenic changes in cardiovascular system, and results in very severe cardiovascular risk. Therefore, diabetes patients with dyslipidemia have much higher prevalence of mortality and morbidity of cardiovascular risks compared to diabetes patients without dyslipidemia. However, there have been a lot of discussions, especially required statins on type 2 diabetes, because statins increase the risk of new-onset type 2 diabetes mellitus [7-9]. Very recent genetic meta-analysis suggested that the increased risk of type 2 diabetes noted with statins is at least partially explained by 3-hydroxy-3-methyl-glutaryl-CoA reductase (HMG-CoA reductase or HMGCR) inhibition [10].

The statins work in the liver to prevent the formation of cholesterol. This class of drugs are most effective at lowering the LDL- cholesterol, but also have modest effects on lowering triglycerides and raising HDL- cholesterol. There are several large cohort studies investigating the effects of statins on cardiovascular risks such as the Scandinavian Simvastatin Survival Study (4S) [11] and the Cholesterol and Recurrent Events (CARE) [12, 13] trial, however, the results are discordant. Some studies showed the drugs to reduce a patient's risk of cardiac events and stroke, outside of their ability to lower cholesterol levels. On the other hand, the statins are known as their side effects including elevation in glucose levels, which is well documented as one of the risk factors for ischemic heart diseases. A number of investigations have shown that people on a high-dose regimen of the cholesterol drug atorvastatin and other cholesterol-lowering drugs may have a slightly increased risk of developing type 2 diabetes, particularly if they have several of the classic diabetes risk factors. Therefore, the American Heart Association (AHA) /The American College of Cardiology (ACC) stated separately the guideline on dyslipidemia in 2013 [14].

This chapter will review *i)* at first, dyslipidemia as a risk factor for cardiovascular diseases, and then *ii)* the benefits and demerits for dyslipidemia treatments in type 2 diabetes using statins based on the data in several large cohort studies. *iii)* Furthermore, the discrepancy, statins can improve dyslipidemia but cannot prevent the new onset of type 2 diabetes, will be discussed.

2. Statins in type 2 diabetes—Friends or Foe?

2.1. Dyslipidemia is one of the criteria of metabolic syndrome, pre-stage of type 2 diabetes

Prevalence of metabolic syndrome has been increasing with prevalence of obesity. The pathophysiology of metabolic syndrome is very complicated, but has been partially understood. It has been well documented metabolic syndrome is an important risk factor for cardiovascular diseases, especially heart diseases including heart failure and ischemic heart disease. Some studies have shown the prevalence of metabolic syndrome in the USA to be an estimated 34% of the adult population [15], and the prevalence increases with age. In addition, weight gain is associated with metabolic syndrome. Central obesity is the most important

http://dx.doi.org/10.5772/59862

confounder of metabolic syndrome, therefore, waist circumference may represent the existence of metabolic syndrome (Table 1). Another key confounder of metabolic syndrome is insulin resistance [20, 21]. Hypertensive patients, even they are nonobese, show high prevalence of insulin resistance, and metabolic syndrome coexists. Usually, people with metabolic syndrome has higher risk of developing cardiac events by twice and diabetes by 5 times compared to individuals who do not have metabolic syndrome. Therefore, hypertensive patients, even not obese, with metabolic syndrome have very high risks of cardiac events and diabetes.

	WHO (16)	**EGIR** (17, 18)	**NCEP AT III (Expert Panel on Detection Evaluation and Treatment of High Blood Cholesterol in Adults)** (3)	**American Heart Association Updated NCEP III** (19)
Insulin resistance	Top 25% of population Distribution	Top 25% of population distribution	Not considered	Not considered
Hyperinsulinemia	Not considered	Top 25% of population	Not considered	Not considered
Fasting glucose (mmol/L)	impaired fasting glucose, or impaired glucose tolerance or diabetes	>6.1, but not diabetic	≥6.1	≥5.6 (100 mg/dL) or medications for hyperglycemia
Hypertension (mmHg)	≥160/≥ 90	≥140/≥ 90 or on medications for hypertension	≥130/85	≥130/85 or medications for hypertension
Central obesity	waist/hip ratio >0.9 (men), >0.85 (women) and/or BMI≥30kg/m^2			
Waist circumference (cm)	Not considered	≥94 (men), ≥ 80 (women)	>102 (men), >88 (women)	≥102 (men), ≥88 (women)
HDL-cholesterol (mmol/L)	<1.0 or medications for dyslipidemia	<1.0 or medications for dyslipidemia	<1.07 (40 mg/dL, men), <1.25 (50 mg/dL , women)	<1.07 (40 mg/dL, men) 25 (50 mg/dL, women)
Triglyceride (mmol/L)	<1.0 or medications for Dyslipidemia	>2.0 or medications for dyslipidemia	≥1.695 (150 mg/dL)	≥1.695 (150 mg/dL)
Micro-albuminemia	Present	Not considered	Not considered	Not considered
Criteria	1 of the first two + 2 of other features	2 of other features	3 of above	3 of above

BMI, body mass index; EGIR, European Group of the study of Insulin Resistance; NCEP ATPIII, 3rd Recommendations of the Adult Treatment Panel of the National Cholesterol Education Program; HDL-cholesterol, high-density lipoprotein cholesterol. Values in NECP definition and American Heart Association/Updated NCEP are approximations of values in mg/dL.

Table 1. Criteria for Metabolic Syndrome including Insulin Resistance (11)

In addition, many epidemiological and clinical studies have shown that insulin resistance may lead to dyslipidemia; Dyslipidemia, especially low HDL-cholesterol and high triglycerides are also important criteria with high glucose levels for the metabolic syndrome (Table 1). Carg [22] hypothesized approximately 20 years ago that insulin resistance might cause dyslipidemia in metabolic syndrome. Ruotolo and Howard [23] suggested that hyperinsulinemia as a compensatory mechanisms of insulin resistance leaded to, at first, very low-density of lipoprotein (VLDL) cholesterol overproduction, then the decreased clearance of fasting and postprandial triglyceride rich lipoproteins (TRLs), and the decreased production of HDL particles [23]. In addition, they suggested that increases in TRLs play major role in metabolic syndrome, and elevated VLDL-cholesterol and decreased HDL-cholesterol may be consequence of TRLs elevation. Very recently, the Framingham study [24] supported the close relationship between dyslipidemia and insulin resistance for the onset of coronary heart disease. The incidence of coronary heart disease risk associated with HDL-cholesterol or triglycerides were significantly increased only in the presence of insulin resistance.

2.2. Dyslipidemia is an atherogenic factor

It is well established that elevation of serum LDL is a major cause of atherosclerosis and coronary heart disease (CHD) [25-29]. Many epidemiological studies have shown that elevated LDL cholesterol level is strongly related to future cardiac events [30, 31]. Therefore, LDL-cholesterol can be used as an important predictor for the future cardiac events in cardiac risk assessments (*i.e.* the Framingham Risk Score) [30, 31]. However, it is also known that other serum lipoproteins, such as triglyceride-rich lipoproteins (TRLs), very low-density lipoproteins (VLDL), chylomicrons, and HDL-cholesterol, are involved. In atherogenic dyslipidemia, the pattern of lipoprotein abnormalities or atherogenic lipoprotein phenotype includes elevations of VLDL levels, increased small LDL particles, and low HDL-cholesterol [32, 33]. The abnormalities usually coexist because they have a common metabolic basis. Grundy summarized and figured the relationship insulin resistance, dyslipidemia and coronary heart disease [34]. Besides the multiple mechanisms for atherogenesis accompanying the lipid triad, atherogenic dyslipidemia commonly is associated with several non-lipid risk factors as part of metabolic syndrome (insulin resistance) [35]. In addition, the prothrombotic state may be accompanied by several abnormalities in the coagulation system in metabolic syndrome; most notable are elevations in fibrinogen and plasminogen activator inhibitor-1 (PAI-1). These phenomena might be related to the onset and development of atherogenic damage in vessels

2.3. Statins can improve dyslipidemia in type 2 diabetes, and result in the prevention for coronary heart diseases or other cardiovascular events.

A number of large cohort clinical studies on the efficacy of statins, especially atorvastatin, have been conducted for the primary and secondary prevention of cardiovascular events in adults with, or at risk of, coronary heart disease (CHD). [36, 37] In primary prevention, CARDS (Collaborative Atorvastatin Diabetes Study) [38] showed that atorvastatin 10 mg/day significantly reduced cardiovascular events compared to placebo (relative risk of the composite primary endpoint; acute CHD events, coronary revascularisation, or stroke) by 37% ($p = 0.001$).

The decrease of cardiovascular events in CARDS study with atorvastatin was similar to those in the ASCOT-LLA (Anglo-Scandinavian Cardiac Outcomes Trial-Lipid Lowering Arm) with atorvastatin [39, 40] and HPS (Heart Protection Study) with simvastatin [41]. However, lipids lowering effects of atorvastatin was observed to be faster compared to simvastatin, 6 months with atorvastatin observed in CARDS [38] versus 15-18 months in simvastatin observed in HPS [41]. The ASCOT-LLA trial [39] conducted in 2,226 hypertensive diabetic patients without previous cardiovascular disease, showed that atorvastatin could decrease the relative risk on primary coronary heart diseases (CHD) by 36% (p=0.0005), and all cardiovascular diseases (CVD) risk by 25% (p = 0.038) compared to placebo. The IDEAL (Incremental Decrease in End Points Through Aggressive Lipid Lowering) [42, 43] and TNT (Treating to New Targets) trials [44, 45] demonstrate that both low (10 mg/day) and high (80 mg/day) doses of atorvastatin reduced the risk of non-fatal myocardial infarction by 17-22% (p < 0.02). [42-45]

Sub-studies of the GREACE (GREek Atorvastatin and Coronary-heart-disease Evaluation) [45-48], TNT (Treating to New Targets) [43, 49-51] and PROVE-IT (PRavastatin Or atorVastatin Evaluation and Infection Therapy) [52-54] trials showed similar results of atorvastatin reduced cardiac events but not only patients without diabetes but also in those with diabetes. Those studies included 15-25% of patients with diabetes.

In the GREACE sub-study, which compared to physicians'standard care [47], atorvastatin significantly reduced the relative risk of total mortality and cardiac moratility and morbidity (coronary mortality, coronary morbidity, and stroke). Furthermore, atorvastatin improved renal function [47] and liver function [46]. Of interest, patients with non-alcoholic fatty liver disease, statins (atorvastatin 24 mg/day) improved liver function, although liver injury was worsen in others without statin treatment for dyslipidemia. This study demonstrated that statin treatment is safe for mild-to-moderate liver injury caused by non-fatty liver disease, and can improve liver injury and reduce cardiovascular morbidity. In addition, statins treatment has benefits for all age groups including old patients. In the older patients, intensive lipids lowering treatments are more effective to reduce cardiovascular risks compared to younger patients when compared to usual lipids lowering treatment. The GREACE study demonstrated that one should not deprive older patients of CVD prevention treatment and lipid target achievement. [48]

Similarly, TNT (Treating to New Targets) trials [49, 50] demonstrate the preventive efficacy of atorvastatin on the reductions of cardiac events in patients with stable CHD. In the TNT sub-study [51] including a total of 9,251 coronary heart disease patients with low-density lipoprotein cholesterol, higher dose of atorvastatin (80 mg/day) over 4.9 years was more effective on the prevention on major cardiovascular events (n=729) such as coronary death, non-fatal myocardial infarction, cardiac arrest, or stroke regardless of fatal or non-fatal, compared to lower dose (10 mg/day). [52] In sub-analysis of TNT trial conducted in 5,584 CHD patients with metabolic syndrome, higher dose of atorvastatin (80mg/day) reduced the major cardiovascular and cerevrovascular events by 29%. In addition, this sub-study also demonstrated that CHD patients with metabolic syndrome had a 44% greater level of absolute cardiovascular risk compared to those without metabolic syndrome, indicating the clinical feasibility of administering intensive lipid-lowering therapy to CHD patients with metabolic syndrome

[53]. In addition, the other sub-analysis [43] demonstrated even in treatment resistant hypertensive patients, who were at high risk of cardiac events, intensive lipid lowering with atorvastatin 80 mg is associated with a significant reduction in cardiovascular events.

In the PROVE-IT (PRavastatin Or atorVastatin Evaluation and Infection Therapy) sub-study [54, 55], a significantly lower incidence of acute cardiac events was reported in patients with atorvastatin compared to pravastatin (21.1% vs. 26.6%; $p = 0.03$). Therefore, an absolute risk reduction of 5.5% was associated with atorvastatin therapy [54-56]. Similarly, the IDEAL trial (the Incremental Decrease in End Points through Aggressive Lipid Lowering trial) [57] compared the effects on cardiovascular risks between atorvastatin 80 mg daily versus simvastatin 20-40 mg daily in post-myocardial infarction patients. The IDEAL trial had smaller statistical power due to the smaller number of patients compared to the PROVE-IT study, but longer follow-up (5 years vs. 2 years). Interestingly, decreases in the relative risk of cardiovascular events at 5 years in group with simvastatin was similar to that in the 2-year follow-up with atorvastatin group, and the decreases in the cardiovascular risk maintained consistently from 2 years to 5 years in atorvastatin group. The 2 treatment regimens (atorvastatin versus simvastatin) were well tolerated. These results indicated that patients with recent myocardial infarction should be on intensive statin therapy with atorvastatin and maintain the high dose of atorvastatin as long as possible, over 2 years.

ASPEN (Atorvastatin Study for Prevention of coronary heart disease Endpoints in Non-insulin-dependent diabetes mellitus) [58] in 2,410 type 2 diabetic patients demonstrated that a 29% lower low-density lipoprotein-cholesterol level was seen with atorvastatin than placebo at endpoint ($p < 0.0001$) over a 4-year period. In sub-analysis in the 505 subjects with prior myocardial infarction or interventional procedure, atorvastatin did not reduce relative risk of a primary end-point (cardiovascular mortality, non-fatal major cardiovascular event, stroke, and unstable angina pectoris, fatal or non-fatal myocardial infaction). Therefore, ASPEN trial failed to confirm the benefit of atorvastatin on cardiocvascular risk in type 2 diabetes [58].

The ALLIANCE (Aggressive Lipid-Lowering Initiation Abates New Cardiac Events) [59-61] and GREACE (GREek Atorvastatin and Coronary-heart-disease Evaluation) [62, 63] trials demonstrated the benefits of treatment with atorvastatin for dyslipidemia compared to usual care with generic statins as the real practical clinic (*i.e.* simvastatin) in patients with stable CHD. Atorvastatin reduced the risk of non-fatal myocardial infarction by 47-59% ($p < 0.0002$) compared to usual dyslipidemia therapy with generic statins as a usual community practice in 2008. The MIRACL (Myocardial Ischemia Reduction with Aggressive Cholesterol Lowering) [64, 65], PROVE-IT [54] and IDEAL-ACS (Acute Coronary Syndromes) [57] studies also recommend the benefits of high-dosage atorvastatin therapy started from early phase after the onset of acute coronary syndrome such as within 24-96 hours observed in the MIRACL trial. When compared to placebo, all statins including pravastatin and simvastatin, atorvastatin are effective to reduce the risk of death or major cardiovascular events by 16-18% ($p = 0.048$). In patients undergoing revascularization procedures, the AVERT (Atorvastatin VErsus Revascularization Treatment) study [66] revealed that administration of atorvastatin 80 mg/day over 18 months had similar benefits on reducing the ischemic cardiac risk to angioplastity plus usual care in low-risk patients with stable coronary artery disease. Furthermore, Arca [62] reviewed that the ARMYDA (Atorvastatin for Reduction in MYocardial DAmage during angioplasty) and ARMYDA-3 trials showed atorvastatin's benefits on myocardial infaction patients; Atorvastatin 40 mg/day over 7 days before coronary intervention significantly reduced the risks of myocardial ischemic damage (ARMYDA), post-procedural acute myocardial infarction (ARMYDA) and atrial fibrillation (ARMYDA-3) versus placebo. In addition, it has been observed that post-myocardial infactionm patients without atorvastatin have significantly higher C-reactive protein levels and higher prevalence of the combined incidence of cardiovascular events (death, MI and target segment revascularization during the 6-month follow-up). In addition, the ATTEMP study (Assessing The Treatment Effect in Metabolic syndrome without Perceptible diabetes) [67] showed atorvastatin improved renal function and reduced serum uric acid levels in metabolic syndrome without cardiovascular diseases. These changes were more prominent in stage 3 chronic kidney diseases patients and might have contributed to the reduction in cardiovascular risk and clinical events.

Overall, therefore, the marked efficacy of atorvastatin in the primary and secondary prevention of cardiovascular events were provided in many large cohort trials not only in relative healthy individuals, but also in diabetes or post-myocardial infarction patients, and the effects were stronger than usual statins such as simvastatin. Atorvastatin has in general cardiovascular disease management including improving renal function, and liver injury with non-alcoholic fatty liver, suggests even greater potential clinical utility for the drug in some clinical settings. [37, 66] The results from the meta-analysis using 31 randomized studies compared statins and placebo or other statins showed in patients with CVD, (or at risk of CVD), statin reduced relative risk of all cause mortality, cardiovascular mortality, coronary heart disease mortality and fatal myocardial infarction, but did not reduce the risk of fatal stroke. Statin could not reduce relative risk of morbidity of non-fatal stroke, non-fatal myocardial infarction, transient ischemic attack (TIA), unstable angina, and coronary revascularization.

The differentiations on the clinical efficacy between statins; atorvastatin, fluvastatin, pravastatin and simvastatin, are almost impossible from the previous large clinical studies, however, there is some evidence from direct comparisons between statins to suggest that atorvastatin may be more effective than pravastatin in patients with symptomatic coronary heart diseases, although there is limited evidence for the effectiveness of statins in different subgroups [67].

2.4. Statins may improve renal function

The comparisons analysis related to renal function [43] from clinical trials with data from 149,882 patient-years of follow-up failed to show an association between high-potency statins and risk of acute kidney injury with statins (10,345 patients on atorvastation, 10-80 mg/day) compared with controls (placebo, 8,945 patients with placebo). In addition, there were no differences in effects on renal function between high-dose versus low-dose. This comparison was performed in the 24 placebo-controlled trials including IDEAL [57], TNT [47], CARDS [69, 70], ASPEN (The Atorvastatin Study for Prevention of coronary heart disease Endopoints in Non-diabeties mellitus) [58], SPARCL (The Stroke Prevention by Aggressive Reduction in Cholesterol Levels) [43, 71], and other large study using placebo with 10,345 patients with atorvastatin and 8945 patients with placebo. [43]

The TNT trial in 10,001 CHD patients with and without pre-existing chronic kidney diseases demonstrated efficacy of atorvastatin (80 mg/day) on reduction of CHD risk as well as improving renal function in both with and without pre-existing renal injury patients. No difference in the incidence of renal-related serious adverse events were observed at 120 days (0.04% in atorvastatin; 0.10% in placebo, $p = 0.162$) [50, 51]. Similarly, the use of a high-potency statin regimen did not increase the risk of kidney injury was observed in 2 large randomized trials of statin therapy in patients with acute coronary syndrome; PROVE IT-TIMI 22 [50, 55] (atorvastatin 80 mg/day) including 4,162 patients, and A-to-Z trial (pravastatin 40 mg/day for 1 month + simvastatin 80 mg/day after 1 month) including 4, 497 patients. [72] As mentioned in the previous section, the ATTEMP (Assessing the treatment Effect in Metabolic syndrome without Perceptible diabetes) study [67] showed that multifactorial intervention in patients with metabolic syndrome without established CVD improved renal function and reduced serum uric acid levels. Of importance, these changes were more prominent in stage 3 chronic kidney diseases patients. PROVE-IT-TIMI 22 sub-study [73] used urinary albumin excretion as an index of renal injury, showed no significant change in urinary albumin concentration from enrollment to end of study in either the standard (pravastatin 40 mg/day) or intensive (atorvastatin 80 mg/day) statin therapy groups in an acute coronary syndrome in statin treated patient. [52] Microalbuminuria may reflect traditional cardiovascular risk factor burden and offer little prognostic information independent of those factors. [52]

2.5. Cost-effectiveness

Cost-effectiveness between statins has been compared in several studies such as the Aggressive Lipid-lowering Initiation Abates New Cardiac Events study (ALLIANCE study) [73], and those observations showed the advantage of atorvastatin in high-risk CVD patients [68] and type 2 diabetes patients [74]. Despite the non-adherence levels observed in actual practice, statin treatment is cost-effective for primary prevention in patients newly diagnosed with type 2 diabetes. Because of large differences in cost-effectiveness according to different risk and age groups, the efficiency of the treatment could be increased by targeting patients with relatively higher cardiovascular risk and higher ages [74]. When the efficacy and cost-effectiveness were compared between rosuvastatin, atorvastatin, pravastatin and simvastatin, rosuvastatin therapy in commonly prescribed doses is most effective for improving hypercholesterolemia and most cost effective in diabetic patients with and without metabolic syndrome. [75] The PROVE IT trial [76] demonstrated that atorvastatin 80 mg/day has stronger efficacy on reducing cardiovascular events compared to pravastatin 40 mg/day in patients with acute coronary syndrome. Genetic investigations in PROVE-IT sub-study showed that the prevalence of event reduction was greater in carriers of the Trp719Arg variant in kinesin family member 6 protein (KIF6) than in non-carriers. Parthan *et al.* [76] assessed the cost effectiveness of testing for the KIF6 variant followed by targeted statin therapy (KIF6 Testing) versus not testing patients, and they found that cost-effectiveness is sensitive to the price of generic atorvastatin and the effect on adherence of knowing KIF6 carrier status.

http://dx.doi.org/10.5772/59862

2.6. The JUPITER trial and meta-analyses show statins increase the risk of new onset of type 2 diabetes

Statins are known as well-tolerated and very rare adverse events reported. Side effects of statins are very rare but still exist such as elevations of liver enzymes, muscle aches, and very rarely, rhabdomyolysis [76]. If people have adverse events, discontinuation is primary as usual procedure to resolve these adverse events similarly to other any medications.. Recently, debate has focused on the possible negative long-term effects of statin treatment on cognitive decline, and the incidence of cancer [78]. Some investigators have documented that statins affect the risk of developing cancer, when they are taken at low doses for managing hypercholesterolaemia. There is some possibility of an increased cancer risk in elderly patients associated with hydrophilic statin use. On the other hand, some recent studies have shown the benefits of statins in modifying the prognosis of cancer, and the decreases in the risks of certain cancers, such as gastric, oesophageal, liver, colorectal and advanced/aggressive prostate cancer. In addition, Jukema *et al.* [78] reported that there was no increased risk of cognitive decline or cancer with statin use. However, regarding the relations between statins and cancer, results remain controversial. Further investigations will be necessary to clarify.

Since the report of the new onset of diabetes during rosuvastatin treatment, as an unexpected finding in the JUPITER trial [7], safety concerns on abnormal glucose metabolisms related to statins have emerged in 2012. The possible association of diabetes with statin therapy has been discussed over several years, but statins' effects on reducing of cardiovasculoar risk has been overweighted than the new onset of diabetes or glucose metabolism impairement. In addition, guidelines of the American Diabetes Association [3], American Heart Association [1, 14], and American Copllege of Cardiology [14] have shown the same direction of overweighting on dyslipidemia control. In addition, several studies and meta-analysis data have shown that statin use is related to a small increased risk of type 2 diabetes mellitus. The JUPITER (Justification for the Use of Statins in Prevention: an Intervention Trial Evaluating Rosuvastatin) trial [79-81] demonstrated new onset of diabetes, although rosuvastatin reduces cardiovascular events and all-cause mortality and concomitant evidence of moderate chronic kidney diseases. The JUPITER finding on impairement of glucose metabolisms was the first data showing the strong relationship between statins and the new onset of diabetes. The JUPITER trial [78, 80]was conducted in 17,603 men and women without histories of cardiovascular diseases or diabetes with randomized, double blind design to evaluate the efficacy of rosuvastatin 20 mg/day over 5 years. In this trial, the participants who had diabetes risk factor (n=11,508), showed developing diabetes more frequently than those without a diabetic risk factor (n=6,095). In individuals with diabetic risk factors, rosuvastatin decreased the cardiovascular risks such as the primary endpoint by 39%, venous thrombosis by 36%, and total mortality by 17%, but increased diabetes risk by 28 %. On the other hand, in the participants without diabetic risk factors, all parameters decreased significantly with larger drops compare dto those with diabetic risk factors (primary endpoint by 52%; venous thrombosis by 53%; total mortality by 22 %). And, importantly, no elevations in the new onset of diabetes or impairment of glucose metabolism were observed. These results suggested that statins may have more stronger benefits on reduction of cardiovascular risks and glucose metabolisms in individuals without diabetes compared to those with diabetes. When compared to placebo, the onset of diabetes needed longer duration by 5,4 weeks in rosuvastatin (rosuvastatin, 84.3 weeks vs placebo, 89.7 weeks). The benefits on cardiovascular risk and total mortality in rosuvastatin group were greater than the hazard of the new onset of diabetes [7].

Furthermore, three recent meta-analyses of large-scale placebo-controlled and standard care-controlled trials [82] showed approximately more than 10% increased risk for incident diabetes associated with statin therapy. [83, 84]

On the other, recently the post hoc analysis of ATTEMPT study assesses the incidence of new-onset diabetes over 3.5 years in patients with metabolic syndrome observed no differences in the new onset of diabetes in patients with statins (statins, 0.83 vs. placebo, 1.00/100 patient-years) from the general population [67, 85], and no differences in the new onset of diabetes between individuals with and without diabetic risk factors [84]. New-onset diabetes incidence and CVD events were negligible and not different from what is expected in the general population. [85]

Park *et al.* [9] analysed the linkage of statins and the new-onset diabetes using meta-analysis in published large cohort studies in MEDLINE from 2000 to October 2013 with the following MESH terms and text key words alone or in combination were included: 3-hydroxy-3-methylglutaryl coenzyme A reductase inhibitors, HMG-CoA reductase inhibitors, statins, incident diabetes, new-onset diabetes, insulin resistance, impaired insulin secretion, meta-analysis, cohort study, and observational study written in English. Results of observational studies and meta-analyses show association of incident diabetes with statin use in patients with concomitant risk factors for diabetes. They concluded a possible association between statin use and incident diabetes in patients with underlying diabetes risk factors in available clinical data. Although study data may be insufficient to change the current practice paradigm, clinicians should vigilantly monitor for incident diabetes in patients on statins. Patients with a low risk of CVD and high risk of diabetes should reconsider statin use and focus on lifestyle management. Each statins has different effects on glucose metabolisms, and women and elderly persons are known at higher risk of diabetes. Therefore, various confounders related to adverse events, especially glucose metabolisms, should be considered

Muscoqiuri, *et al.* [86] discussed the effects of statins on insulin sensitivity or insulin secretion, because statins deteriorates glycemic control may accelerate progression to diabetes via molecular mechanisms that impact insulin sensitivity and secretion. The weight of clinical evidence suggests a worsening effect of statins on insulin resistance and secretion, but basic science studies could not find a clear molecular explanation from searches of computerized databases, providing conflicting evidence regarding both the beneficial and the adverse effects of statin therapy on insulin sensitivity.

A number of meta-analyses conducted in recent years have demonstrated that the association is real but causality has not yet been proved [8]. And the underlying mechanisms for this association remain unclear.

In summary, although many clinical studies have demonstrated that statins worsen glucose metabolism or cause the new onset of diabetes, the cardiovascular benefits of statin therapy overweigh the risk of impairment of glucose metabolism. Clinical practice for statin therapy should not be changed on the basis of the most recent Food and Drug Administration informational warnings in 2012. Therefore, the data suggest the need to treat dyslipidemia and to make patients aware of the possible risk of developing type 2 diabetes or, if they already are diabetic, of worsening their metabolic control.

3. Conclusions

In 2014, Simic and Reiner [87] summarized benefits and side effects of stastins as follow; 1) reduction in cardiovascular mortality and morbidity even in patients with very high risk of cardiovascular disease; 2) myopathy and rhabdomyolysis as most important side effects; 3) liver injury as a side effects, which occurs occasionally but is reversible. On the other hand, statins also improve hepatic steatosis and liver injury in fatty liver diseases; 4) similarly, renal injury as a side effect, but also statins showed protective effects on renal injury [69] and majority of data have shown the beneficial effects on renal function [33, 50-53, 67. 72]. 5) statins increase the incidence of type 2 diabetes, especially in individuals with diabetic risk factors [78]. But the cardiovascular benefits of such a treatment by far exceed this risk. Therefore, currently many guidelines for treatments for dyslipidemia, diabetes concluded that the cardiovascular benefits of statins by far outweight non-cardiovascular harms in patients with cardiovascular risk. However, it should be needed to treat dyslipidemia and to make patients aware of the possible risk of developing type 2 diabetes or, if they already are diabetic, of worsening their metabolic control.

Author details

Kazuko Masuo*

Address all correspondence to: kazuko.masuo@bakeridi.edu.au

Baker IDI Heart & Diabetes Institute, Melbourne, Victoria, Australia

The author declares no conflict of interest.

References

[1] US Department of Health and Human Services. National Institutes of Health National Heart, Lung, and Blood Institute. JNC 7 Express. The Seventh Report of Joint National Committee on Prevention, Detection, Evaluation, and Treatment of High Blood Pressure. 2003. http://www.nhlbi.nih.gov/files/docs/guidelines/express.pdf.

[2] Ogihara T, Kikuchi K, Matsuoka H, Fujita T, et al. Japanese Society of Hypertension Committee. The Japanese Society of Hypertension Guidelines for the Management of Hypertension (JSH 2009). Hypertens Res. 2009 Jan;32(1):3-107.

[3] Third report of the National Cholesterol Education Program (NCEP) Expert Panel on Detection, Evaluation, and Treatment of High Blood Cholesterol in Adults (Adult Treatment Panel III) final report. Circulation. 2002; 106: 3143-3121.

[4] American Diabetes Association. Standards of medical care in diabetes—2013. Diabetes Care. 2013 Jan;36 Suppl 1:S11-66. doi: 10.2337/dc13-S011

[5] Carmena R, Betteridge DJ. Statins and diabetes. Semin Vasc Med. 2004; 4: 321-332.

[6] Asselbergs FW, Guo Y, van Iperen EP, Sivapalaratnam S, Tragante V, Lanktree MB, et al. Large-scale gene-centric meta-analysis across 32 studies identifies multiple lipid loci. Am J Hum Genet. 2012; 91: 823-838. doi: 10.1016/j.ajhg.2012.08.032.

[7] Ridker PM, Pradhan A, MacFadyen JG, Libby P, Glynn RJ. Cardiovascular benefits and diabetes risks of statin therapy in primary prevention: an analysis from the JUPITER trial. Lancet. 2012; 380: 565-571. doi: 10.1016/S0140-6736(12)61190-8.

[8] Aiman U, Najmi A, Khan RA. Statin induced diabetes and its clinical implications. J Pharmacol Pharmavother. 2014; 5: 181-184. doi: 10.4103/0976-500X.136097.

[9] Park ZH, Juska A, Dyakov D, Patel RV. Statin-associated incident diabetes: a literature review. Consul Pharm. 2014; 29: 317-334. doi: 10.4140/TCP.n.2014.317.

[10] Swerdlow DI, Preiss D, et al. HMG-coenzyme A reductase inhibition, type 2 diabetes, and bodyweight: evidence from genetic analysis and randomised trials. Lancet. 2014 Sep 24. pii: S0140-6736(14)61183-1. doi: 10.1016/S0140-6736(14)61183-1.

[11] Huskey J, Lindenfeld J, Cook T, Targher G, Kendrick J, Kjekshus J, Pedersen T, Chonchol M. Effect of simvastatin on kidney function loss in patients with coronary heart disease: findings from the Scandinavian Simvastatin Survival Study (4S). Atherosclerosis. 2009; 205: 202-206. doi: 10.1016/j.atherosclerosis.2008.11.010.

[12] Sheng X, Murphy MJ, MacDonald TM, Wei L. The comparative effectiveness of statin therapy in selected chronic diseases compared with the remaining population. BMC Public Health. 2012; 12: 712. doi: 10.1186/1471-2458-12-712.

[13] Miyazaki T, Chiuve S, Sacks FM, Ridker PM, Libby P, Aikawa M. Plasma pentraxin 3 levels do not predict coronary events but reflect metabolic disorders in patients with coronary artery disease in the CARE trial. PLoS One. 2014; 9: e94073. doi: 10.1371/journal.pone.0094073. eCollection 2014.

[14] Stone NJ, Robinson J, et al. Expert panel Members, and ACC/AHA Task Force Members. 2013 ACC/AHA Guideline on the Treatment of Blood Cholesterol to Reduce Atherosclerotic Cardiovascular Risk in Adults. A Report of the American College of Cardiology/American Heart Association Task Force on Practice Guidelines. at VA

MED CTR BOISE on December 24, 2014. http://circ.ahajournals.org/ (Download at VA MED CTR BOISE on December 24 2014).

[15] Ford ES, Giles WH, Dietz WH. Prevalence of metabolic syndrome among US adults: findings from the third National Health and Nutrition Examination Survey. JAMA 2002; 287: 356–359. doi:10.1001/jama.287.3.356. PMID 11790215.

[16] Alberti KG, Zimmet PZ. Definition, diagnosis and classification of diabetes mellitus and its complications. Part 1: diagnosis and classification of diabetes mellitus provisional report of a WHO consultation. Diabet Med. 1998; 15: 539-553.

[17] Balkau B, Charles MA. Comment on the provisional report from the WHO consultation. European Group for the study of Insulin Resistance (EGIR). Diabet Med. 1999; 16: 442-443.

[18] Balkau B, Charles MA, Drivsholm T, et al. European Group for the study of Insulin Resistance (EGIR). Frequency of the WHO metabolic syndrome in European Cohorts, and an alternative definition of an insulin resistance syndrome. Diabetes Metab. 2002; 28: 364-376.

[19] Grundy SM, Brewer HB, Cleeman JI, Smith SC Jr, Lenfant C, The American Heart association, the National Heart, Lung, and Blood Institute : Definition of metabolic syndrome: Report of the National Heart, Lung, and Blood Institute/American Heart association conference on scientific issues related to definition. Circulation. 2004; 109: 433-438.

[20] DeFronzo RA, Ferrannini E. Insulin resistance. A multifaceted syndrome responsible for NIDDM, obesity, hypertension, dyslipidemia, and atherosclerotic cardiovascular disease. Diabetes Care. 1991; 14: 173-194.

[21] Ferrannini E. Definition of intervention points in prediabetes. Lancet Diabetes Endocrinol. 2014; 2: 667-675. doi: 10.1016/S2213-8587(13)70175-X.

[22] Carg A. Insulin resistance in the pathogenesis of dyslipidemia. Diabetes Care. 1996; 19: 387-389.

[23] Robins SJ, Lyass A, Zachariah JP, Massaro JM, Vasan RS. Insulin resistance and the relationship of a dyslipidemia to coronary heart disease: The Framingham Heart Study. Arterioscler Thromb Vasc Biol. 2011; 31: 1208-1214.

[24] Ruotolo G, Howard G. Dyslipidemia in the metabolic syndrome. Curr Cardiolo Rep. 2004; 4: 494-500]

[25] Expert Panel on Detection, Evaluation, and Treatment of High Blood Cholesterol in Adults. National Cholesterol Education Program: second report of the Expert Panel on Detection, Evaluation, and Treatment of high blood cholesterol (Adult Treatment Panel II). Circulation. 1994; 89: 1329-1445.

[26] Stamler J, Wentworth D, Neaton JD. Is the relationship between serum cholesterol and risk of premature death from coronary heart disease continuous and graded?

Findings in 356,222 primary screenees of the Multiple Risk Factor Intervention Trial (MRFIT). JAMA. 1986; 256: 2823-2828.

[27] Scandinavian Simvastatin Survival Study Group. Randomised trial of cholesterol lowering in 4444 patients with coronary heart disease: the Scandinavian Simvastatin Survival Study (4S). Lancet. 1994; 344: 1383-1389.

[28] The Long-Term Intervention with Pravastatin in Ischaemic Disease (LIPID) Study Group. Prevention of cardiovascular events and death with pravastatin in patients with coronary heart disease and a broad range of initial cholesterol levels. N Engl J Med. 1998; 339: 1349-1357.

[29] Shepherd J, Cobbe SM, Ford I, et al, for the West of Scotland Coronary Prevention Study Group. Prevention of coronary heart disease with pravastatin in men with hypercholesterolemia. N Engl J Med. 1995; 333: 1301-1307.

[30] hah RV, Goldfine AB. Statins and risk of new-onset diabetes mellitus. Circulation. 2012; 126: e282-e284. doi: 10.1161/CIRCULATIONAHA.112.122135

[31] Cobain M, Massaro J, Kannel W. General cardiovascular risk profile for use in primary care: the Framingham Heart Study. Circulation. 2008;117:743–753.

[32] Grundy SM. Atherogenic dyslipidemia: lipoprotein abnormalities and implications for therapy. Am J Cardiol. 1995; 75: 45B-52B.

[33] Grundy SM. Small LDL, atherogenic dyslipidemia, and the metabolic syndrome. Circulation. 1997; 95: 1-4.

[34] Grundy SM. MedScape Diabetes & Endocrinology. http://www.medscape.com/viewarticle/412684_2

[35] Grundy SM. Hypertriglyceridemia, atherogenic dyslipidemia, and the metabolic syndrome. Am J Cardiol. 1998; 81: 18B-25B.

[36] Ward S, Lloyd JM, Pandor A, Holmes M, Ara R, et al. A systemic review and economic evaluation of statins for the prevention of coronary events. Health Technol Assess. 2007; 11: 1-160, iii-iv.

[37] Arca M. Ateovastatin efficacy in the prevention of cardiovascular events in patients with diabetes mellitus and/or metabolic syndrome. Drugs 2007; 67 Suppl 1: 43-54.

[38] Newman CB, Szarek M, Colhiun HM, Betteridge DJ, et al. The safety and tolerability of atorvastatin 10 mg in the Collaborative Atorvastatin Diabetes Study (CASRDS). Diab Vasc Dis Res. 2008; 5: 177-183. doi: 10.3132/dvdr.2008.029.

[39] Sever PS, Chang CL, Gupta AK, Whitehouse A, Poulter NR; ASCOT Investigators. The Anglo-Scandinavian Cardiac Outcomes Trial: 11-year mortality follow-up of the lipid-lowering arm in the U.K. Eur Heart J. 201; 32: 2525-2532. doi: 10.1093/eurheartj/ehr333.

[40] Chapman N, Chang CL, Caulfield M, Dahlöf B, Feder G, Sever PS, Poulter NR. Ethnic variations in lipid-lowering in response to a statin (EVIREST): a substudy of the Anglo-Scandinavian Cardiac Outcomes Trial (ASCOT). Ethn Dis. 2011; 21: 150-157.

[41] Heart Protection Study Collaborative Group, Bulbulia R, Bowman L, Wallendszus K, Parish S, et al. Effects on 11-year mortality and morbidity of lowering LDL cholesterol with simvastatin for about 5 years in 20,536 high-risk individuals: a randomised controlled trial. Lancet. 2011; 378: 2013-2020. doi: 10.1016/S0140-6736(11)61125-2.

[42] Arsenault BJ, Boekholdt SM, Hovingh GK, Hyde CL, et al. TNT and IDEAL Investigators.The 719Arg variant of KIF6 and cardiovascular outcomes in statin-treated, stable coronary patients of the treating to new targets and incremental decrease in end points through aggressive lipid-lowering prospective studies. Circ Cardiovasc Genet. 2012; 5: 51-57. doi: 10.1161/CIRCGENETICS.111.960252.

[43] Bangalore S, Fayyad R, Hovingh GK, Laskey R, et al. Treating to New Targets Steering Committee and Investigators. Statin and the risk of renal-related serious adverse events: Analysis from the IDEAL, TNT, CARDS, ASPEN, SPARCL, and other placebo-controlled trials. Cardiol. 2014; 113: 2018-2020. doi: 10.1016/j.amjcard.2014.03.046.

[44] Arsenault BJ, Boekholdt SM, Mora S, DeMicco DA, et al. Impact of high-dose atorvastatin therapy and clinical risk factors on incident aortic valve stenosis in patients with cardiovascular disease (from TNT, IDEAL, and SPARCL). Am J Cardiol. 2014; 113:1378-1382. doi: 10.1016/j.amjcard.2014.01.414.

[45] Athyros VG, Tziomalos K, Gossios TD, Griva T, et al. GREACE Study Collaborative Group. Safety and efficacy of long-term statin treatment for cardiovascular events in patients with coronary heart disease and abnormal liver tests in the Greek Atorvastatin and Coronary Heart Disease Evaluation (GREACE) Study: a post-hoc analysis. Lancet. 2010; 376: 1916-1922. doi: 10.1016/S0140-6736(10)61272-X.

[46] Athyros VG, Kakafika AI, Papageorgiou AA, Paraskevas KI, et al. Effects of statin treatment in men and women with stable coronary heart disease: a subgroup analysis of the GREACE Study. Curr Med Res Opin. 2008; 24:1593-1599. doi: 10.1185/03007990802069563.

[47] Athyros VG, Kakafika AI, Papageorgiou AA, Pagourelias ED, et al. Statin-Induced Increase in HDL-C and Renal Function in Coronary Heart Disease Patients. Open Cardiovasc Med J. 2007; 1: 8-14. doi: 10.2174/1874192400701010008.

[48] Athyros VG, Katsiki N, Tziomalos K, Gossios TD, et al. GREACE Study Collaborative Group. Statins and cardiovascular outcomes in elderly and younger patients with coronary artery disease: a post hoc analysis of the GREACE study. Arch Med Sci. 2013; 9: 418-426. doi: 10.5114/aoms.2013.35424.

[49] Ong KL, Waters DD, Messig M, DeMicco DA, Rye KA, Barter PJ. Effect of change in body weight on incident diabetes mellitus in patients with stable coronary artery dis-

ease treated with atorvastatin (from the treating to new targets study). Am J Cardiol. 2014; 113: 1593-1598. doi: 10.1016/j.amjcard.2014.02.011.

[50] LaRosa JC, Deedwania PC, Shepherd J, Wenger NK, Greten H, DeMicco DA, Breazna A; TNT Investigators. Comparison of 80 versus 10 mg of atorvastatin on occurrence of cardiovascular events after the first event (from the Treating to New Targets [TNT] trial). Am J Cardiol. 2010; 105: 283-287. doi: 10.1016/j.amjcard.2009.09.025.

[51] Ho JE, Waters DD, Kean A, Wilson DJ, Demicco DA, Breazna A, Wun CC, Deedwania PC, Khush KK. TNT Investigators. Relation of improvement in estimated glomerular filtration rate with atorvastatin to reductions in hospitalizations for heart failure (from the Treating to New Targets [TNT] study). Am J Cardiol. 2012; 109:1761-1766. doi: 10.1016/j.amjcard.2012.02.019.

[52] Deedwania P, Barter P, Carmena R, Fruchart JC, et al. Treating to New Targets Investigators. Reduction of low-density lipoprotein cholesterol in patients with coronary heart disease and metabolic syndrome: analysis of the Treating to New Targets study. Lancet. 2006 Sep 9;368(9539):919-28.

[53] Arca M. Atorvastatin efficacy in the prevention of cardiovascular events in patients with diabetes mellitus and/or metabolic syndrome. Drugs. 2007;67 Suppl 1:43-54

[54] Gibson CM, Pride YB, Hochberg CP, Sloan S, Sabatine MS, Cannon CP; TIMI Study Group. Effect of intensive statin therapy on clinical outcomes among patients undergoing percutaneous coronary intervention for acute coronary syndrome. PCI-PROVE IT: A PROVE IT-TIMI 22 (Pravastatin or Atorvastatin Evaluation and Infection Therapy-Thrombolysis In Myocardial Infarction 22) Substudy. J Am Coll Cardiol. 2009; 54: 2290-22955. doi: 10.1016/j.jacc.2009.09.010.

[55] Murphy SA, Cannon CP, Wiviott SD, McCabe CH, Braunwald E. Reduction in recurrent cardiovascular events with intensive lipid-lowering statin therapy compared with moderate lipid-lowering statin therapy after acute coronary syndromes from the PROVE IT-TIMI 22 (Pravastatin or Atorvastatin Evaluation and Infection Therapy-Thrombolysis In Myocardial Infarction 22) trial. J Am Coll Cardiol. 2009; 54: 2358-2362. doi: 10.1016/j.jacc.2009.10.005.

[56] sley WL1; PROVE-IT-TIMI 22. What did PROVE-IT prove?. Diabetes Technol Ther. 2004 Dec;6(6):864-867.

[57] Pedersen TR, Cater NB, Faergeman O, Kastelein JJ, et al. Comparison of atorvastatin 80 mg/day versus simvastatin 20 to 40 mg/day on frequency of cardiovascular events late (five years) after acute myocardial infarction (from the Incremental Decrease in End Points through Aggressive Lipid Lowering [IDEAL] trial). Am J Cardiol. 2010; 106: 354-359. doi: 10.1016/j.amjcard.2010.03.033.

[58] Knopp RH, d'Emden M, Smilde JG, Pocock SJ. Efficacy and safety of atorvastatin in the prevention of cardiovascular end points in subjects with type 2 diabetes: the

Atorvastatin Study for Prevention of Coronary Heart Disease Endpoints in non-insulin-dependent diabetes mellitus (ASPEN). Diabetes Care. 2006; 29:1478-1485.

[59] Isaacsohn JL, Davidson MH, Hunninghake D, Singer R, McLain R, Black DM. Aggressive Lipid-Lowering Initiation Abates New Cardiac Events (ALLIANCE)-rationale and design of atorvastatin versus usual care in hypercholesterolemic patients with coronary artery disease. Am J Cardiol. 2000; 86: 250-252.

[60] Koren MJ. Statin use in a "real-world" clinical setting: aggressive lipid lowering compared with usual care in the Aggressive Lipid-Lowering Initiation Abates New Cardiac Events (ALLIANCE) trial. Am J Med. 2005; 118 Suppl 12A: 16-21.

[61] Koren MJ, Davidson MH, Wilson DJ, Fayyad RS, Zuckerman A, Reed DP; ALLIANCE Investigators. Focused atorvastatin therapy in managed-care patients with coronary heart disease and CKD. Am J Kidney Dis. 2009; 53: 741-750. doi: 10.1053/j.ajkd.2008.11.025.

[62] Mikhailidis DP, Wierzbicki AS. The GREek Atorvastatin and Coronary-heart-disease Evaluation (GREACE) study. Curr Med Res Opin. 2002; 18: 215-219.

[63] Athyros VG, Mikhailidis DP, Papageorgiou AA, Bouloukos VI, et al. Effect of statins and aspirin alone and in combination on clinical outcome in dyslipidaemic patients with coronary heart disease. A subgroup analysis of the GREACE study. Platelets. 2005; 16: 65-71.

[64] Kinlay S, Schwartz GG, Olsson AG, Rifai N, Bao W, Libby P, Ganz P; Myocardial Ischemia Reduction with Aggressive Cholesterol Lowering (MIRACL) Study Investigators. Endogenous tissue plasminogen activator and risk of recurrent cardiac events after an acute coronary syndrome in the MIRACL study. Atherosclerosis. 2009; 206: 551-555. doi: 10.1016/j.atherosclerosis.2009.03.020.

[65] Zamani P, Schwartz GG, Olsson AG, Rifai N, Bao W, Libby P, Ganz P, Kinlay S; Myocardial Ischemia Reduction with Aggressive Cholesterol Lowering (MIRACL) Study Investigators. Inflammatory biomarkers, death, and recurrent nonfatal coronary events after an acute coronary syndrome in the MIRACL study. J Am Heart Assoc. 2013; 2: e003103. doi: 10.1161/JAHA.112.003103.

[66] Arca M, Gaspardone A. Atorvastatin efficacy in the primary and secondary prevention of cardiovascular events. Drugs. 2007;67 Suppl 1:29-42.

[67] Athyros VG, Karagiannis A, Ganotakis ES, Paletas K, et al. Assessing The Treatment Effect in Metabolic syndrome without Perceptible diabetes (ATTEMPT) Collaborative Group. Curr Med Res Opin. 2011; 27: 1659-1668. doi: 10.1185/03007995.2011.595782.

[68] Plosker GL, Lyseng-Williamson KA. Atrovastatin. a pharmacoeconomic review of its use in the primary and secondary prevention of cardiovascular events. Pharmacoeconomics. 2007; 25: 1031-1053.

[69] Hawa MI, Buchan AP, Ola T, Wun CC, et al. LADA and CARDS: a prospective study of clinical outcome in established adult-onset autoimmune diabetes. Diabetes Care. 2014; 37: 1643-1649. doi: 10.2337/dc13-2383.

[70] olse H, Sternhufvud C, Andy Schuetz C, Rengarajan B, Gandhi S. Impact of switching treatment from rosuvastatin to atorvastatin on rates of cardiovascular events. Clin Ther. 2014; 36: 58-69. doi: 10.1016/j.clinthera.2013.12.003.

[71] Amarenco P, Callahan A 3rd, Campese VM, Goldstein LB, et al. Effect of High-Dose Atorvastatin on Renal Function in Subjects With Stroke or Transient Ischemic Attack in the SPARCL Trial. Stroke. 2014; 45: 2974-82. doi: 10.1161/STROKEAHA.114.005832.

[72] arma A, Cannon CP, de Lemos J, Rouleau JL, et al. The incidence of kidney injury for patients treated with a high-potency versus moderate-potency statin regimen after an acute coronary syndrome. J Am Heart Assoc. 2014; 3: e000784. doi: 10.1161/JAHA. 114.000784.

[73] Mullins CD, Rattinger GB, Kuznik A, Koren MJ. Cost-effectiveness of intensive atorvastatin treatment in high-risk patients compared with usual care in a postgeneric statin market: economic analysis of the Aggressive Lipid-lowering Initiation Abates New Cardiac Events (ALLIANCE) study. Clin Ther. 2008;30 Pt 2:2204-16. doi: 10.1016/j.clinthera.2008.12.007.

[74] Annemans L, Marbaix S, Webb K, Van Gaal L, Scheen A. Cost effectiveness of atrovastatin in patients in type 2 diabetes mellitus: a pharmacoeconomic analysis of the collaborative atrovastatin diabetes study in the Belgian population. Clin Drug Investig. 2010; 30: 133-142. Doi: 10.2165/1153910-000000000-00000.

[75] Bener A, Dogan M, Barakat L, Al-Hamag AO. Comparison of cost-effectiveness, safety, and efficacy of rosuvastatin versus atrvastatin, pravastatin, and simbastatin in dyslipidemic diabetic patients with or without metabolic syndrome. J Prim Care Community Health. 2014; 11: 180-187.

[76] Parthan A, Leahy KJ, O'Sullivan AK, Iakoubova OA, et al. Cost effectiveness of targeted high-atorvastatin therapy following genotype testing in patients with acute coronary syndrome. Pharmacoeconomics. 2013; 31: 519-531. doi: 10.1007/s40273-013-0054-5.

[77] Silva MA, Swanson AC, Gandhi PJ, Tataronis GR. Statin-related adverse events: a meta-analysis. Clin Ther. 2006; 28: 26-35.

[78] Jukema JW, Cannon CP, de Craen AJ, Westendorp RG, Trompet S. The controversies of statin therapy: weighing the evidence. J Am Coll Cardiol. 2012; 40: 875-881. doi: 10.1016/j.jacc.2012.07.007.

[79] Sondermeijer BM, Boekholdt SM, Rana JS, Kastelein JJ, Wareham NJ, Khaw KT. Clinical implications of JUPITER in a contemporary European population: the EPIC-Nor-

folk prospective population study. Eur Heart J. 2013; 34: 1350-1357. doi: 10.1093/eurheartj/eht047.

[80] Teng JF, Gomes T, Camacho X, Grundy S, Juurlink DN, Mamdani MM. Impact of the JUPITER trial on statin prescribing for primary prevention. Pharmacotherapy. 2014; 34:9-18. doi: 10.1002/phar.1340.

[81] Khera AV, Everett BM, Caulfield MP, Hantash FM, Wohlgemuth J, Ridker PM, Mora S. Lipoprotein(a) concentrations, rosuvastatin therapy, and residual vascular risk: an analysis from the JUPITER Trial (Justification for the Use of Statins in Prevention: an Intervention Trial Evaluating Rosuvastatin). Circulation. 2014; 129: 635-642. doi: 10.1161/CIRCULATIONAHA.113.004406.

[82] Rajpathak SN, Kumbhani DJ, Crandall J, Brazilai N, Alderman M, Ridker PM. Statin therapy and risk of developing type 2 diabetes: a meta-analysis. Diabetes Care. 2009; 32: 1924-1929. doi: 10.2337/dc09-0738.

[83] Sampson UK, Linton MF, Fazio S. Are statins diabetogenic? Curr Opin Cardiol. 2011; 26: 342-347. doi: 10.1097/HCO.0b013e3283470359.

[84] Waters DD, Ho JE, DeMicco DA, Breazna A, Arsenault BJ, Wun CC, Kastelein JJ, Colhoun H, Barter P. Predictors of new-onset diabetes in patients treated with atorvastatin: results from 3 large randomized clinical trials. J Am Coll Cardiol. 2011; 57: 1535-1545. doi: 10.1016/j.jacc.2010.10.047

[85] Athyros VG, Elisaf MS, Alexandrides T, Achimastos A, et al. Assessing the Treatment Effect in Metabolic Syndrome Without Perceptible Diabetes (ATTEMP) Collaborative Group. Long-term impact of multifactorial treatment on new-onset diabetes and related cardiovascular events in metabolic syndrome: a post-hoc ATTEMPT analysis. Angiology. 2012; 63: 358-366. doi: 10.1177/0003319711421341.

[86] Muscoqiuri G, Sarno G, Gastaldelli A, Savastano S, Ascione A, et al. The good and bad effects of statins on insulin sensitivity and secretion. Endocr Res. 2014; 30: 137-143. doi: 10.3109/07435800.2014.952018.

[87] Simic I, Reiner Z. Adverse effects of statins-Myths and reality.Curr Pharm Des. 2014 Oct 13. [Epub ahead of print].

[88] Vidt DG, Ridker PM, Monyak JT, Schreiber MJ, Cressman MD. Longitudinal assessment of estimated glomerular filtration rate in apparently healthy adults: a posy hoc analysis from the JUPITER study (justification for the use of statins in prevention: an intervention trial evaluating rosuvastatin. Clin Ther. 2011; 33: 717-725. doi: 10.1016/.clinthera.2011.05.004.

Chapter 11

Incretin System in the Pathogenesis of Type 2 Diabetes and the Role of Incretin Based Therapies in the Management of Type 2 Diabetes

Ayse Nur Torun and Derun Taner Ertugrul

Additional information is available at the end of the chapter

http://dx.doi.org/10.5772/59241

1. Introduction

Discovery of incretin hormones and their role on glucose metabolism and pathogenesis of type 2 diabetes mellitus (T2 DM) are current interests of diabetology. Incretin hormones are secreted from intestinal endocrine cells in response to food ingestion and potentiate pancreatic insulin secretion when compared with iv glucose administration. Since malfunction of incretin hormones has been found to have role in T2 DM pathogenesis, incretin based therapies have been developed. Incretin effect, incretine hormones, functions, their role in pathogenesis of T2 DM and management of T2 DM with incretin-based drugs are discussed in this chapter.

2. Incretin effect, incretin hormones, secretion and functions

2.1. The incretin effect

Pancreas secrete insulin in response to the food content in the gastrointestinal lumen. Endocrine pancreas senses food ingestion via incretin hormones, nerve inputs and substrates to secrete insulin. This chain of secretion which starts with food ingestion and result with insulin secretion by endocrine pancreas is called enteroinsulinar axis [1, 2]. The first definition of incretin effect depend on the fact that, much more insulin secretion is induced by oral glucose than with iv glucose administration. So two-to three fold augmented insulin response to oral glucose compared with iv glucose is known as the incretin effect [3].

A duodenal exctract has been found to reduce glucosuria first in early 20th century before the discovery of this phenomenon. The elements of the incretin effect were recognised much more before their insulinotropic effects. Glucagon like insulinotropic peptide (GIP) is the first, which was discovered in 1973 by its inhibitory effect on gastric acid secretion and insulinotropic effect was defined later. This discovery was followed by the definiton of another intestinal peptide called glucagon like peptide 1 (GLP-1) ten years later. Discovery of incretin system, and its pathogenetic role in T2 DM caused an important evolution in pathogenesis and management of diabetes. This discovery pointed the role of gastrointestinal system and derived peptides on insulin secretion and glucose metabolism, which has not been taken into account for a very long time.

Postprandial rate of insulin secretion is assumed to be solely affected by the stimulatory effect of incretin hormones, and the role of gastrointestinal motility seems not to be accounted. Passage rate of the ingested foods through the gastrointestinal tract directly affects the secretion rate, secretion amount and the type of incretin hormone [4-6]. These mentioned gastrointestinal motility dependent events play an important role on postprandial glucose homeostasis. Effect of gastrointestinal motor function on glucose metabolism, pathogenesis of diabetes and glycemic regulation still need to be further evaluated.

2.2. Incretin hormones

There are two incretin hormones known to function on postprandial insulin secretion, which called GIP and GLP-1. Their malfunction and malsecretion have been shown to have role in the pathogenesis of T2 DM.

GIP is a large peptide hormone which is processed from a larger prohormone. Expression of GIP is widely distributed in the body, but the functions are not well understood at these locations. GIP is secreted from enteroendocrine, so called K cells, which predominantly located in the proximal duodenal mucosa but may be seen anywhere in the entire intestinal mucosa [7].

The other incretine hormone GLP-1 is derived from proglucagon peptide. Proglucagon gene is dominantly expressed in pancreatic alpha cells, brain stem and distal intestinal mucosal endocrine, so called L cells [8]. Posttranslational processing of proglucagon peptide differ between pancreatic alpha, brain and intestinal cells, resulting with different endproducts [9-10]. Proglucagon peptide contains two proglucagon peptides named glicentin and major proglucagon fragment. Pancreas contains these two proglucagon peptides in one molecule and secrete glucagon along with major proglukagon fragment. Pancreas processes glicentin to glicentin related pancreatic polypeptide (GRPP), glucagon, and intervening peptide 1 (IP-1), while major proglucagon fragment is not further processed in pancreas. Intestinal L cells secrete these two glucagon like peptide seperately. Unlike alpha cells, intestinal cells have the ability to process major proglucagon fragment to GLP-1, GLP-2 and IP-2. Glicentin is not cleaved or partly cleaved into GRPP and oxyntomodulin in the intestinal cells [Figure 1].

Mechanism of organ spesific posttranslational progulcagon processing is not fully determined. Several factors have been defined to have role in organ spesific processing. Transcription factor named pax6 and the other novel regulator is β-catenin, which is the major effector in Wnt signalisation system are among these regulators. T cell factor 4 (TCF-4 or known as TCF7L2) has been discovered to mediate the Wnt pathway, and shown to induce proglucagon gene

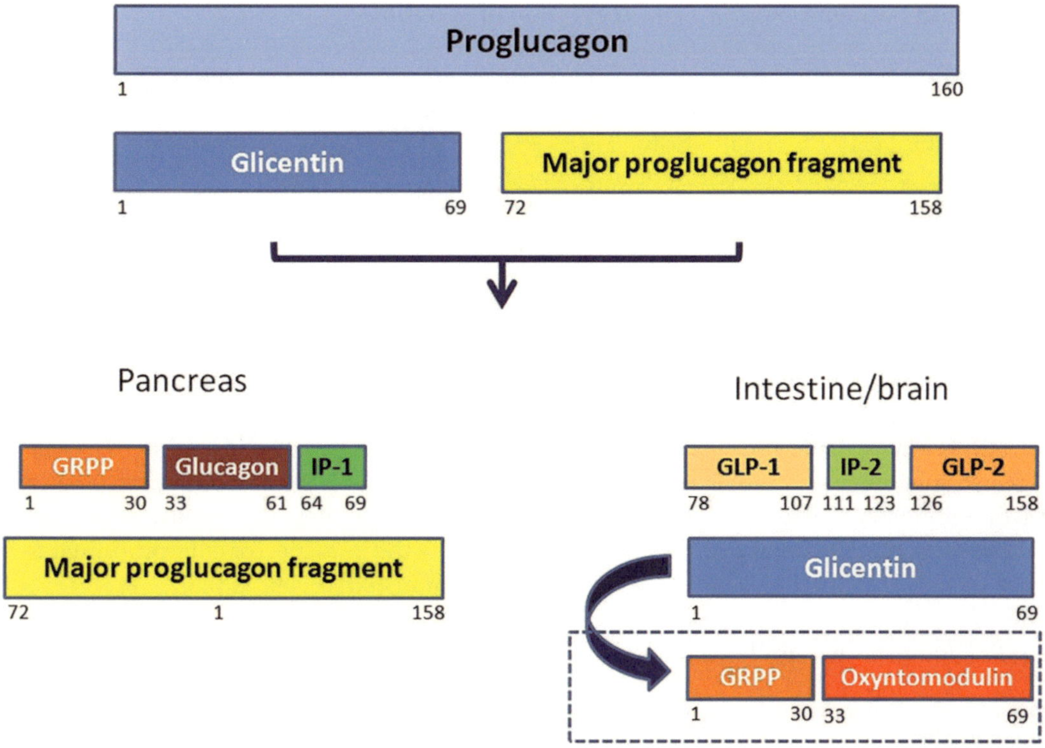

Figure 1. Post-translational processing of proglucagon peptide in pancreas, intestine and brain (GRPP: Glicentin related polypeptide, IP-1: intervening peptide 1).

expression to produce GLP-1 in the intestinal endocrine cells, but not in alpha cells [11, 12]. Later a TCF-4 gene polymorphism has been found to be involved in susceptibity to T2 DM. This is an important evidence which proved a link between disrupted incretin effect and development of T2 DM.

Active forms of GLP-1 are GLP-1 (7-36) and GLP-1 (7-37). Lower than %25 of total amount of active form secretion leaves intestine, then 40-50% of this degraded in the liver. In conclusion a very low amount of active GLP-1 reaches into the systemic circulation [13, 14]. GLP-1 (7-36) is cleaved by dipeptidylpeptidase 4 (DPP-4) to GLP-1 (9-36). This enzyme is highly expressed in the brush border of the enterocytes and also in the endothelial cells of the enteric vasculature [15]. Inactive GLP-1 (9-36) and active GLP-1 (7-36) are also degraded by neutral endopeptidase 24.11 (NEP 24,11) to form another inactive form named GLP-1 (28-36) [16]. Although GLP-1 (9-36) and GLP-1 (28-36) are known as inactive forms, it has been shown that they may be as beneficial as their active counterparts on glucose metabolism [17, 18]. Active GLP-1 and its metabolites are cleared from kidneys [19].

Both incretin hormones has been shown to be important in food induced insulin secretion but their potency and molar secretion amounts differ. GIP is secreted into the circulation 10-fold higher amount than GLP-1, but the potency of GLP-1 exceeds GIP [20].

2.3. Incretin hormone secretion and regulation of secretion

Both incretin hormones are secreted from gastrointestinal endocrine cells response to food ingestion. Although it is very low in amount, incretins are also has been shown to secreted during fasting [21]. Proximal intestinal cells secrete GIP, while GLP-1 is secreted from distal ileal and colonic L cells. It is the amount of ingested foods and the gastric emptying rate which effect the type of incretin hormone secreted [22, 23]. For example small amounts of food and a rapid gastric emptying induce GIP secretion, while slow gastric emptying and large complex food portions induce GLP-1 secretion. The exact mechanism of how food components induce the selective secretion of incretin hormones are still not clear. Elements of glucose transport system, such as sodium glucose transporter 1 (SGLT-1) and G protein coupled long chain fatty acid receptors on L cells has been shown to mediate the pathways which induce enteric endocrine cells to secrete incretin hormones in a selective manner [24, 25]. In conclusion incretin hormone levels are very low during fasting state, they are secreted in response to ingested glucose and lipids. Food ingestion is the trigger which starts enteroinsulinar axis result with insulin secretion from pancreatic β-cells. Although neuronal pathways modulate insulin secretion, neuronal pathways do not have role in the induction of enteroinsulinar axis, since GLP-1 does not increase during cephalic phase of insulin secretion [26].

2.4. Functions of incretin hormones

The incretin GIP shows its actions via a G protein coupled membrane receptor which belongs to the secretin-glucagon receptor family [27, 28]. The other incretin GLP-1 also shows its effects on target cells via a G protein coupled GLP-1 receptor (GLP-1R), which is widely expressed in the body unlike limited secretion sites of GLP-1 [29]. Only one type GLP-1R has been defined in the body, and the organ spesific effects of GLP-1 is believed to be determined by the difference in the glycosilation of the receptor. Wide distribution of the receptor such as endocrine pancreas, brain, heart, gastrointestinal system and kidney, is responsible for the extrapancreatic and extraintestinal effects of the peptide.

Because GIP has been reported to be nearly not affected in diabetic patients, and there is a clear evidence of diminished GLP-1 secretion in T2 DM, this chapter will mention GLP-1 as a representative of incretine hormones [30, 31].

1. **Effects of GLP-1 on β-cells:**

   It has been shown that GLP-1 has insulinomimetic, insulinotropic and insulinotrophic effects, which mean insulin-like, insulin secretory and regenerative and proliferative effects respectively.

   Insulin-like effect of GLP-1 has been shown in several studies, in which GLP-1 inhbibited hepatic glucose output [32, 33]. The mechanisms of inhibition of hepatic glucose output and involving receptors need to be clarified, since hepatocytes do not express GLP-1R.

   Insulin secretion is potentiated by GLP-1 only in the presence of glucose. This effect starts with the interaction between the GLP-1 and its G protein coupled membrane receptor. GLP-1 induces insulin secretion only in the presence of glucose in the β-cell [34]. GLP-1 and glucose both increase intracellular cAMP levels sinergistically, then cAMP induces protein kinase A (PKA) and cAMP regulated guanine nucleotide exchange factor II (cAMP-GEF II), also known as Epac2. These two system induce β-cells to secrete insulin by several mechanisms. Closure of ATP sensitive potassium channel and activation of calcium channels both cause depolarisation of β-cell, and then insulin secretion occurs. Both calcium derived from intracellular stores and extracellular space contribute in increase in intracellular calcium levels. Increase in intracellular calcium further stimulate insulin secretion via granule exocytosis. The latter calcium dependent insulin secretion may contribute to >70 % of overall GLP-1 induced insulin secretion. Induction of insulin secretion is not the only effect of GLP-1 on β-cells. Insulin gene promoter region which is mediated with PKA and possibly mitogen activated protein (MAP) kinase pathway are also modulated by GLP-1 [35]. Pancreatic duodenal homeobox-1 (PDX-1), which is a key regulator of developing pancreas, and essential for β-cell growth and insulin gene transcription in adulthood, has been shown to be regulated by GLP-1 [36]. Intracellular glucose concentration depends on the function of glucose transporter system, predominantly GLUT-2, and β-cells sense the presence of high glucose levels by the action of the enzyme glucokinase. These two effectors modulate insulin secretion and GLP-1 upregulates the transcription of glucose transporter and glucokinase genes [37].

Research on carcinogenesis and embryogenesis revealed an important intracellular signaling pathway named wnt. Insulinotropic, pancreatic and extrapanceratic insulinomimetic effects of GLP-1 and possibly its metabolites, has shown to be mediated by the activation of wnt pathway. Role of GLP-1 metabolites and GLP-1R in the induction of wnt pathway are not clear [38]. The pathway starts with a wnt ligand and LRP5/6-frizzled receptor complex interaction. The cytosolic effector of pathway is β-catenin (β-cat) and is tightly regulated by a phophorylation-destruction complex. This complex is formed by glycogene synthase kinase 3β (GSK-3β), casein kinase 1 (CK-1), axin/conductin, adenomatosis poliposis coli (APC), and phosphorylated extracellular signal-regulated kinase (pERK) [Figure 2]. When the receptor complex is stimulated by a wnt ligand, phosphorylation complex which stimulate the degredation of β-cat by phosphorylation is disrupted. So β-cat escapes from phosphorylation and remains free. Free β-cat then enter to the nucleus and make complex with nuclear coactivator transcription factor named TCF-7. This β-cat-TCF-7 complex induce the target gene expression. Effector β-cat is degraded due to phosphorylation when the receptor is not stimulated. TCF-7 remain free when β-cat does not reach into the nucleus and free TCF-7 regulates the repression of target genes. The most attractive function of GLP-1 is its insulinotrophic effect, which means a regenerative effect on β-cells and progenitor cells of pancreas [39]. Regeneration of β-cells is maintained by stimulation of β-cell proliferation and differentiation of ductal epithelial progenitor cells into β-cells by GLP-1 [40-44]. GLP-1 increases free β-cat in β-cells, which then induce wnt pathway to show its insulinotrophic effects and decreasing glucotoxicity on β-cells. Anti-apoptotic effect of GLP-1 on β-cells has been currently defined and may be a promising cure for diabetes [45]. Oxidative stress, which play role in β-cell death is another possible target of GLP-1. Thioredoxin (TRX), the thiol oxidoreductase is an important intracellular anti-oxidant. The function of TRX is downregulated by a binding protein, called TRX binding protein-2 (TBP-2). This binding protein has been shown to induce β-cell apoptosis, by increasing intracellular oxidative stress. Intracellular levels of TBP-2 closely correlate with blood glucose level [46, 47]. Several studies have found that GLP-1 decreases TBP-2 levels, which in turn increases intracellular TRX and decreases oxidative stress, and further β-cell damage [47, 48].

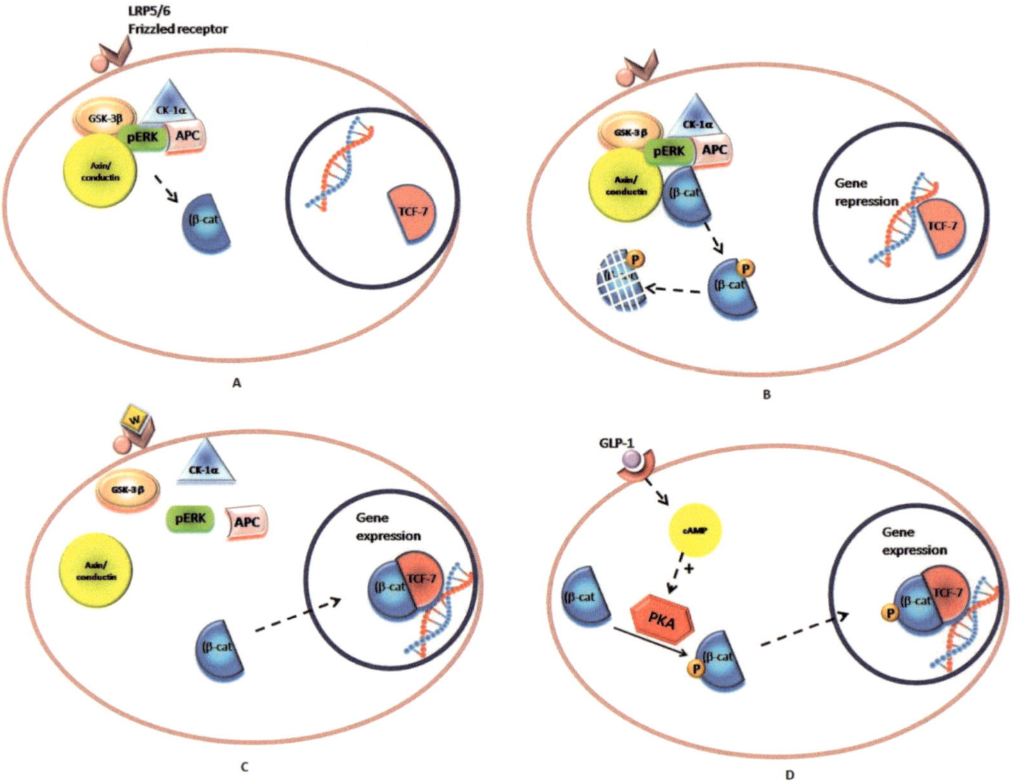

Figure 2. The wnt pathway and the role of GLP-1 on wnt pathway (APC:adenomatosis polyposis coli, CK-1: casein kinase 1, pERK: phosphorylated extracellular signal-regulated kinase, GSK-3β: glycogene synthase kinase 3β, β-cat:beta catenin, TCF-7: T cell like factor 7) (A and B: Inactive wnt pathway, C: Activation of wnt pathway by a wnt ligand, D: Activation of wnt pathway by GLP-1).

2. **Effects of GLP-1 on alpha cells**:

Glucagon plays an important role in pathogenesis of T2 DM. Glucagon hypersecretion has been shown during both fasting and postprandial states in patients with diabetes [49]. GLP-1 decrease glucagon secretion. The exact mechanism of this inhibition is not yet elucidated, but the most possible mechanism is the induction of pancreatic somatostatin secretion, which inhibit the glucagon secretion by paracrine manner [50, 51].

3. **Effects of GLP-1 on gastrointestinal system**:

   Gastrointestinal system has a central role in nutrient metabolism with its absorption and endocrine functions. GLP-1 inhibits gastrointestinal system motility, gastrin induced gastric acid and exocrine pancreatic secretions, which lead to a physiological malabsorption state [52, 53]. This malabsorbtive state contributes to alleviation of postprandial glucose excursions in diabetic patients.

4. **Effects of GLP-1 on central nervous system and satiety**:

   Low levels of GLP-1 in the systemic circulation may not reach to the central nervous system, but it has been shown that GLP-1 mediated vagal stimulation may play role in decreased gastrointestinal motility. The effect of GLP-1 on vagal afferent sensorial neurons may be a local effect, which in turn these afferent neurons transmit the inputs to solitary tract nucleus, then inhibit the gastrointestinal motility [54, 55]. GLP-1 decreases food intake by inducing satiety. Hypotalamic satiety centers, predominantly arcuate nucleus has been shown to express GLP-1 receptors. But the exact mechanism of how peripheral GLP-1 stimulate these central receptors is not yet elucidated.

5. **Pleitropic effects of GLP-1**

   Nontraditional (pleitropic) effects of GLP-1 and its metabolites is an evolving area of research. Wide expression of GLP-1R mediate the widespread action of the peptide. Insulin like effects of GLP-1 has been shown in heart and vasculature. Since cardiovascular diseases are the major contributor of mortality and morbidity in patients with T2 DM, scientific concerns about cardiovascular effects of GLP-1 and based therapies are growing. Preclinical and clinical studies revealed several cardioprotective effects of GLP-1. There are two possible mechanism of action of GLP-1 on cardivascular system, one via GLP-1R, and the other one is receptor-independent [56]. Preliminary cinical studies show that GLP-1 decreases post-ischemic left ventricular dysfunction in patients with coronary heart disease [57, 58].

   Invitro studies revealed that GLP-1 improves endothelial dysfunction via decreasing TNF-α, PAI-1 and cellular adhesion molecules [59]. But these observations need to be suggested by clinical studies.

   A study with an insulin resistant patient population showed that GLP-1 increases renal sodium and fluid excretion, which is oppose to the mechanism of hypertension in T2 DM [60]. This finding raise the possible blood pressure lowering and renoprotective effect of GLP-1 and based thearpies. Improved endothelial function and anti-oxidant effects of GLP-1 may be another contributory effect in their renoprotective action.

   Favorable effects on lipids is another important metabolic action of GLP-1. Preliminary studies reveal that GLP-1 decreases triglyceride, apo B-48 and cholesterol levels [61].

   GLP-1 is proposed to be a new therapeutic option for neurodegenerative diseases with its neuroprotective effects which has been shown in animal studies [62].

3. Contribution of incretin system in the pathogenesis of diabetes

Diabetes is the state of compromised insulin secretion which resulted with hyperglycemia. Incretin effect is reduced or almost absent in T2 DM [63]. Although the secretion of GIP is nearly normal, its insulinotropic effect has been shown to be lost in T2 DM [27]. Secretion of GLP-1 is decreased in contrast to GIP, but its favorable effects on endocrine pancreas and extrapanceratic sites are preserved in T2 DM [20, 64]. In conclusion, detoriation of both the effect and secretion of incretin hormones are involved in the pathogenesis of T2 DM. It is not clear wheter the detoriation of incretin effect is a primary defect in the pathogenesis of diabetes or not. Studies suggest that incretin hormone detoriation is a secondary defect during progression of diabetes. Another important fact is the restoration of insulin secretion with GLP-1 replacement is possible and improve hyperglycemia [65, 66].

There are several mechanisms of action of GLP-1 in T2 DM. The first one is the augmentation of glucose induced insulin secretion, resulting with improvement in hyperglycemia. Near-normal improvement in β-cell response to glucose, improvement in the first phase insulin secretion and completely normalisation of second phase insulin secretion by GLP-1 has been exactly defined [67]. Although the induction of insulin secretion is lost during chronic GLP-1 administration, glucose lowering action with maintained insulin levels tend do persist. Reduction in glucagon secretion is another mechanism of antiglycemic effect of GLP-1 [68]. Administration of GLP-1 delays gastric emptying significantly, and results with reduced postprandial glucose levels [69, 70]. The latter mechanism seems to be lost in chronic fashion. Based upon these mentioned antiglycemic effects of GLP-1, several pharmacological agents are developed for the treatment of diabetes, which will be talked about elswhere in this chapter.

4. Incretin based therapies and their role in the management of type 2 diabetes

Effects of incretin hormones on glucose metabolism and contribution of incretins in the pathogenesis of T2 DM, make these hormones ideal therapeutical targets. Decrease in apetite, reduction of body weight, improvement in insulin secretion and delay in gastric emptying are among several favorable effects of GLP-1 infusion [71]. Rapid degradation of bioactive GLP-1 by DPP-4 shortens half life, and limits anti-diabetic effects of GLP-1 [73]. Two treatment strategies has been developed to overcome this problem, first to develop DPP-4 resistant GLP-1 analogs, and the second to inhibit the degrading enzyme DPP-4. These two groups of medications will be discussed in detail.

4.1. Dipeptydyl peptidase-4 inhibitors

These oral agents are approved for treatment of diabetes whose hyperglycemia do not improve with monotherapy with sullphonylurea, tiazolidinedione and metformin or their dual combinations. They exert their effects by inhibiting the enzyme which cleaves the incretins and increase GIP and GLP-1 levels. Sitagliptin, saxagliptin, linagliptin and alogliptin are available in US, and vildagliptin is used in outside US. They have the advantage of being weight neutral and do not cause hypoglycemia except for combinations with sulphonylureas. They have been shown to be effective and safe when combined with sulphonylurea, tiazolidinedione or metformin in patients with T2 DM [73]. Usual dose of sitagliptin is 100 mg once daily, and renal dysfunction necessitate dose reduction (50 mg for patients who have glomerular filtration rate 50 mL/min and 25 mg for patients with <30 mL/min) [74]. Saxagliptin is used 2.5-5 mg once a day and the dose should be reduced to 2.5 mg for moderate renal insufficiency. It is also an effective agent in combinations like sitagliptin [75, 76]. Vildagliptin is used 50 mg twice daily in T2 DM. Dose adjustment is not necessary in mild renal insufficency, 50 mg daily dose is suggested in case of modarate and severe renal dysfunction. Linagliptin is used 5 mg daily, and it differs from other DPP-4 inhibitors with its completely hepatic elimination, which makes it possible to use in renal dysfunction. Efficacy and safety of linagliptin have been proven in monotherapy and combination studies [78-80]. Alogliptin is used 25 mg daily and dose adjustment is necessary in renal dysfunction. It has similar efficacy and safety profiles with other DPP-4 inhibitors [80].

All of the members of DPP-4 inhibitors seem to have similar efficacy, but their enzymatic affinity may be different [81, 82]. Their side effects include headache, increased risk of nasopharyngitis, urinary tract infection, and skin reactions [83]. There are reports about hepatic dysfunction with alogliptin and vildagliptin. Although the incidence of pancreatitis is not increased, a population based data suggested an increased frequency of hospitalisation for pancreatitis among sitagliptin users [84]. There is concern about whether DPP-IV inhibitors cause panceratic cancer development or not, but a causal relationship has not been established yet.

Cardiovascular safety of DPP-4 inhibitors is the matter of concern, since cardiovascular diseases are the most common cause of death in T2 DM patient population and there are several antidiabetic drugs which have been withdrawn from marketing due to their cardivascular safety problems. In a study which cardiovascular events was an endpoint, saxagliptine and metformin showed similar cardiovascular safety pattern, but patients in saxagliptin group hospitalised more frequently for heart failure when compared with metformin group [85]. Two other studies showed that neither alogliptin, nor sitagliptin have beneficial or adverse cardiovascular effects in short term use [86, 87]. Although these studies showed increased or decreased risks for cardiovascular events with DPP-4 inhibitors in short term use, their long term cardiovascular safety need to be further evaluated in long term clinical trials.

4.2. GLP-1 receptor agonists

There are two approved synthetic GLP-1R agonist molecules in the marketing. First one is Exenatide and the second one is Liraglutide. They are approved for T2 DM as an add-on drug for patients whom glycemic regulation is failed with one or two oral anti-diabetic medication [88]. Lower hypoglycemia risk is an important advantage of these molecules, which make them an excellent choice of therapy in patients whom hypoglycemia is of concern. Although they are as effective as other older anti-diabetic agents in comparison trials, data about their long term safety, effects on mortality and weight reduction is lacking [89]. Their effects on weight reduction has been proven by several studies, in which weight reducion was a secondary endpoint [90].

4.3. Exenatide

It is the synthetic analog of GLP-1, and it naturally occurs in the saliva of Gila monster (Heloderma spectum) as Exendin-4. It has 53% aminoacid homology with original GLP-1 molecule and has a long half-life beacuse of its resitance to DPP-4 mediated degradation. It is approved for T2 DM, as single or an add-on agent with other oral anti-diabetics in US. It can be combined with all of the oral anti-diabetics except for DPP-4 inhibitors.

It binds to GLP-1R and shows insulinotropic effects of GLP-1 on β-cells in the presence of glucose. It slows gastric emptying, lowers plasma glucose levels and reduces weight by inducing satiety like GLP-1 [91, 92]. Insulinotrophic effects has been shown in animal models [93, 94].

Beneficial effects on hyperglycemia, weight reduction, lipids and blood pressure has been shown with clinical trials, which has less than 30 weeks of duration [71, 95-99]. Exenatide reduces a1c levels by aproximately 1%, has lower hypoglycemia risk and hypoglycemia risk is increased with concurrent use of sulphonylurea. Exenatide causes a significant weight loss, which seems independent from its nausea inducing effect. Of note, patients experience nause lose more weight compared with patients who do not have [83, 100]. Preceding type of of drug is another important factor on weight loss during exenatide use. Patients using metformin show much more weight loss when compared with patients using sulphonylurea and tiazolidinedions [100-103].

The most common side effect of exenatide is gastrointestinal, predominantly nausea and rarely vomitting, which wane with ongoing therapy. Starting with 5 mcg and increasing the dose after one month to 10 mcg help to overcome nausea. Although risk of pancreatitis among patients who use incretin based drugs has been shown to be similar to the diabetic patients who do not use incretin based therapy, hospitalisation for acute pancreatitis may be increased [84, 104-106]. Insulinotrophic effects of GLP-1 raised concerns about the possibilty of pancreatic cancer and neuroendocrine tumor risk among patients using incretin-based therapies [107-110]. There is no data which prove or unprove these issues, so it is suggested to monitor patients for possible adverse effects affecting pancreas [111]. Although acute renal failure following exenatide use has been reported, it is difficult to prove direct relationship with exenatide use and renal failure in this patient population, which is prone to develop acute renal failure because of concurrent use of nephrotoxic drugs and underlying diabetic nephropathy [112]. Exenatide is conraindicated in severe renal impairment (creatinine clearance below 30 mL/min), and close follow up for serum creatinine is suggested when initiating therapy and after the dose titration from 5 to 10 mcg in patients with moderate renal impairment (creatinine clearance 30-50 mL/min. Gastroparesis and history of past acute pancreatitis are the other contraindications for exenatide use.

Although Exendin-4 is a GLP-1R analog, it shares a %53 homology with human GLP-1, which leads to development of anti-exendin antibody. It has been shown that anti-exenatide antibody development occur in about %40-57 of treated group [103, 113]. In one study the frequency of anti-exenatide antibody was reported to be more than %70 at the end of 24 weeks, and %40 of these antibody positive patients did not show further a1c reduction [114].. Although these mentioned studies have some limitations, ineffectiveness of exenatide due to blocking antibodies in long term use is possible.

The usual administarion schedule is starting with 5 mcg sc twice a day within 1 hours before breakfast and diner, and titration to 10 mcg twice a day 1 month later. Exenatide once weekly sc formulation is also available in US and Europe, and efficacy on hyperglycemia has been shown [115]. There are studies which compare the efficacy of daily and weekly formulations of exenatide. The improvement in a1c level seem to be better achieved with weekly formulation when compared with daily formulation, with similar body weight reduction [116, 117].

4.4. Liraglutide

Liraglutide is a GLP-1 analog which is produced by a recombinant DNA technology. Substitution of lysine at position 34 by arginine, and attachment of palmitic acid side chain to lysine group at position 26 of original GLP-1 produce liraglutide. The lipid side chain lead to formation of a non-covalent bond with albumin, which in turn slows degredation of the molecule, allowing it to be used once a day sc. Liraglutide shares 97% aminoacid homology with GLP-1.

Clinical indications are similar with exenatide. Once daily administration of 0.6 mg sc for one week reduce gastrointestinal side effects. The dose should be increased to 1.2 mg once daily for one week, and to 1.8 mg once daily if blood glucose remains above the goals [118]. Liraglutide monotherapy and comibination with one or two oral agents are efficacous in reducing blood glucose and a1c, causing significant weight reduction compared with placebo, glimepride and sitagliptin [119-121].

Nausea, vomiting and diarrhea are the most common adverse events [119]. The relationship between liraglutide use and pancreatitis is controversial. Animal studies have shown a relationship between liraglutide use and benign and malligant parafollicular C-cell tumors [122]. It may be a species specific effect and GLP-1R expression of human C-cell has been shown to be very low [122]. Short term human studies did not show any elevation in calcitonin levels with liraglutide, but this issue need further evaluation, since it takes a long time for a malligant transformation. Liraglutide is not recommended for use in patients who have medullary thyroid carcinoma or a related syndrome, or a family history of these diseases.

4.5. Is one GLP-1 receptor agonist superior to the other?

In a 26 week trial comparing the effects of liraglutide and exenatide showed a beter glycemic control with liraglutide compared with exenatide, with similar weight loss and adverse effects [123]. In another study the effects of both analogs on hyperglycemia was similar, with slightly better weight reduction in liraglutide group [124]. One potential superiority of liraglutide to exenatide may be its molecular homology to GLP-1, which is not associated with development of blocking antibodies causing drug ineffectiveness during chronic use.

Besides their beneficial effects like weight reduction and low frequency of hypoglycemia, long-term safety data, effect on diabetic macro and microvascular complications and mortality of these GLP-1R analogs are still lacking.

5. Summary

The role of comperatively older drugs such as insulin, insulin secretagogues, metformin, thiazolidinediones and alpha glucosidase inhbitors in the management of diabetes are familiar aspects of diabetes therapy. These medications target insulin secretion, insulin sensitivity and glucose absorption, which may be intrepreted as having limited targets in the pathogenesis of diabetes. Definition of incretin hormones and their role on β-cell function and survival are the new aspects of the pathogenesis of diabetes, and management of hyperglycemia. Besides the novelty of incretin based therapies in the management of diabetes, their roles on β-cell function and regeneration, which are really promising effects for an anti-diabetic agent are so interesting and need to be observed in long term clinical practice. Possible effects of these drugs that is associated with their pleitropic effects, which have been shown in invitro studies on diabetes related complications are the new era in diabetology. In our opinion the role of incretin besed therapies in the progression of diabetes and diabetic complications will be determined in the future, although fovarable or not.

Author details

Ayse Nur Torun[1*] and Derun Taner Ertugrul[2]

*Address all correspondence to: aysenurizol@yahoo.com

1 Department of Endocrinology and Metabolism, Baskent University, Medical school, Adana Research and Training Center, Adana, Turkey

2 Department of Endocrinology and Metabolism, Kecioren Research and Training Center, Ankara, Turkey

References

[1] Creutzfeldt W. Entero-insular axis and diabetes mellitus. Horm Metab Res. 1992; Suppl 26:13-18.

[2] Unger RH and Eisentraut AM. Entero-insular axis. Arch Intern Med. 1969;123: 261-5.

[3] Nauck MA, Homberger E, Siegel EG, Allen RC, Eaton RP, Ebert R, and Creutzfeldt W. Incretin effects of increasing glucose loads in man calculated from venous insulin and C-peptide responses. J Clin EndocrinolMetab. 1986;63: 492-8.

[4] Horowitz M, Edelbroek MA, Wishart JM, Straathof JV. Relationship between oral glucose tolerance and gastric emptying in normal healthy subjects. Diabetologia. 1993;36:857-62.

[5] Jones KL, Horowitz M, Carney BI, Wishart JM, Guha S, Green L. Gastric emptying in early noninsulin-dependent diabetes mellitus. Journal of Nuclear Medicine. 1996;37:1643-8.

[6] Gonlachanvit S, Hsu CW, Boden GH, Knight LC, Maurer AH, Fisher RS, et al. Effect of altering gastric emptying on postprandial plasma glucose concentrations following a physiologic meal in type-II diabetic patients. Digestive Diseases and Sciences. 2003;48:488-97.

[7] Mortensen K, Christensen LL, Holst JJ, and Orskov C. GLP-1 and GIP are colocalized in a subset of endocrine cells in the small intestine. Regul Pept. 2003;114:189-96.

[8] Mojsov S, Heinrich G, Wilson IB, Ravazzola M, Orci L, and Habener JF. Preproglucagon gene expression in pancreas and intestine diversifies at the level of post-translational processing. J Biol Chem. 1986;261:11880-9.

[9] Holst JJ, Bersani M, Johnsen AH, Kofod H, Hartmann B, Orskov C. Proglucagon processing in porcine and human pancreas. J Biol Chem. 1994;269:18827-33.

[10] Orskov C, Holst JJ, Knuhtsen S, Baldissera FG, Poulsen SS, Nielsen OV. Glucagon-like peptides GLP-1 and GLP-2, predicted products of the glucagon gene, are secreted separately from pig small intestine but not pancreas. Endocrinology. 1986;119:1467-75.

[11] Trinh DK, Zhang K, Hossain M, Brubaker PL, Drucker DJ. Pax-6 activates endogenous proglucagon gene expression in the rodent gastrointestinal epithelium. Diabetes. 2003; 52:425-33.

[12] Yi F, Brubaker PL, Jin T. TCF-4 mediates cell type-specific regulation of proglucagon gene expression by beta-catenin and glycogen synthase kinase-3. 2005;J Biol Chem. 280:1457-64.

[13] Hansen L, Hartmann B, Bisgaard T, Mineo H, Jorgensen PN, Holst JJ. Somatostatin restrains the secretion of glucagon-like peptide-1 and 2 from isolated perfused porcine ileum. Am J Physiol Endocrinol Metab. 2000;278:E1010-E1018.

[14] Deacon CF, Pridal L, Klarskov L, Olesen M, Holst JJ. Glucagon-like peptide 1 undergoes differential tissue-specific metabolism in the anesthetized pig. Am J Physiol Endocrinol Metab. 1996;271:E458-E464.

[15] Hansen L, Deacon CF, Orskov C, Holst JJ. Glucagon-like peptide-1-(7–36)amide is transformed to glucagon-like peptide-1-(9–36)amide by dipeptidyl peptidase IV in

the capillaries supplying the L cells of the porcine intestine. Endocrinology. 1999;140:5356-63.

[16] Hupe-Sodmann K, McGregor GP, Bridenbaugh R, Göke R, Göke B, Thole H, et al. Characterisation of the processing by human neutral endopeptidase 24.11 of GLP-1(7-36) amide and comparison of the substrate specificity of the enzyme for other glucagon-like peptides. Regul Pept. 1995; 58:149-56.

[17] Ban K, Kim KH, Cho CK, Sauve M, Diamandis EP, Backx PH, et al. Glucagon-like peptide (GLP)-1(9-36)amide-mediated cytoprotection is blocked by exendin(9-39) yet does not require the known GLP-1 receptor. Endocrinology. 2010;151:1520-31.

[18] Liu Z, Stanojevic V, Brindamour LJ, Habener JF. GLP1-derived nonapeptide GLP1(28-36)amide protects pancreatic β-cells from glucolipotoxicity. J Endocrinol. 2012;213:143-54.

[19] Meier JJ, Nauck MA, Kranz D, Holst JJ, Deacon CF, Gaeckler D, Schmidt WE, Gallwitz B. Secretion, degradation, elimination of glucagon-like peptide 1 and gastric inhibitory polypeptide in patients with chronic renal insufficiency and healthy control subjects. Diabetes. 2004;53:654-62.

[20] Nauck MA, Heimesaat MM, Orskov C, Holst JJ, Ebert R,Creutzfeldt W. Preserved incretin activity of glucagon-like peptide 1 [7–36 amide] but not of synthetic human gastric inhibitory polypeptide in patients with type-2 diabetes mellitus. J Clin Invest. 1993;91: 301-7.

[21] Mari A, Sallas WM, He YL, Watson C, Ligueros-Saylan M, Dunning BE, et al. Vildagliptin, a dipeptidyl peptidase-IV inhibitor, improves model-assessed –cell function in patients with type 2 diabetes. J Clin Endocrinol Metab. 2005;90:4888-94.

[22] Vilsboll T, Krarup T, Sonne J, Madsbad S, Volund A, Juul AG, Holst JJ. Incretin secretion in relation to meal size and body weight in healthy subjects and people with type 1 and type 2 diabetes mellitus. J Clin Endocrinol Metab. 2003;88: 2706-13.

[23] Miholic J, Orskov C, Holst JJ, Kotzerke J, Meyer HJ. Emptying of the gastric substitute, glucagon-like peptide-1 (GLP-1), reactive hypoglycemia after total gastrectomy. Dig Dis Sci. 1991;36:1361-70.

[24] Gribble FM, Williams L, Simpson AK, Reimann F. A novel glucose-sensing mechanism contributing to glucagon-like peptide-1 secretion from the GLUTag cell line. Diabetes. 2003;52:1147-54.

[25] Hirasawa A, Tsumaya K, Awaji T, Katsuma S, Adachi T, Yamada M, et al. Free fatty acids regulate gut incretin glucagon-like peptide-1 secretion through GPR120. Nat Med. 2005;11: 90-4.

[26] Hansen L, Lampert S, Mineo H, Holst JJ. Neural regulation of glucagon-like peptide-1 secretion in pigs. Am J Physiol Endocrinol Metab. 2004;287:E939-E947.

[27] Vilsboll T, Krarup T, Madsbad S, and Holst JJ. Defective amplification of the late phase insulin response to glucose by GIP in obese Type II diabetic patients. Diabetologia. 2002;45:1111-9.

[28] Mayo KE, Miller LJ, Bataille D, Dalle S, Goke B, Thorens B, et al. The glucagon receptor family. Pharmacol Rev. 2003;55:167-94.

[29] Wei Y, Mojsov S. Tissue-specific expression of the human receptor for glucagon-like peptide-I: brain, heart and pancreatic forms have the same deduced amino acid sequences. FEBS Lett. 1995;358:219-24.

[30] Krarup T. Immunoreactive gastric inhibitory polypeptide. Endocr Rev. 1988;9:122-34.

[31] Toft-Nielsen MB, Damholt MB, Madsbad S, Hilsted LM, Hughes TE, Michelsen BK, et al. Determinants of the impaired secretion of glucagon-like peptide-1 in type 2 diabetic patients. J Clin Endocrinol Metab. 2001;86: 3717-23.

[32] Egan JM, Meneilly GS, Habener JF, Elahi D. Glucagon-like peptide-1 augments insulin-mediated glucose uptake in the obese state. J Clin Endocrinol Metab. 2002;87:3768-73.

[33] Elahi D, Egan JM, Shannon RP, Meneilly GS, Khatri A, Habener JF, et al. GLP-1 (9-36) amide, cleavage product of GLP-1 (7-36) amide, is a glucoregulatory peptide. Obesity (Silver Spring). 2008;16:1501-9.

[34] Holst JJ, Gromada J. Role of incretin hormones in the regulation of insulin secretion in diabetic and nondiabetic humans. Am J Physiol Endocrinol Metab. 2004;287:E199-E206.

[35] Kemp DM, Habener JF. Insulinotropic hormone glucagon-like peptide 1 (GLP-1) activation of insulin gene promoter inhibited by p38 mitogen-activated protein kinase. Endocrinology. 2001;142:1179-87.

[36] Li Y, Cao X, Li LX, Brubaker PL, Edlund H, Drucker DJ. Cell Pdx1 expression is essential for the glucoregulatory, proliferative, cytoprotective actions of glucagon-like peptide-1. Diabetes.2005;54: 482-91.

[37] Buteau J, Roduit R, Susini S, Prentki M. Glucagon-like peptide-1 promotes DNA synthesis, activates phosphatidylinositol 3-kinase and increases transcription factor pancreatic and duodenal homeobox gene 1 (PDX-1) DNA binding activity in beta (INS-1)-cells. Diabetologia. 1999;42:856-64.

[38] Xiong X, Shao W, Jin T. New insight into the mechanisms unedrlying the function of the incretin hormone glucagon-like peptide-1 in pancreatic β-cells. Involvement of the Wnt signaling pathway effector β-catenin. Islets. 2012;4(6):359-65.

[39] Egan JM, Bulotta A, Hui H, Perfetti R. GLP-1 receptor agonists are growth and differentiation factors for pancreatic islet beta cells. Diabetes Metab Res Rev. 2003;19:115-23.

[40] Edvell A, Lindstrom P. Initiation of increased pancreatic islet growth in young normoglycemic mice (Umea _/?). Endocrinology. 1999;140:778-83.

[41] Farilla L, Hui H, Bertolotto C, Kang E, Bulotta A, Di MU, et al. Glucagon-like peptide-1 promotes islet cell growth and inhibits apoptosis in Zucker diabetic rats. Endocrinology. 2002;143:4397-408.

[42] Stoffers DA, Kieffer TJ, Hussain MA, Drucker DJ, Bonner-Weir S, Habener JF, et al. Insulinotropic glucagon-like peptide 1 agonists stimulate expression of homeodomain protein IDX-1 and increase islet size in mouse pancreas. Diabetes. 2000;49: 741-8.

[43] Xu G, Stoffers DA, Habener JF, Bonner-Weir S. Exendin-4 stimulates both beta-cell replication and neogenesis, resulting inincreased beta-cell mass and improved glucose tolerance in diabetic rats. Diabetes. 1999;48:2270-6.

[44] Zhou J, Wang X, Pineyro MA, Egan JM. Glucagon-like peptide 1 and exendin-4 convert pancreatic AR42J cells into glucagon-and insulin-producing cells. Diabetes. 1999;48:2358-66.

[45] Butler AE, Janson J, Bonner-Weir S, Ritzel R, Rizza RA, Butler PC. Beta-cell deficit and increased beta-cell apoptosis in humans with type 2 diabetes. Diabetes. 2003;52:102-10.

[46] Spindel ON, World C, Berk BC. Thioredoxin interacting protein: redox dependent and independent regulatory mechanisms. Antioxid Redox Signal. 2012;16:587-96.

[47] Chen J, Couto FM, Minn AH, Shalev A. Exenatide inhibits beta-cell apoptosis by decreasing thioredoxin-interacting protein. Biochem Biophys Res Commun. 2006; 346:1067-74.

[48] Chen J, Hui ST, Couto FM, Mungrue IN, Davis DB, Attie AD, et al. Thioredoxin-interacting protein deficiency induces Akt/Bcl-xL signaling and pancreatic beta-cell mass and protects against diabetes. FASEB J. 2008;22:3581-94.

[49] Shah P, Vella A, Basu A, Basu R, Schwenk WF, Rizza RA. Lack of suppression of glucagon contributes to postprandial hyperglycemia in subjects with type 2 diabetes mellitus. J Clin Endocrinol Metab. 2000;85:4053-59.

[50] Fehmann HC, Goke R, Goke B. Cell and molecular biology of the incretin hormones glucagon-like peptide-I and glucose-dependent insulin releasing polypeptide. Endocr Rev. 1995;16:390-410.

[51] De Heer J, Hoy M, Holst JJ. GLP-1, but not GIP, inhibits glucagon secretion via somatostatin in the perfused rat pancreas. Diabetologia. 2005;48 Suppl 1:A64.

[52] Nauck MA, Niedereichholz U, Ettler R, Holst JJ, Orskov C, Ritzel R, et al. Glucagon-like peptide 1 inhibition of gastric emptying outweighs its insulinotropic effects in healthy humans. Am J Physiol Endocrinol Metab. 1997;273:E981-E988.

[53] Wettergren A, Schjoldager B, Mortensen PE, Myhre J, Christiansen J, Holst JJ. Truncated GLP-1 (proglucagon 78–107-amide) inhibits gastric and pancreatic functions in man. Dig Dis Sci. 1993;38:665-73.

[54] Wettergren A, Petersen H, Orskov C, Christiansen J, Sheikh SP, Holst JJ. Glucagon-like peptide-1 7–36 amide and peptide YY from the L-cell of the ileal mucosa are potent inhibitors of vagally induced gastric acid secretion in man. Scand J Gastroenterol. 1994;29:501-5.

[55] Wettergren A, Wojdemann M, Meisner S, Stadil F, Holst JJ. The inhibitory effect of glucagon-like peptide-1 (GLP-1) 7–36 amide on gastric acid secretion in humans depends on an intact vagal innervation. Gut. 1997;40:597-601.

[56] Ban K, Noyan-Ashraf MH, Hoefer J, Bolz SS, Drucker DJ, Husain M. Cardioprotective and vasodilatory actions of glucagon-like peptide 1 receptor are mediated through both glucagon-like peptide 1 receptor-dependent and-independent pathways. Circulation. 2008;117:2340-50.

[57] Nikolaidis LA, Mankad S, Sokos GG, Miske G, Shah A, Elahi D, et al. Effects of glucagon-like peptide-1 in patients with acute myocardial infarction and left ventricular dysfunction after successful reperfusion. Circulation. 2004;109:962-5.

[58] Read PA, Khan FZ, Dutka DP. Cardioprotection against ischaemia induced by dobutamine stress using glucagonlike peptide-1 in patients with coronary artery disease. Heart. 2012;98:408-13.

[59] Liu H, Hu Y, Simpson RW, Dear AE. Glucagon-like peptide-1 attenuates tumour necrosis factor-alpha-mediated induction of plasminogen [corrected] activator inhibitor-1 expression. J Endocrinol. 2008;196:57-65.

[60] Gutzwiller JP, Tschopp S, Bock A, Zehnder CE, Huber AR, Kreyenbuehl M, et al. Glucagon-like peptide 1 induces natriuresis in healthy subjects and in insulin-resistant obese men. J Clin Endocrinol Metab. 2004;89:3055-61.

[61] Hsieh J, Longuet C, Baker CL, Qin B, Federico LM, Drucker DJ, et al. The glucagon-like peptide 1 receptor is essentialfor postprandial lipoprotein synthesis and secretion in hamsters and mice. Diabetologia. 2010;53:552-61.

[62] Perry TA, Greig NH. A new Alzheimer's disease interventive strategy: GLP-1. Curr Drug Targets. 2004;5: 565-71.

[63] Nauck M, Stockmann F, Ebert R, Creutzfeldt W. Reduced incretin effect in type 2 (non-insulin-dependent) diabetes. Diabetologia. 1986;29:46-52.

[64] Kjems LL, Holst JJ, Volund A, Madsbad S. The influence of GLP-1 on glucose-stimulated insulin secretion: effects on beta-cell sensitivity in type 2 and nondiabetic subjects. Diabetes. 2003;52 (2):380-6.

[65] Nauck MA, Holst JJ, Willms B. Glucagon-like peptide 1 and its potential in the treatment of non-insulin-dependent diabetes mellitus. Horm Metab Res. 1997;29:411-6.

[66] Toft-Nielsen MB, Madsbad S, Holst JJ. Determinants of the effectiveness of glucagon-like peptide-1 in type 2 diabetes. J Clin Endocrinol Metab. 2001;86: 3853-60.

[67] Hucking K, Kostic Z, Pox C et al. Alpha-Glucosidase inhibition (acarbose) fails to enhance secretion of glucagon-like peptide 1 (7–36 amide) and to delay gastric emptying in type 2 diabetic patients. Diabetic Medicine. 2005; 22:470-6.

[68] Nauck MA, Kleine N, Orskov C, Holst JJ, Willms B, Creutzfeldt W. Normalization of fasting hyperglycaemia by exogenous glucagon-like peptide 1 (7–36 amide) in type 2 (non-insulindependent) diabetic patients. Diabetologia. 1993; 36:741-4.

[69] Willms B, Werner J, Holst JJ, Orskov C, Creutzfeldt W, Nauck MA. Gastric emptying, glucose responses, and insulin secretion after a liquid test meal: effects of exogenous glucagon-like peptide-1 (GLP-1)-(7–36) amide in type 2 (noninsulin-dependent) diabetic patients. J Clin Endocrinol Metab. 1996;81:327-32.

[70] Kendall DM, Kim D, Maggs D. Incretin mimetics and dipeptidyl peptidase-IV inhibitors: a review of emerging therapies for type 2 diabetes. Diabetes Technol Ther. 2006;8: 385-96.

[71] Buse JB, Bergenstal RM, Glass LC, Heilmann CR, Lewis MS, Kwan AY, et al. Use of twice-daily exenatide in Basal insulin-treated patients with type 2 diabetes: a randomized, controlled trial. Ann Intern Med. 2011;154(2):103-12.

[72] Arnolds S, Dellweg S, Clair J, Dain MP, Nauck MA, Rave K, et al. Further improvement in postprandial glucose control with addition of exenatide or sitagliptin to combination therapy with insulin glargine and metformin: a proof-of-concept study. Diabetes Care. 2010;33(7):1509-15.

[73] Fonseca V, Schweizer A, Albrecht D, Baron MA, Chang I, Dejager S. Addition of vildagliptin to insulin improves glycaemic control in type 2 diabetes. Diabetologia. 2007;50(6):1148-55.

[74] Bergman AJ, Cote J, Yi B, Marbury T, Swan SK, Smith W, et al. Effect of renal insufficiency on the pharmacokinetics of sitagliptin, a dipeptidyl peptidase-4 inhibitor. Diabetes Care. 2007;30(7):1862-4.

[75] Chacra AR, Tan GH, Apanovitch A, Ravichandran S, List J, Chen R, CV181-040 Investigators. Saxagliptin added to a submaximal dose of sulphonylurea improves glycaemic control compared with uptitration of sulphonylurea in patients with type 2 diabetes: a randomised controlled trial. Int J Clin Pract. 2009;63(9):1395-406.

[76] DeFronzo RA, Hissa MN, Garber AJ, Luiz Gross J, Yuyan Duan R, Ravichandran S, et al. Saxagliptin 014 Study Group. The efficacy and safety of saxagliptin when added to metformin therapy in patients with inadequately controlled type 2 diabetes with metformin alone. Diabetes Care. 2009;32(9):1649-55.

[77] Del Prato S, Barnett AH, Huisman H, Neubacher D, Woerle HJ, Dugi KA. Effect of linagliptin monotherapy on glycaemic control and markers of β-cell function in patients with inadequately controlled type 2 diabetes: a randomized controlled trial. Diabetes Obes Metab. 2011;13(3):258-67.

[78] Forst T, Uhlig-Laske B, Ring A, Graefe-Mody U, Friedrich C, Herbach K, et al. Linagliptin (BI 1356), a potent and selective DPP-4 inhibitor, is safe and efficacious in combination with metformin in patients with inadequately controlled Type 2 diabetes. Diabet Med. 2010;27(12):1409-19.

[79] Taskinen MR, Rosenstock J, Tamminen I, Kubiak R, Patel S, Dugi KA, et al. Safety and efficacy of linagliptin as add-on therapy to metformin in patients with type 2 diabetes: a randomized, double-blind, placebo-controlled study. Diabetes Obes Metab. 2011;13(1):65-74.

[80] Seino Y, Miyata Y, Hiroi S, Hirayama M, Kaku K. Efficacy and safety of alogliptin added to metformin in Japanese patients with type 2 diabetes: a randomized, double-blind, placebo-controlled trial with an open-label, long-term extension study. Diabetes Obes Metab. 2012 Oct;14(10):927-36.

[81] Scheen AJ, Charpentier G, Ostgren CJ, Hellqvist A, Gause-Nilsson I. Efficacy and safety of saxagliptin in combination with metformin compared with sitagliptin in combination with metformin in adult patients with type 2 diabetes mellitus. Diabetes Metab Res Rev. 2010;26(7):540-9.

[82] Richter B, Bandeira-Echtler E, Bergerhoff K, Lerch CL. Dipeptidyl peptidase-4 (DPP-4) inhibitors for type 2 diabetes mellitus. Cochrane Database Syst Rev. 2008 Apr 16;(2):CD006739. doi:10.1002/14651858.CD006739.pub2.

[83] Amori RE, Lau J, Pittas AG. Efficacy and safety of incretin therapy in type 2 diabetes: systematic review and meta-analysis. JAMA. 2007;298(2):194-206.

[84] Singh S, Chang HY, Richards TM, Weiner JP, Clark JM, Segal JB. Glucagon like peptide 1-based therapies and risk of hospitalization for acute pancreatitis in type 2 diabetes mellitus: a population-based matched case-control study. JAMA Intern Med. 2013;173(7):534-9.

[85] Scirica BM, Bhatt DL, Braunwald E, Steg PG, Davidson J, Hirshberg B, et al;. SAVOR-TIMI 53 Steering Committee and Investigators. Saxagliptin and cardiovascular outcomes in patients with type 2 diabetes mellitus. N Engl J Med. 2013;369(14):1317-26.

[86] White WB, Cannon CP, Heller SR, Nissen SE, Bergenstal RM, Bakris GL, et al; EXAMINE Investigators. Alogliptin after acute coronary syndrome in patients with type 2 diabetes. N Engl J Med. 2013;369(14):1327-35.

[87] Eurich DT, Simpson S, Senthilselvan A, Asche CV, Sandhu-Minhas JK, McAlister FA. Comparative safety and effectiveness of sitagliptin in patients with type 2 diabetes: retrospective population based cohort study. BMJ. 2013;346:f2267.

[88] Riddle MC, Drucker DJ. Emerging therapies mimicking the effects of amylin and glucagon-like peptide 1. Diabetes Care. 2006;29(2):435-49.

[89] Shyangdan DS, Royle P, Clar C, Sharma P, Waugh N, Snaith A. Glucagon-like peptide analogues for type 2 diabetes mellitus. Cochrane Database Syst Rev. 2011 Oct 5;(10):CD006423

[90] Vilsboll T, Christensen M, Junker AE, Knop FK, Gluud LL. Effects of glucagon-like peptide-1 receptor agonists on weight loss: systematic review and meta-analyses of randomised controlled trials. BMJ. 2012;344:d7771

[91] Egan JM, Clocquet AR, Elahi D. The insulinotropic effect of acute exendin-4 administered to humans: comparison of nondiabetic state to type 2 diabetes. J Clin Endocrinol Metab. 2002;87(3):1282-90.

[92] Kolterman OG, Buse JB, Fineman MS, Gaines E, Heintz S, Bicsak TA, et al. Synthetic exendin-4 (exenatide) significantly reduces postprandial and fasting plasma glucose in subjects with type 2 diabetes. J Clin Endocrinol Metab. 2003;88(7):3082-9.

[93] Xu G, Stoffers DA, Habener JF, Bonner-Weir S. Exendin-4 stimulates both beta-cell replication and neogenesis, resulting in increased beta-cell mass and improved glucose tolerance in diabetic rats. Diabetes. 1999;48(12):2270-6.

[94] Stoffers DA, Desai BM, DeLeon DD, Simmons RA. Neonatal exendin-4 prevents the development of diabetes in the intrauterine growth retarded rat. Diabetes. 2003;52(3):734-40.

[95] Riddle MC, Henry RR, Poon TH, Zhang B, Mac SM, Holcombe JH, et al. Exenatide elicits sustained glycaemic control and progressive reduction of body weight in patients with type 2 diabetes inadequately controlled by sulphonylureas with or without metformin. Diabetes Metab Res Rev. 2006;22(6):483-91.

[96] Ratner RE, Maggs D, Nielsen LL, Stonehouse AH, Poon T, Zhang B, et al. Long-term effects of exenatide therapy over 82 weeks on glycaemic control and weight in overweight metformin-treated patients with type 2 diabetes mellitus. Diabetes Obes Metab. 2006;8(4):419-28.

[97] Heine RJ, Van Gaal LF, Johns D, Mihm MJ, Widel MH, Brodows RG, GWAA Study Group. Exenatide versus insulin glargine in patients with suboptimally controlled type 2 diabetes: a randomized trial. Ann Intern Med. 2005;143(8):559-69.

[98] Gallwitz B, Guzman J, Dotta F, Guerci B, Simor R, Basson BR, et al. Exenatide twice daily versus glimepiride for prevention of glycaemic deterioration in patients with type 2 diabetes with metformin failure (EUREXA): an open-label, randomised controlled trial. Lancet. 2012 Jun;379(9833):2270-8.

[99] Arnolds S, Dellweg S, Clair J, Dain MP, Nauck MA, Rave K, et al. Further improvement in postprandial glucose control with addition of exenatide or sitagliptin to com-

bination therapy with insulin glargine and metformin: a proof-of-concept study. Diabetes Care. 2010;33(7):1509-15.

[100] DeFronzo RA, Ratner RE, Han J, Kim DD, Fineman MS, Baron AD. Effects of exenatide (exendin-4) on glycemic control and weight over 30 weeks in metformin-treated patients with type 2 diabetes. Diabetes Care. 2005;28(5):1092-100.

[101] Buse JB, Henry RR, Han J, Kim DD, Fineman MS, Baron AD. Exenatide-113 Clinical Study Group. Effects of exenatide (exendin-4) on glycemic control over 30 weeks in sulfonylurea-treated patients with type 2 diabetes. Diabetes Care. 2004;27(11): 2628-35.

[102] Kendall DM, Riddle MC, Rosenstock J, Zhuang D, Kim DD, Fineman MS, et al. Effects of exenatide (exendin-4) on glycemic control over 30 weeks in patients with type 2 diabetes treated with metformin and a sulfonylurea. Diabetes Care. 2005;28(5): 1083-91.

[103] Zinman B, Hoogwerf BJ, Duran Garcia S, Milton DR, Giaconia JM, Kim DD, et al. The effect of adding exenatide to a thiazolidinedione in suboptimally controlled type 2 diabetes: a randomized trial. Ann Intern Med. 2007;146(7):477-85.

[104] Garg R, Chen W, Pendergrass M. Acute pancreatitis in type 2 diabetes treated with exenatide or sitagliptin: a retrospective observational pharmacy claims analysis. Diabetes Care. 2010;33(11):2349-54.

[105] Girman CJ, Kou TD, Cai B, Alexander CM, O'Neill EA, Williams-Herman DE, et al. Patients with type 2 diabetes mellitus have higher risk for acute pancreatitis compared with those without diabetes. Diabetes Obes Metab. 2010;12(9):766-71.

[106] Gonzalez-Perez A, Schlienger RG, Rodriguez LA. Acute pancreatitis in association with type 2 diabetes and antidiabetic drugs: a population-based cohort study. Diabetes Care. 2010;33(12):2580-5.

[107] Elashoff M, Matveyenko AV, Gier B, Elashoff R, Butler PC. Pancreatitis, pancreatic, and thyroid cancer with glucagon-like peptide-1-based therapies. Gastroenterology. 2011;141(1):150-6.

[108] Halfdanarson TR, Pannala R. Incretins and risk of neoplasia. BMJ. 2013;346:f3750.

[109] Cohen D. Has pancreatic damage from glucagon suppressing diabetes drugs been underplayed? BMJ. 2013;346:f3680.

[110] Butler AE, Campbell-Thompson M, Gurlo T, Dawson DW, Atkinson M, Butler PC. Marked expansion of exocrine and endocrine pancreas with incretin therapy in humans with increased exocrine pancreas dysplasia and the potential for glucagon-producing neuroendocrine tumors. Diabetes. 2013;62(7):2595-604.

[111] Egan AG, Blind E, Dunder K, de Graeff PA, Hummer BT, Bourcier T, et al. Pancreatic safety of incretin-based drugs--FDA and EMA assessment. N Engl J Med. 2014 Feb; 370(9):794-7.

[112] Weise WJ, Sivanandy MS, Block CA, Comi RJ. Exenatide-associated ischemic renal failure. Diabetes Care. 2009;32(2):e22-3.

[113] Gedulin BR, Smith P, Prickett KS, Tryon M, Barnhill S, Reynolds J, et al. Dose-response for glycaemic and metabolic changes 28 days after single injection of longacting release exenatide in diabetic fatty Zucker rats. Diabetologia. 2005;48:1380-5.

[114] Faludi P, Brodows R, Burger J, Ivanyi T, Braun DK. The effect of exenatide re-exposure on safety and efficacy. Peptides. 2009;30:1771-4

[115] Diamant M, Van Gaal L, Stranks S, Northrup J, Cao D, Taylor K, et al. Once weekly exenatide compared with insulin glargine titrated to target in patients with type 2 diabetes (DURATION-3): an open-label randomised trial. Lancet. 2010;375(9733): 2234-43.

[116] Drucker DJ, Buse JB, Taylor K, Kendall DM, Trautmann M, Zhuang D, et al, DURATION-1 Study Group. Exenatide once weekly versus twice daily for the treatment of type 2 diabetes: a randomised, open-label, non-inferiority study. Lancet. 2008;372(9645):1240-50.

[117] Blevins T, Pullman J, Malloy J, Yan P, Taylor K, Schulteis C, et al. DURATION-5: exenatide once weekly resulted in greater improvements in glycemic control compared with exenatide twice daily in patients with type 2 diabetes. J Clin Endocrinol Metab. 2011 May; 96(5):1301-10.

[118] lbrond B, Jakobsen G, Larsen S, Agerso H, Jensen LB, Rolan P, et al. Pharmacokinetics, pharmacodynamics, safety, and tolerability of a single-dose of NN2211, a long-acting glucagon-like peptide 1 derivative, in healthy male subjects Diabetes Care. 2002;25(8):1398-404.

[119] Garber A, Henry R, Ratner R, Garcia-Hernandez PA, Rodriguez-Pattzi H, Olvera-Alvarez I, et al. LEAD-3 (Mono) Study Group. Liraglutide versus glimepiride monotherapy for type 2 diabetes (LEAD-3 Mono): a randomised, 52-week, phase III, double-blind, parallel-treatment trial. Lancet. 2009;373(9662):473-81.

[120] Marre M, Shaw J, Brandle M, Bebakar WM, Kamaruddin NA, Strand J, et al. LEAD-1 SU study group. Liraglutide, a once-daily human GLP-1 analogue, added to a sulphonylurea over 26 weeks produces greater improvements in glycaemic and weight control compared with adding rosiglitazone or placebo in subjects with Type 2 diabetes (LEAD-1 SU). Diabet Med. 2009;26(3):268-78.

[121] Russell-Jones D, Vaag A, Schmitz O, Sethi BK, Lalic N, Antic S, et al. Liraglutide vs insulin glargine and placebo in combination with metformin and sulfonylurea therapy in type 2 diabetes mellitus (LEAD-5 met+SU): a randomised controlled trial. Lira-

glutide Effect and Action in Diabetes 5 (LEAD-5) met+SU Study Group. Diabetologia. 2009;52(10):2046-55.

[122] Bjerre Knudsen L, Madsen LW, Andersen S, Almholt K, de Boer AS, Drucker DJ, et al. Glucagon-like Peptide-1 receptor agonists activate rodent thyroid C-cells causing calcitonin release and C-cell proliferation. Endocrinology. 2010;151(4):1473-86.

[123] Buse JB, Rosenstock J, Sesti G, Schmidt WE, Montanya E, Brett JH, et al. LEAD-6 Study Group. Liraglutide once a day versus exenatide twice a day for type 2 diabetes: a 26-week randomised, parallel-group, multinational, open-label trial (LEAD-6). Lancet. 2009;374(9683):39-47.

[124] Buse JB, Nauck M, Forst T, Sheu WH, Shenouda SK, Heilmann CR, et al. Exenatide once weekly versus liraglutide once daily in patients with type 2 diabetes (DURATION-6): a randomised, open-label study. Lancet. 2013; 381(9861):117-24.

Chapter 12

Anti-Obesity Effects of Androgens, Dehydroepiandrosterone (DHEA) and Testosterone

Kazuo Kajita, Ichiro Mori, Masahiro, Takahide Ikeda,
Hiroyuki Morita and Tatsuo Ishizuka

Additional information is available at the end of the chapter

http://dx.doi.org/10.5772/59604

1. Introduction

Despite considerable research, the relationships between obesity and metabolic disorders have yet to be fully understood. Recent evidence has revealed that fat depots, rather than the volume of fat, are essential in determining systemic insulin sensitivity. Adipose tissue is classified into visceral adipose tissue, including epididymal, mesenteric and perirenal fat, and subcutaneous adipose tissue according to its anatomical location. Increases in visceral adipose tissue are considered to be linked to insulin resistance [1, 2]. Especially, mesenteric fat is postulated to relate more closely to metabolic disorders, as mesenteric fat secretes free fatty acids and other substances directly into the portal vein [3]. Although the mechanisms regulating fat distribution remain obscure, sex hormones are unquestionably one of the determinants.

Since men tend to accumulate much more visceral fat than women, androgens have been postulated to promote insulin resistance. In practice, low serum testosterone levels promote obesity. Numerous studies have demonstrated that androgen deprivation therapy (ADT) increases the risk of obesity, metabolic syndrome, type 2 diabetes and cardiovascular disease in patients with prostate cancer [4-8]. Basaria *et al*, pointed out that high fat mass, as well as low bone density and anemia, was observed in men with prostate cancer treated with ADT compared with ones treated without it. They concluded that patients receiving ADT are at enhanced risk for insulin resistance and cardiovascular disease. Katznelson *et al*, reported that percent body fat was greater in acquired hypogonadal men compared with eugonadal controls, which was improved by testosterone replacement therapy [9].

Recently, a high prevalence of hypogonadism in men with obesity, metabolic syndrome and type 2 diabetes has been recognized. Dhindsa *et al*, reported that total testosterone and free testosterone inversely relate to BMI and fat mass [10] in type 2 diabetic men. Kapoor *et al*, in a cross-sectional study of 355 type 2 diabetic subjects, found overt and borderline hypogonadism in 42%, with 42 of these men having free testosterone levels <0.255 nM [11]. Although the Framingham Heart Study concluded that sex hormone-binding globulin (SHBG), but not testosterone, is significantly associated with metabolic syndrome [12], both low SHBG and low free testosterone may contribute to low serum total testosterone level in obese and diabetic men [13]. Another issue currently of interest is whether low testosterone is a cause or result [13, 14]. Weight loss induced by diet or surgery has been demonstrated to increase testosterone level and sexual function [15-17]. Probably, low testosterone and metabolic disorders worsen each other. The results of clinical studies of testosterone replacement therapy were reviewed by Grossmann [13]. RTC was performed in 10 trials in obese men with borderline low testosterone levels. Although reduced fat mass was commonly observed, improved insulin sensitivity was detected in only 2 trials. Six RCTs in diabetic patients similarly demonstrated beneficial changes in body composition. However, reduction of HOMA-R was detected in 3 trials, and decreased HbA1c in one. These data suggested the limited efficacy of testosterone replacement. Although only one meta-analysis noted that combined prostate events including prostate cancer, elevated PSA and prostate biopsies were more frequent in testosterone-treated men [18], there is no clear evidence that testosterone replacement increases the incidence of prostate cancer. However, the possibility remains that the study was too small to detect significant results. In contrast, a significantly increased risk of cardiovascular events has been associated with testosterone therapy [19, 20], emphasizing that its potential risks should not be ignored.

Dehydroepiandrosterone (DHEA) and its sulfate ester, dehydroepiandrostrone-sulphate (DHEA-S) are referred as a weak androgen produced in adrenal gland (90%) and testis (10%) in men [21]. DHEA is an intermediate product, which is synthesized from pregnenolone, and converted to testosterone and estrogen. DHEA is one of the most abundantly secreted steroids, although its precise physiological roles remain uncertain. DHEA exerts 0.1-2% of the activity of testosterone on the genital organs [22], and 42% on bone formation in mice [23]. Since no specific nuclear receptor for DHEA or DHEA-S has been identified, these hormones are regarded as precursors of more active androgens, such as testosterone and 5α-dihydrotestosterone (DHT), or estrogens. In addition, DHEA and DHEA-S can be converted to more active forms subcellularly in target tissues, the underlying mechanism of which was referred to as "intracine" by Labrie [24].

Both serum DHEA and testosterone levels decline during the aging process [25, 26]. Hence, low serum DHEA level has been assumed to be involved in the development of age-related diseases and shortening of the life span. Such studies suggest an association between high serum DHEA-S level and longevity. However, numerous studies have reported that serum DHEA(-S) exhibits positive, negative or no relation to adiposity, cardiovascular disease and mortality in men and women [27]. Recent longitudinal and cross sectional studies support the favorable effects of DHEA-S on cardiovascular disease and all-cause mortality in both sexes [28-30].

Like the case of testosterone, inconsistent results of DHEA replacement have been published. DHEA replacement decreased fat mass and elevated bone mineral density (BMD) [31], whereas, opposite results were obtained [32] in elderly men and women with DHEA deficiency. Recently, Corona *et al*, conducted a meta-analysis study of 25 RTC trials of DHEA supplementation in elderly men. They observed no significant effects on the levels of glucose, insulin, total cholesterol or BMD with DHEA, while a small but significant reduction of fat mass was detected in the supplemented group [33].

Production of testosterone in the testis is regulated by gonadotropin, while that of DHEA in the adrenal gland is by ACTH. Low free testosterone is correlated positively with LH in diabetic men, and therefore, hypogonadotropic hypogonadism is common in these patients [34]. However, the pathogenesis of low DHEA level has been unclear. Both serum testosterone and DHEA levels decline with aging. Although some studies have published data on testosterone and DHEA in elderly persons [35, 36], to our knowledge, no research has focused on individual relationships among testosterone, DHEA and metabolic disorders. Theoretically, low testosterone level might be compensated for by DHEA via an intracrine mechanism in men having low testosterone and normal DHEA level. The opposite can also be supposed. Therefore, we speculate that severe metabolic impairment might be observed in men with low testosterone and low DHEA levels. Further study is necessary to help clarify this issue.

In animal studies, extensive research has elucidated the physiological and pharmacological roles of androgens. However, few papers have compared testosterone and DHEA. The hormonal actions of testosterone and DHEA are mediated via the androgen receptor (AR), and so the difference in biological activity between these hormones may be caused by the efficacy of steroid converting enzymes mediated by an intracrine mechanism. In addition, numerous cell surface receptors for testosterone and DHEA have been identified [37, 38]. Differences in the biological responses to testosterone and DHEA may be derived from these membrane receptors. Anagnostopoulou *et al*, reported opposite effects of DHEA and testosterone on the apoptosis of prostate and colon cancer [39]. They concluded that the differential effects of these hormones on nerve growth factor receptors in cancer cells accounted for these results. Piñeiro *et al*, showed that DHT, DHEA-S, stanozolol (non-aromatizable androgen), and androstenedion, but not testosterone, suppressed leptin secretion in cultured adipocytes sampled from female omental adipose tissue [40]. The authors presumed that aromatization of testosterone might result in effects opposite to those of other androgens. Sato *et al*, considered that testosterone increased the expression level of Glut4 more potently than DHEA in cultured skeletal muscle, which was abrogated by a DHT inhibitor [41]. These results suggested that DHT, a metabolite of testosterone and DHEA, finally acts as an androgen in skeletal muscle. In this article, we outline our research investigating the impact of androgens, testosterone and DHEA, on adiposity and glucose metabolism, and the results of our recent study.

2. Materials and Methods

2.1. Animals

Male Wistar rats and C57/black mice at 8 wk of age were fed with or without (control) 0.4% testosterone or 0.4% DHEA containing food in CE2 powder (carbohydrate 51.4%, protein 24.9%, fat 4.6%, fiber 3.7%) for 4 wk. Individual food consumption was determined by subtracting the food remaining from that supplied every 2-3 days, with the averages of these values in one week expressed as the weekly food consumption. The animals were housed in a specific pathogen-free facility with a 12-h light/12-h dark cycle. After sacrifice white adipose tissue (epididymal fat), skeletal muscle (gastrocnemius muscle) brown adipose tissue (BAT) and liver were collected. All procedures for animal care were carried out in accordance with protocols approved by the University of Gifu's Institutional Animal Care Committee.

O_2 consumption (VO_2), CO_2 production (VCO_2) and locomotor activity in mice were measured individually by indirect calorimetry using an Oxymax apparatus (Columbus Instruments, Columbus, OH) as described previously [42]. Respiratory exchange rate (RER) was calculated as VCO_2/VO_2. Heat generation was calculated as caloric value (3.815+1.232 × RER) × VO_2.

2.2. Cell culture

3T3-L1 preadipocytes were cultured in Dulbecco's modified Eagle's medium (DMEM) supplemented with 10% fetal bovine serum, 100 U/mL penicillin, and 0.1 mg/mL streptomycin. Upon confluence, 3T3-L1 preadipocytes were differentiated with differentiation medium containing insulin, dexamethasone and IBMX for 3 days followed by incubation with DMEM again. At 5 days after the differentiation, cells were stimulated with 50 nM DHEA or 50 nM testosterone for 48 hr. The content of triglyceride was visualized with Oil Red O (Santa Cruz Biotechnology, Santa Cruz, CA) according to the manufacturer's instruction.

F442A preadipocytes were cultured in DMEA with supplement as described above. When confluence was reached (0d), 50 nM DHEA or testosterone was added to the medium to evaluate the effects of these hormones on spontaneous differentiation of F442A cells into mature adipocytes without differentiation medium.

C_2C_{12} myoblasts were cultured in DMEM supplemented with 10% fetal bovine serum, 100 U/mL penicillin, and 0.1 mg/mL streptomycin. When cells reached 90% confluence, the medium was exchanged for DMEM containing 4% horse serum (differentiation medium). After incubation with the differentiation medium for 7 days, cells were morphologically determined to complete the differentiation into C_2C_{12} myotubes, and then these cells were treated with various concentrations of testosterone for 48 hr

2.3. Real time PCR

Real time PCR was performed to measure mRNA expression levels of PPARγ, fatty acid binding protein 4 (FABP4), lipoprotein lipase (LPL), adiponectin, SREBP-1, fatty acid synthase

http://dx.doi.org/10.5772/59604

(FAS) and glyceraldehyde 3-phosphate dehydrogenase (G3PDH) in 3T3-L1 adipocytes, and PGC1α, cytochrome C and G3PDH in C_2C_{12} myotubes, as described previously [43-45]. All data were normalized to the expression level of G3PDH.

2.4. Triglyceride content in liver and skeletal muscle

Liver and gastrocunemius muscle were homogenized in KRP buffer, and the triglyceride in the homogenate was extracted with chloroform-methanol, and assayed using a LabAssay Triglyceride kit (Wako Pure Chemical Industries, Ltd, Osaka, Japan) as described previously [43].

2.5. Western blot

The cell lysate was mixed with Laemmli sample buffer and boiled for 3 min. Equal amounts of cell lysate were subjected to SDS-PAGE, and transferred onto nitrocellulose paper. The paper was blocked with 1% BSA, and incubated with anti-PPARγ antibody, anti-adiponectin antibody or anti-actin antibody (Santa Cruz). Protein bands were visualized with an ECL system.

2.6. Statistics

All experimental results were calculated as means ± SE. Statistical comparisons were performed by Student's t-test or ANOVA. Significance was defined as $P < 0.05$.

3. Results

3.1. Body weight and plasma glucose level

Treatment with testosterone or DHEA containing food reduced weight gain in both rats (Fig. 1A) and mice (Fig. 1B). Administration of testosterone and DHEA reduced body weight equivalently. The dose response study showed that food containing both testosterone and DHEA at 0.4% significantly suppressed body weight gain (Fig.1C). Our previous study [43] indicated that treatment with 0.4% testosterone for 4 wk resulted in an increase of serum testosterone and DHEA-S levels up to 674% and 1040%, respectively (note that serum DHEA-S level is very low in rodents due to the lack of 17α hydroxylase in adrenal glands), whereas treatment with DHEA increased testosterone and DHEA-S levels up to 310% and 6420%, respectively. The fact that these androgens are convertible to each other, partially explains the similar results obtained with administration of these hormones. Administration of testosterone and DHEA did not influence fasting plasma glucose level in rats (Fig. 1D), while testosterone suppressed it a little but significantly in mice (Fig. 1E). Food consumption was not influenced by the administration of either hormone in rats (Fig. 1F).

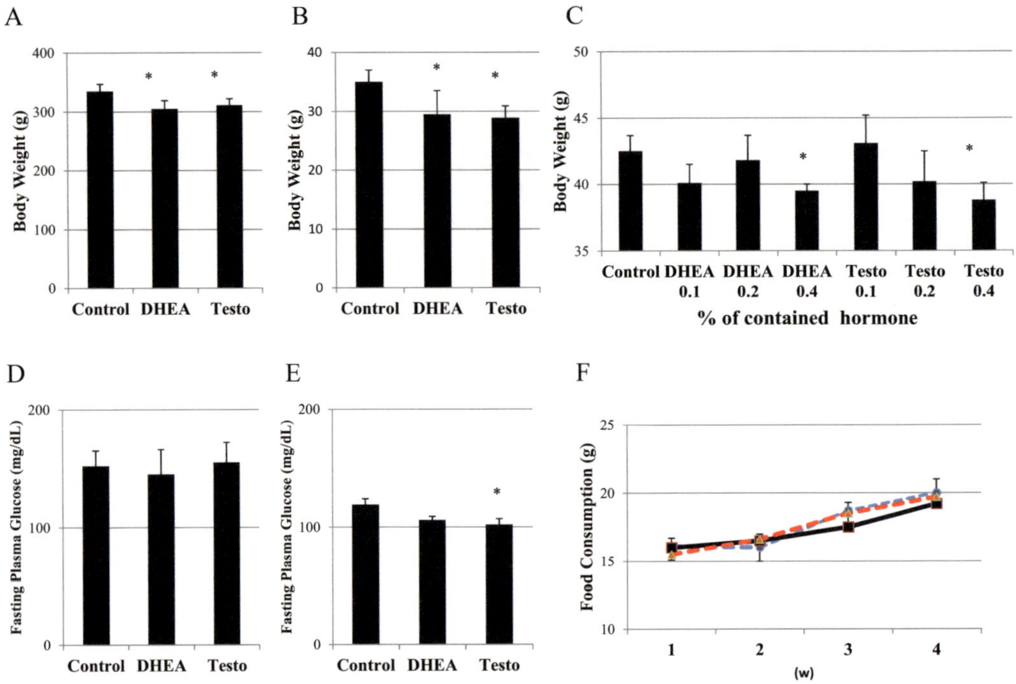

Figure 1. Effects of administration of DHEA and testosterone on body weight. Effects of treatment with 0.4% DHEA or testosterone containing food for 4wk on body weight in Wistar rats (n=6) (A) and C56/black mice (n=4) (B) at 8 wk of age are shown. *: p<0.05 vs control. Effects of 0.1%-0.4% DHEA or testosterone containing food for 4wk on body weight in C57/black mice (n=4) (C) are shown. *: p<0.05 vs control. Effects of treatment with 0.4% DHEA or testosterone containing food for 4wk on fasting plasma glucose level in Wistar rats (n=6) (D) and C56/black mice (n=4) (E) are shown. *: p<0.05 vs control. Effects of DHEA or testosterone administration on food consumption in mice (n=4) are shown. Black solid line: Control, Red broken line: DHEA, Blue broken line: testosterone. *: p<0.05 vs control.

3.2. Effect of DHEA and testosterone on adipocytes

Administration of DHEA or testosterone suppressed fat weight, including that of subcutaneous, epididymal and mesenteric fat (Fig. 2A). In addition, both DHEA and testosterone decreased adipocyte size equivalently (Fig. 2B). We found that treatment with DHEA reduced the expression of PPARγ in adipocytes in both *in vivo* and *in vitro* [42]. Treatment with DHEA and testosterone similarly reduced the expression level of PPARγ in adipose tissue isolated from Wistar rats and 3T3-L1 adipocytes (Fig. 2C, D). Genes regulated by PPARγ, such as FABP 4, LPL and adiponectin were equally down-regulated by DHEA and testosterone in 3T3-L1 adipocytes. Neither hormone influenced the expression levels of genes, which are not directly regulated by PPARγ, such as SREBP-1 and FAS (data not shown). Administration of DHEA or testosterone decreased triglyceride content in liver and skeletal muscle to the same degree in rats (Fig. 2 E, F).

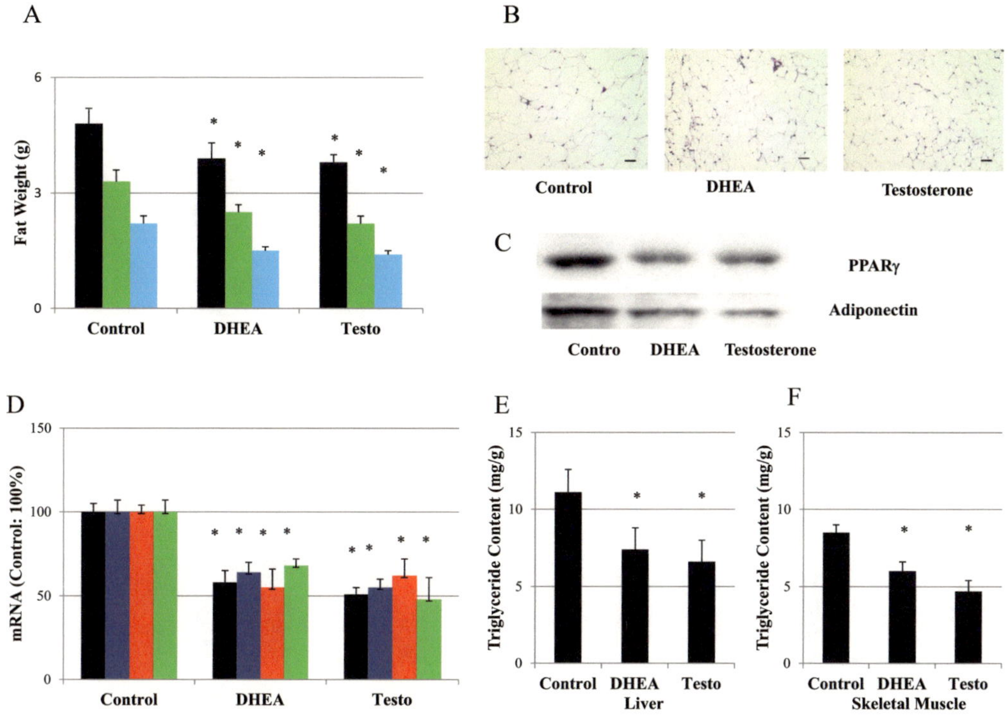

Figure 2. Effects of administration of DHEA and testosterone on adipocytes. Effects of treatment with DHEA or testosterone for 4wk on fat weight (black: subcutaneous, green: epididymal, blue: mesenteric fat, n=6) (A), and histological findings (B) are shown. *: $p<0.05$ vs each control. Effects of treatment with DHEA or testosterone on the protein level of PPARγ and adiponectin in adipose tissue in Wistar rats were evaluated. A typical result was shown (C). Effects of treatment with DHEA or testosterone on the expression of adipocyte specific genes in 3T3-L1 adipocytes are shown (D). Fully differentiated 3T3-L1 adipocytes were incubated with 50 nM DHEA or testosterone for 48 hr. Expression levels of PPARγ (black), FABP4 (blue), LPL (red), adiponectin (green) were shown (n=6). *: $p<0.05$ vs each control. Effects of treatment with DHEA or testosterone on triglyceride content in liver (n=5) (E) and skeletal muscle (n=5) (F) in Wistar rats are presented. *:$p<0.05$ vs control.

Next, we examined the effects of these hormones on adipocyte differentiation. We observed the differentiation of F442A cells, since they spontaneously differentiate into mature adipocytes when they reach confluence. DHEA and testosterone suppressed the accumulation of triglyceride (Fig. 3A) and the appearance of PPARγ and FABP4 mRNA during the differentiation process. These data indicated that DHEA and testosterone similarly suppress adipocyte differentiation.

3.3. Effect of DHEA and testosterone on mitochondrial biogenesis

As noted above, since the administration of neither DHEA nor testosterone influenced food consumption, we speculated that these hormones elevate energy expenditure. Hence we examined the effects of testosterone administration on energy production. Mice were treated with or without testosterone for 4 wk, and then, oxygen consumption and locomotor activity were measured by indirect calorimetry. O_2 consumption and CO_2 production were increased

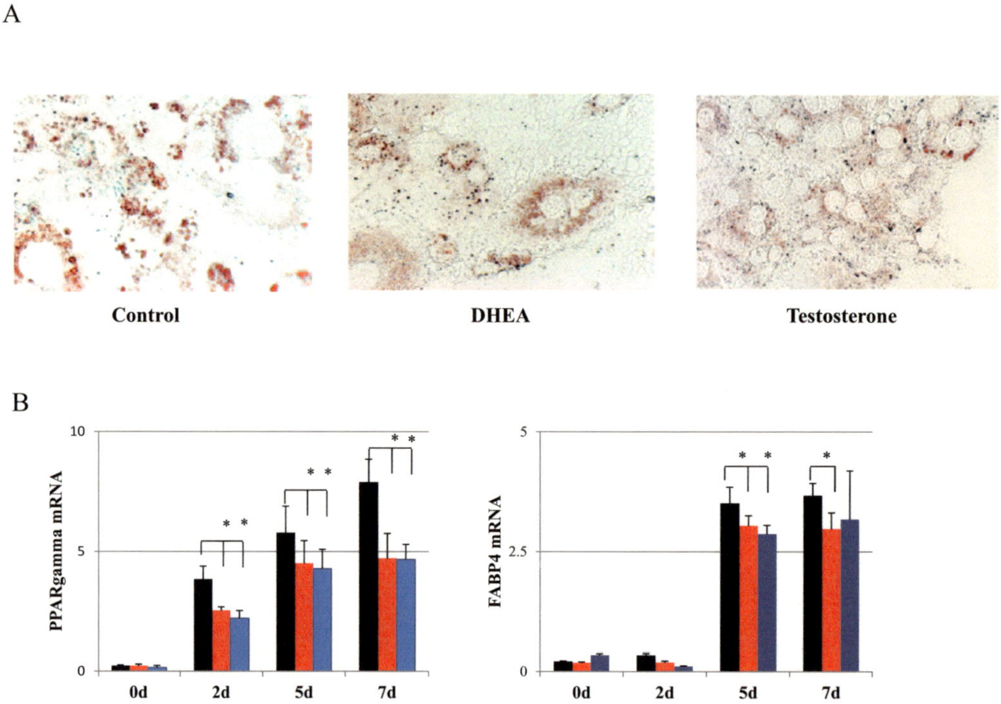

Figure 3. Effect of treatment with DHEA and testosterone on the differentiation of F442A adipocytes. F442A preadipocytes were cultured in DMED. When cells reached confluence as judged by the morphological findings (0d), 50nM DHEA or testosterone was added to the medium, followed by subsequent incubation for the indicated period. Triglyceride accumulation was assessed with oil-Red staining at 7d (A). Expression levels of PPARγ and FABP4 were measured with real time PCR on the indicated day (n=4) (B). *:$p<0.05$ vs each control.

significantly in testosterone-treated mice, regardless of whether the values were normalized by body weight or not (Fig. 4B-E). In addition, heat production, the values of which were normalized by body weight, was elevated in testosterone-treated mice (Fig. 4G). No difference was detected in respiratory exchange rate between control and testosterone-treated mice (Fig. 4H). To our surprise, administration of testosterone suppressed locomotor activity (Fig. 4I).

These results indicate that administration of testosterone increases the basal metabolic rate. Therefore, we evaluated the effects of administration of these androgens on mitochondrial biogenesis and its upstream regulator, PGC1α. Expression of mitochondrial protein, Cox4, and PGC1α was elevated in skeletal muscle, but not brown BAT or liver, isolated from testosterone-treated rats (Fig. 5A). The increase of Cox4 in skeletal muscle induced by DHEA administration was less than that induced by testosterone (Fig. 5B). The testosterone-induced increases in mRNA levels of PGC1α and cytochrome C were greater than the DHEA-induced ones in C_2C_{12} myotubes (Fig. 5C). These results show that increased mitochondrial biogenesis by these hormones leads to up-regulation of energy expenditure, which may result in reduced adiposity.

http://dx.doi.org/10.5772/59604

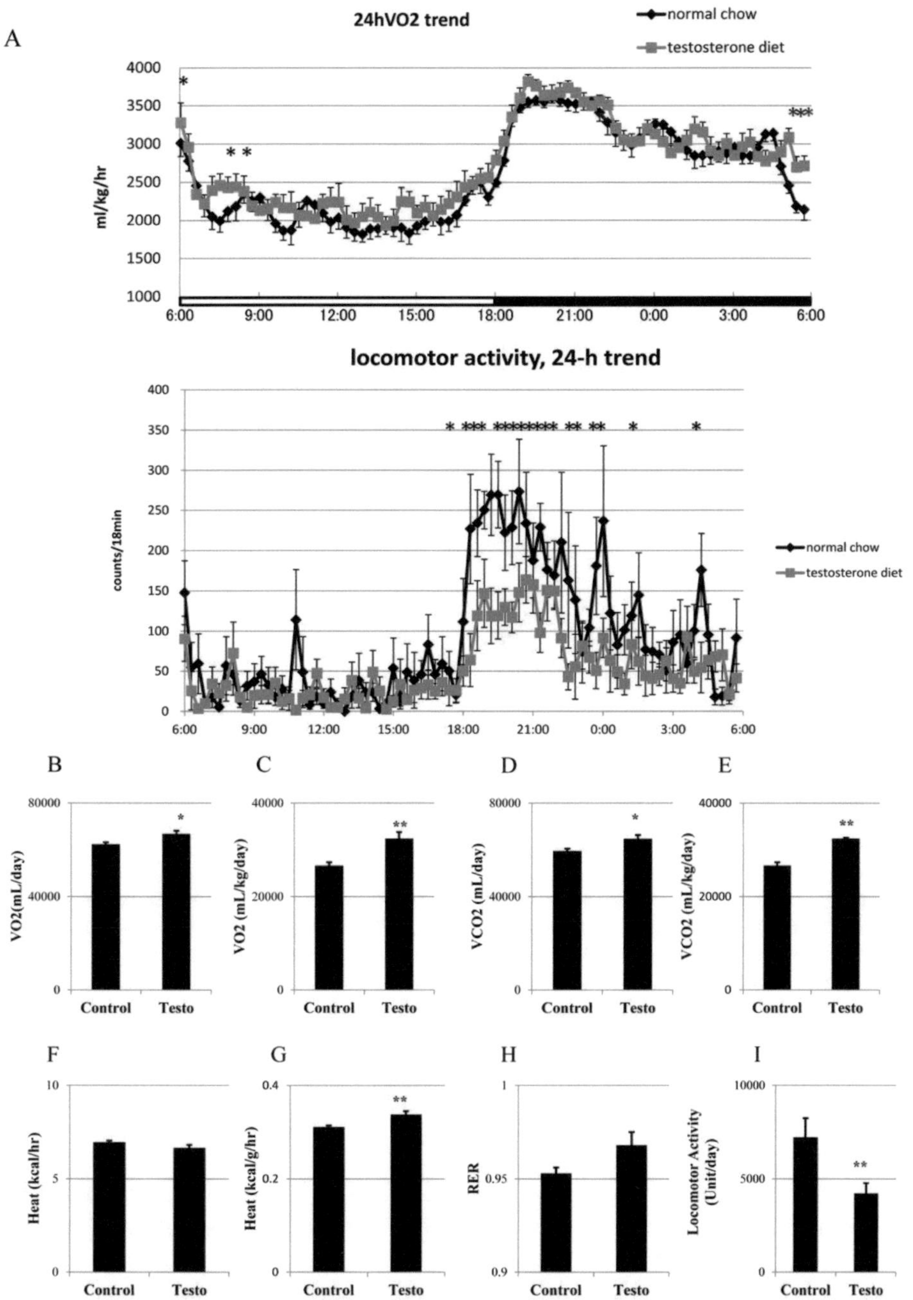

Figure 4. Effects of treatment with testosterone on oxygen consumption, heat production and locomotor activity. C56/ black mice at 8 wk of age were treated with testosterone for 4 wk, and individual oxygen consumption and locomotor activity were determined by indirect calorimetry (A). Cumulative O_2 consumption for 24 hr (B) and normalized values by body weight (C), CO2 production (D) and normalized values by body weight (E), heat production for 24 hr (F) and normalized values by body weight (G) are shown. Values of RER (H) and locomotor activity (I) for 24 hr are also shown. *: $p<0.05$ vs control, **: $p<0.01$ vs control

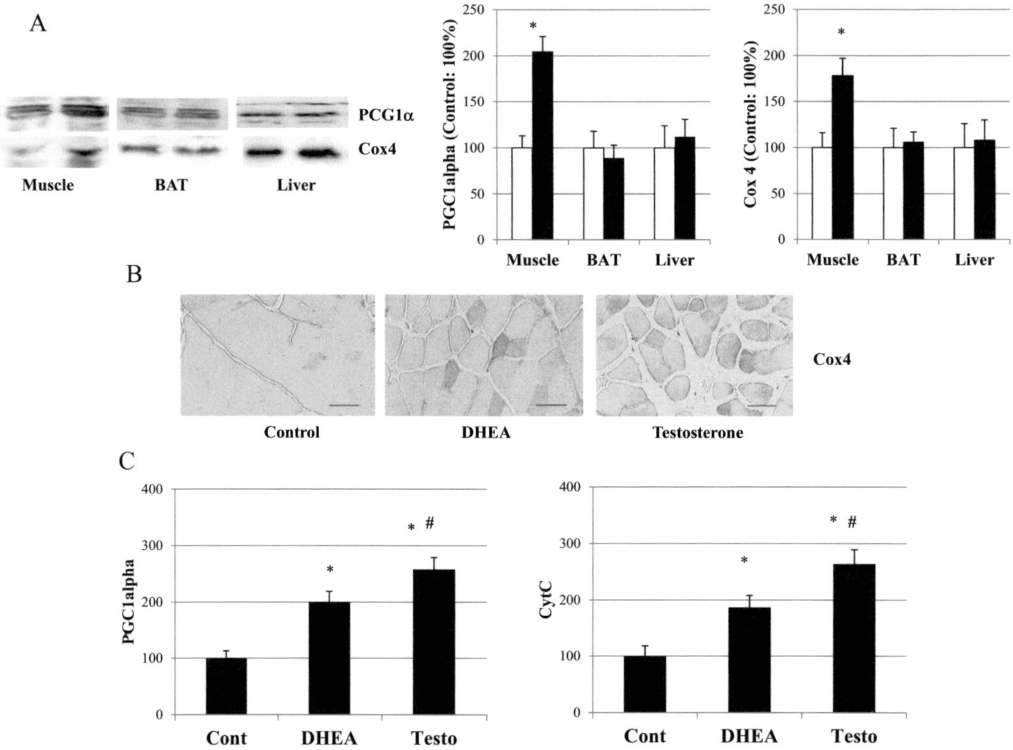

Figure 5. Effect of treatment with DHEA and testosterone on mitochondrial biogenesis. Wistar rats were treated with DHEA or testosterone for 4 wk. Effects of treatment with testosterone on the expression of PGC1α and Cox4 in skeletal muscle, BAT and liver are shown (A). Typical results of western blot are shown in the left panel, and quantified results are shown in the right (n=4). White: Control, Black: Testosterone-treated. *:p<0.05 vs control. Representative image of immunohistochemistry of skeletal muscle isolated from control, DHEA-treated and testosterone-treated rats are shown (B). Effects of incubation with 10 nM DHEA or testosterone for 48 hr on the expression of PGC1α and cytochrome C mRNA in C_2C_{12} myotubes (n-4) are shown (C). *: p<0.05 vs control, #: p<0.05 vs DHEA.

4. Discussion

Coleman *et al.*, demonstrated that administration of DHEA reduces blood glucose level in db/db mice [46]. We found that administration of DHEA improved blood glucose in OLETF rats, a model of obese diabetes, but not GK rats, a model of lean diabetes [47]. Accordingly, we presumed that DHEA-induced weight reduction might contribute to improving blood glucose levels. Although administration of DHEA consistently suppresses body weight and fat weight, significant improvement of blood glucose is detected only in extremely obese animals [44]. We noted that DHEA and testosterone reduce the expression of PPARγ in adipocytes [43, 44]. Heterozygous PPARγ deficient mice are protected from insulin resistance under a high-fat diet [48], and reduced receptor activity of PPARγ by Pro12Ala substitution leads to lower body mass index in man [49], suggesting that modest suppression of PPARγ activity may help to

http://dx.doi.org/10.5772/59604

prevent obesity and resultant insulin resistance. However, the production and secretion of adiponectin are positively regulated by PPARγ in adipocytes [50], and inhibition of PPARγ may result in insulin resistance due to low plasma adiponectin level. In this study, we showed that DHEA and testosterone decrease PPARγ, as well as adiponectin (Fig. 2C, D). This result is consistent with the fact that despite their obese phenotype, glucose homeostasis remained intact because of a high plasma adiponectin level in androgen receptor null mice (ARKO) [51]. These data explain the results of the numerous clinical studies described above in which administration of DHEA or testosterone consistently reduced adiposity, despite which numerous studies have failed to find proof of any beneficial effect on glucose metabolism.

This study confirmed that administration of DHEA and testosterone reduced body weight and fat weight equally, as described in our previous study [44]. If this conclusion is applied to men for weight reduction, supplementation of DHEA would be more desirable than that of testosterone given the smaller possibility of adverse effects. Our study also reveals that DHEA and testosterone attenuate proliferation of 3T3-L1 preadipocytes in a similar concentration dependent manner [44]. In addition, we showed that these hormones decrease the expression levels of PPARγ, LPL and FABP4, but not SREBP-1, at common concentrations and in a time dependent manner [44]. The possibility that fat content increased in other organs in compensation for the decrease in fat mass, was ruled out by the fact that fat content in liver and skeletal muscle decreased similarly both in DHEA and testosterone-treated rats [44], which was confirmed in this experiment. The findings that neither DHEA nor testosterone increased glycerol release in 3T3-L1 adipocytes and administration of these hormones decreased serum free fatty acid concentration in rats, rule out the possibility that these hormones reduce adiposity by increased lipolysis [41]. In this study, we revealed that both DHEA and testosterone suppress differentiation of adipocytes using F442A. Both DHEA and testosterone equivalently inhibited spontaneous differentiation of cells. Recently, concurrent results have been published with regard to 3T3-L1 preadipocytes, C3H 10T1/2 pluripotent cells and human preadipocytes [52-55]. Singh *et al,* reported that formation of androgen receptor/β-catenin and T-cell factor 4 complex and activation of Wnt signaling are involved in androgen-induced inhibition of adipogenesis [54].

To clarify the mechanisms underlying androgen-induced weight reduction, we analyzed the effect of testosterone administration on energy expenditure. Administration of both DHEA and testosterone increased the rectal temperature in rats [44]. Although an abnormally high body temperature was not detected, elevated O_2 consumption and CO_2 production was observed in testosterone-treated mice (Fig. 4A-D). Although heat production was increased in testosterone-treated mice, it was not significant when these values were not normalized by body weight (Fig. 4E). We have no data on lean body mass or water. If lean body mass is not influenced by testosterone, testosterone-induced reduction of adiposity could not result from an increase in energy expenditure. On the other hand, our results indicate that basal metabolic rate increases in testosterone-treated mice since heat production in these mice did not decreas despite suppressed locomotor activity. The result of suppressed locomotor activity in testosterone-treated mice was unexpected, since lower locomotor activity was also reported in

ARKO [51]. We are not yet able to explain this discrepancy, probably because change in locomotor activity may not occur in parallel with an androgen signal.

Next, we speculated that testosterone might increase mitochondrial activity to explain the increased basal metabolic rate. As shown in Fig. 5A, increased Cox4, a mitochondrial protein, as well as PGC1α, an up-stream regulator of mitochondrial biogenesis, was recognized in skeletal muscle isolated from testosterone-treated rats. Similar results were noted in mice [45]. In addition, treatment with testosterone up-regulates the expression levels of genes contributing to mitochondrial biogenesis, such as nuclear respiratory factor-1 (NRF-1), NRF-2 and mitochondrial transcriptional factor A (Tfam), as well as mitochondrial DNA (mitDNA) in skeletal muscle [44]. Although DHEA and testosterone exhibit similar effects on adipocytes, administration of DHEA resulted in less increase in Cox4 than that of testosterone in skeletal muscle. This result was confirmed by the experiment showing that the testosterone-induced increase in mRNA of PGC1α and cytochrome C was greater than the DHEA-induced ones (Fig. 5C) in C_2C_{12} myotubes. These results are consistent with data published by Sato *et al.* [41]. These differences in the response to DHEA and testosterone between adipocytes and myocytes may be attributable to differences in the efficacy of subcellular steroid converting enzymes. Although we did not assess the effect of androgens on total skeletal muscle volume, androgens have been reported to enhance the differentiation into skeletal muscle [53]. Therefore, the conclusion derived from our experiment should be further explored by increasing the whole skeletal muscle mass. In addition, we found that expression of PGC1α and mitochondrial genes was reduced in skeletal muscle isolated from ARKO [45].

The results of our studies were summarized in Fig. 6. DHEA and testosterone equally suppressed proliferation of preadipocytes, differentiation of adipocytes and expression of PPARγ and its down-stream genes including adiponectin in adipocytes. Both DHEA and testosterone up-regulated PGC1α and mitochondrial biogenesis, more actively in the latter than the former in skeletal muscle. Which organ plays the main role in the androgens-induced reduction of adiposity remains an interesting problem. Our results suggest that reduced adiposity in testosterone-treated animals may be derived from decreased expression of PPARγ and suppressed differentiation into adipocytes. Moderate suppression of PPARγ activity by its antagonist HX531 resulted in decreased fat mass and increased oxygen consumption [56], and therefore androgen-induced reduction of PPARγ expression may be able to influence systemic energy metabolism.

Whole body silencing of AR results in late-onset obesity [51, 56]. Recent technology has facilitated the generation of organ specific deletion of a gene. Adipocyte specific AR deficient mice showed identical body weight and adiposity with wild type at 20 wk of age in one study, although the authors did not show the data of older mice [57]. Since late obesity after 20 wk of age is the distinguishing feature in ARKO, this point is important. Conversely, mice lacking AR in the central nervous system develop late onset obesity and insulin resistance [59]. Although several investigations have reported that myocyte specific AR knockdown did not influence body weight and adiposity [60, 61], myocyte specific AR overexpression resulted in an increased metabolic rate and fat body mass [62]. These results suggest that skeletal muscle and brain might be responsible organs for androgen-induced reduction of adiposity. However,

http://dx.doi.org/10.5772/59604

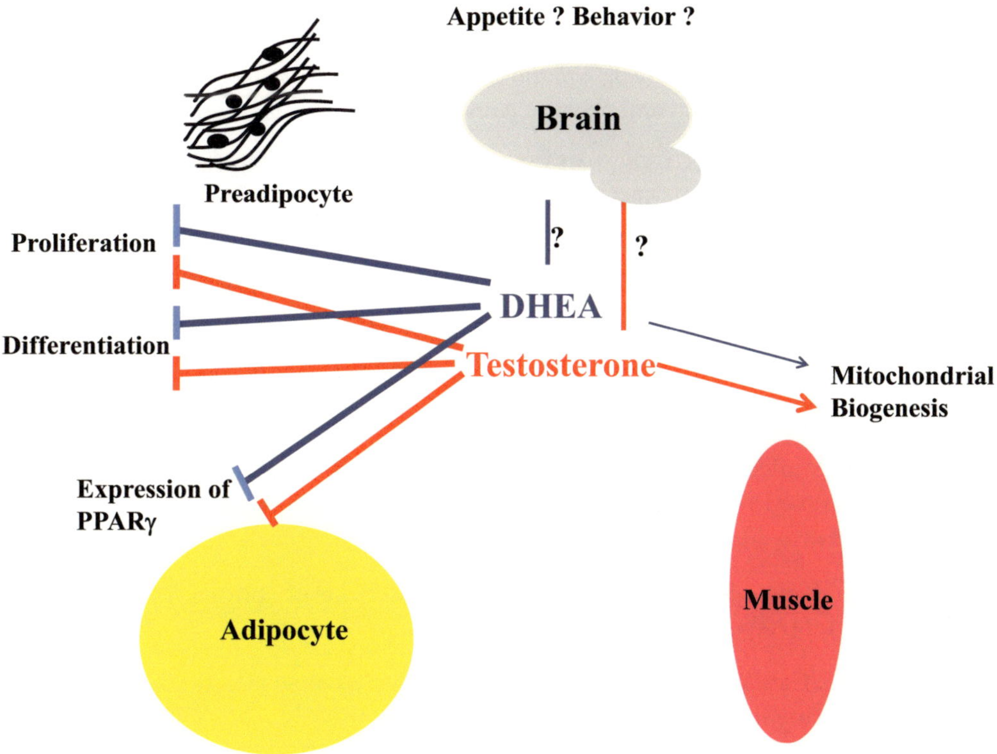

Figure 6. Effect of DHEA and testosterone on brain, adipocytes and skeletal muscle

the role of AR in adipocytes in systemic insulin sensitivity cannot be ruled out at present. Further experiments will be required to help clarify these issues.

Author details

Kazuo Kajita[1*], Ichiro Mori[1], Masahiro[1], Takahide Ikeda[1], Hiroyuki Morita[1] and Tatsuo Ishizuka[2]

*Address all correspondence to: kkajita@gifu-u.ac.jp

1 Department of General Internal Medicine, Gifu University Graduate School of Medicine, 1-1 Yanagido, Gifu, Japan

2 Department of General Internal Medicine and Rheumatology, Gifu Municipal Hospital, 7-1 Kashima-cho, Gifu, Japan

References

[1] Matsuzawa Y, Shimomura I, Nakamura T, Keno Y, Tokunaga K, Pathophysiology and pathogenesis of visceral obesity. Ann N Y Acad Sci (1995)., 17, 399-406

[2] Carey DG, Jenkins AB, Campbell LV, Freund J, Chisholm DJ, Abdominal fat and insulin resistance and overweight women: Direct measurements reveal a strong relationship in subjects at both low and high risk of NIDDM. Diabetes (1996)., 45, 633-638

[3] Björntrop, "Portal" adipose tissue as a generator of risk factors for cardiovascular disease and diabetes. Arteriosclerosis (1990) 10, 493-496

[4] Basaria S et al. Long term effects of androgen deprivation therapy in prostate cancer patients. Clin Endocrinol (2002)., 56, 779-786

[5] Basaria S, Muller DC, Carducci MA, Egan J, Dobs AS, Hyperglycemia and insulin resistance in men with prostate carcinoma who receive androgen deprivation therapy. Cancer (2006),. 106, 581-588.

[6] Hakimian P et al. Metabolic and cardiovascular effects of androgen deprivation therapy. BJU Int (2008),. 102, 1509-1514

[7] Taylor LG, Canfield SE, Du XL, Review of major adverse effects of androgen-deprivation therapy in men with prostate cancer. Cancer (2009)., 115, 2388-2399.

[8] Cleffi S et al. Androgen deprivation therapy and morbid obesity: Do they share cardiovascular risk through metabolic syndrome? Actas Urol Exp (2011),. 35, 259-265

[9] Katznelson L et al. Increase in bone density and lean body mass during testosterone administration in men with acquired hypogonadism. J Clin Endocrinol Metab (1996)., 81, 4358-4365

[10] Dhindsa S et al. The effects of hypogonadism on body composition and bone mineral density in type 2 diabetic patients. Diabetes Care (2007)., 30, 1860-1861

[11] Kapoor D et al. Clinical and biological assessment of hypogonadism in men with clinical and biological assessment of hypogonadism in men with type 2 diabetes. Diabetic Care (2007)., 30, 911-917

[12] Bhasin S et al. Sex hormone-binding globulin, but not testosterone, is associated prospectively and independently with metabolic syndrome in men. Diabetic Care (2011)., 34, 2464-2470

[13] Grossmann M, Testosterone and glucose metabolism in men: current concepts and controversies. J Endocrinol (2014)., 220, R37-R55

[14] Grossmann M, Low testosterone in men with type 2 diabetes: significance and treatment. J Clin Endocrinol Metab (2011)., 96, 2341-2353

[15] Stanik S et al. The effect of weight loss on reproductive hormones in obese men. J Clin Endocrinol Metab (1981)., 53, 828-832

[16] Khoo J, Piantadosi C, Worthley S, Wittert GA, Effects of a low energy diet on sexual function and lower urinary tract symptoms in obese men. Int J Obes (2010)., 34, 1396-1403

[17] Hammoud H et al. Effect of Roux-en-Y gastric bypass surgery on the sex steroids and quality of life in obese men. C Clin Endocrinol Metab 94, 1329-1332

[18] Calof OM et al. Adverse events associated with testosterone replacement in middle-aged ond older men: a meta-analysis of randomized, placebo-controlled trials. J Gerontol A Biol Sci Med Sci (2005)., 60, 1451-1457

[19] Vigen R et al. Association of testosterone therapy with mortality, myocardial infarction, and stroke in men with low testosterone levels. JAMA (2013)., 310, 1829-1836

[20] Xu L et al. Testosterone therapy and cardiovascular events among men: a systemical review and meta-analysis of placebo-controlled randomized trials. BMC Med (2013)., 11, 108-119

[21] Kaufman JM, Vermeulen A, The decline of androgen levels in elderly men and its clinical and therapeutic implications. Endocr Rev (2005)., 26, 1138-1147

[22] Howard E, Dehydroepiandrosterone and testosterone: comparative androgenic potencies and contrasting actions. Endocrinology (1963)., 72, 19-27

[23] Howard E, Steroids and bone maturation in infant mice: Relative actions of dehydroepiandrosterone and testosterone. Endocrinology (1962)., 70, 131-141

[24] Labrie F, Intracrinology. Mol Cell Endocrinol (1991)., 78, C113-C118

[25] Roth GS et al. Biomarkers of caloric restriction may predict longevity in humans. Science (2002)., 297, 2002

[26] Barrett-Connor E, Khaw KT, Yen SS, A prospective study of dehydroepiandrosterone sulfate, mortality, and cardiovascular disease. N Engl J Med (1986)., 315, 1519-1524

[27] Tchernof A, Labrie F, Dehydroepiandrosterone, obesity and cardiovascular disease risk: a review of human studies. Eur J Endocrinol (2004)., 151, 1-14

[28] Ohlsson C et al. Low serum levels of dehydroepiandrosterone sulfate predict all-cause and cardiovascular mortality in elderly Swedish men. J Clin Endocrinol Metab (2010)., 95, 4406-4414

[29] Shufelt C et al. DHEA-S levels and cardiovascular disease mortality in postmenopausal women: Results from the National Institute of Health-national Heart, Lung, and Blood Institute (NHLBI)-sponsored women's ischemia syndrome evaluation (WISE). J Clin Endocrinol Metab (2010)., 95, 4985-4992

[30] Mori I et al. Comparison of biochemical data, blood pressure and physical activity between longevity and non-longevity districts in Japan. Circ J (2008) 72, 1680-1684

[31] Villareal DT, Holloszy JO, Kohrt WM, Effect of DHEA replacement on bone mineral density and body composition in elderly women and men. Clin Endocrinol (2000)., 53, 561-568

[32] Callies F et al. Dehydroepiandrosterone replacement in women with adrenal insufficiency: Effects on body composition, serum leptin, bone turnover, and exercise capacity. J Clin Endrcrinol Metab (2001)., 86, 1968-1972

[33] Corona G et al. Dehydroepiandrosterone supplementation in elderly men: a meta-analysis study of placebo-controlled trials. J Clin Endocrinol Metab (2013)., 98, 3615-3626

[34] Dhindsa S et al. Frequent occurrence of hypogonadotropic hypogonadism in type 2 diabetes. J Clin Endocrinol Metab (2004)., 89, 5462-5468

[35] Vaidya D, Association of baseline sex hormone levels with baseline and longitudinal changes in waist-to-hip ratio: multi-ethnic study of atherosclerosis. Int J Obes (2012)., 36: 1578-1584

[36] Haring R et al. Clinical correlates of sex steroids and gonadotropins in men over the late adulthood: the Framingham Heart Study. Int J andorol (2012)., 35, 775-782

[37] Webb SJ, Geoghegan TE, Prough RA, The biological action of dehydroepiandrosterone involves multiple receptors. Drug Metab Rev (2006)., 38, 89-116

[38] Papadopoulou N et al. Membrane androgen receptor activation triggers down-regulation of PI-3K/AKT/NF-κB activity and induces apoptotic responses via Bad, FasL and caspase-3 in DU145 prostate cancer cells. Mol Cancer (2008)., 7: 88

[39] Anagnostopoulou V et al. Differential effects of dehydroepiandrosterone and testosterone in prostate and colon cancer cell apoptosis: the role of nerve growth factor (NGF) receptors. Endocrinology (2013)., 154, 2446-2456

[40] Piñeiro V et al. Dehydrotestosterone, stanozolol, androstenedione and dehydroepiandrosterone sulphate inhibit leptin secretion in female but not male samples of omental adipose tissue in vitro: lack of effect of testosterone. J Endocrinol (1999)., 160, 425-432

[41] Sato K, Iemitsu M, Aizawa K, Ajisaka R, Testosterone and DHEA activate the glucose metabolism-related signaling pathway in skeletal muscle. Am J Physiol Endocrinol Metab (2008)., 294, E961-E968

[42] Lee YS et al. Hypothalamic ATF3 is involved in regulating glucose and energy metabolism in mice. Diabetologia (2013)., 56, 1383-1393

[43] Kajita K et al. Dehydroepiandrosterone down-regulates the expression of peroxisome-activated receptor gamma in adipocytes. Endocrinology (2003)., 144, 253-259

[44] Fujioka K et al. Dehydroepiandrosterone reduces preadipocyte proliferation via androgen receptor. Am J Physiol Endocrinol Metab (2012)., 15, E694-E704

[45] Usui T et al. Elevated mitochondrial biogenesis in skeletal muscle is associated with testosterone-induced body weight loss in male mice. Febs Lett (2014) 588, 1935-1941

[46] Coleman DL, Leiter EH, Schwizer RW, Therapeutic effects of dehydroepiandrosterone (DHEA) in diabetic mice. Diabetes (1982)., 31, 830-833

[47] Ishizuka et al. DHEA improves glucose uptake via activation of protein kinase C and phosphatidylinositol 3-kinase. Am J Physiol (1999)., 276, E196-E203

[48] Kubota N et al. PPARgamma mediates high-fat diet-induced adipocyte hypertrophy and insulin resistance. Mol Cell (1999)., 4, 597-609

[49] Deeb SS et al. A Pro12Ala substitution in PPARgamma2 associated with decreased receptor activity, lower body mass index and improved insulin sensitivity. Nat Genet (1998)., 20, 284-287

[50] Maeda N et al. PPARg ligands increase expression and plasma concentration of adiponectin, an adipose-derived protein. Diabetes (2001)., 50, 2094-2099

[51] Fan W et al. Androgen receptor null male mice develop late-onset obesity caused by decreased energy expenditure and lipolytic activity but show normal insulin sensitivity with high adiponectin secretion. Diabetes (2005),. 54, 1000-1008

[52] Lea-Currie YR, Wen P, McIntish MK, Dehydroepiandrosterone reduces proliferation and differentiation of 3T3-L1 preadipocytes. Biochem Biophys Rec Commun (1998)., 248, 497-504

[53] Singh R et al. Androgens stimulate myogenic differentiation and inhibit adipogenesis in C3H 10T1/2 pluripotent cells through an androgen receptor-mediated pathway. Endocrinology (2003)., 144, 5081-5088

[54] Singh R et al. Testosterone inhibits adipogenic differentiation in 3T3-L1 cells: nuclear translocation of androgen receptor complex with β-catenin and T-cell factor 4 may bypass canonical wnt signaling to down-regulate adipogenic transcription factors. Endocrinology (2006)., 147, 141-154

[55] Veilleux A et al. Glucocorticoid-induced androgen inactivation by aldo-keto reductase 1C2 promotes adipogenesis in human preadipocytes. Am J Physiol Endocrinol Metab (2012)., 302, E941-E949

[56] Yamauchi T et al, Inhibition of RXR and PPARg ameliorates diet-induced obesity and type 2 diabetes. J Clin Invest (2001)., 108, 1001-1013

[57] Sato T et al. Late onset of obesity in male androgen receptor-deficient (AR-KO) mice. Biochem Biophys Res Commun (2003)., 300, 167-17

[58] Yu IC et al. Hyperleptinemia without obesity in male mice lacking androgen receptor in adipose tissue. Endocrinology (2008)., 149, 2361-2368

[59] Yu IC et al. Neuronal androgen receptor regulates insulin sensitivity via suppression of hypothalamic NF-kB-mediated PTP1B expression. Diabetes (2013)., 62, 411-423

[60] Ophoff J et al. Androgen signaling in myocytes contributes to the maintenance of muscle mass and fiber type regulation but not to muscle strength or fatigue. Endocrinology (2009)., 150, 3558-3566

[61] Dubois V et al. A satellite cell-specific knockout of androgen receptor reveals myostatin as a direct androgen target in skeletal muscle. FASEB J (2014)., 28, 2979-2994

[62] Fernando SM et al. Myocyte androgen receptors increase metabolic rate and improve body composition by regulating fat mass. Endocrinology (2010)., 151, 3125-3132